T0362273

Imaging of Cerebrovascular Disease

Editors

JAVIER M. ROMERO
MAHMUD MOSSA-BASHA

RADIOLOGIC CLINICS OF NORTH AMERICA

www.radiologic.theclinics.com

Consulting Editor
FRANK H. MILLER

May 2023 • Volume 61 • Number 3

ELSEVIER

1600 John F. Kennedy Boulevard • Suite 1800 • Philadelphia, Pennsylvania, 19103-2899

http://www.theclinics.com

RADIOLOGIC CLINICS OF NORTH AMERICA Volume 61, Number 3
May 2023 ISSN 0033-8389, ISBN 13: 978-0-323-94009-2

Editor: John Vassallo (j.vassallo@elsevier.com)
Developmental Editor: Karen Solomon

Radiologic Clinics of North America (ISSN 0033-8389) is published bimonthly by Elsevier Inc., 360 Park Avenue South, New York, NY 10010-1710. Months of issue are January, March, May, July, September, and November. Periodicals postage paid at New York, NY and additional mailing offices. Subscription prices are USD 544 per year for US individuals, USD 1107 per year for US institutions, USD 100 per year for US students and residents, USD 643 per year for Canadian individuals, USD 1415 per year for Canadian institutions, USD 739 per year for international individuals, USD 1415 per year for international institutions, USD 100 per year for Canadian students/residents, and USD 315 per year for international students/residents. To receive student and resident rate, orders must be accompanied by name of affiliated institution, date of term and the signature of program/residency coordinatior on institution letterhead. Orders will be billed at individual rate until proof of status is received. Foreign air speed delivery is included in all *Clinics* subscription prices. All prices are subject to change without notice. **POSTMASTER:** Send address changes to *Radiologic Clinics of North America*, Elsevier Health Sciences Division, Subscription Customer Service, 3251 Riverport Lane, Maryland Heights, MO63043. **Customer Service: Telephone: 1-800-654-2452** (U.S. and Canada); **1-314-447-8871** (outside U.S. and Canada). **Fax: 1-314-447-8029. E-mail: journalscustomerservice-usa@elsevier.com (for print support); journalsonlinesupport-usa@elsevier.com (for online support)**.

Reprints. For copies of 100 or more of articles in this publication, please contact the Commercial Reprints Department, Elsevier Inc., 360 Park Avenue South, New York, New York 10010-1710. Tel.: +1-212-633-3874; Fax: +1-212-633-3820; E-mail: reprints@elsevier.com.

Radiologic Clinics of North America also published in Greek Paschalidis Medical Publications, Athens, Greece.

Radiologic Clinics of North America is covered in *MEDLINE/PubMed (Index Medicus), EMBASE/Excerpta Medica, Current Contents/Life Sciences, Current Contents/Clinical Medicine, RSNA Index to Imaging Literature, BIOSIS, Science Citation Index,* and *ISI/BIOMED*.

Contributors

CONSULTING EDITOR

FRANK H. MILLER, MD, FACR, FSAR, FSABI
Lee F. Rogers, MD Professor of Medical
Education, Chief, Body Imaging Section,
Medical Director, MRI, Professor, Department
of Radiology, Northwestern Memorial Hospital,
Northwestern University Feinberg School of
Medicine, Chicago, Illinois, USA

EDITORS

JAVIER M. ROMERO, MD
Associate Professor of Radiology, Harvard
Medical School, Massachusetts General
Hospital, Director, Vascular Ultrasound
Services, Director, RH Ackerman
Neurovascular Lab, Boston, Massachusetts,
USA

MAHMUD MOSSA-BASHA, MD
Professor of Radiology, Vice Chair of Clinical
Research, Co-Director of the Research
Vascular Imaging Lab, Department of
Radiology, Adjunct Professor of Neurology and
Electrical Engineering, University of
Washington School of Medicine, Director of the
Vascular Imaging Lab, University of
Washington, Seattle, Washington, USA

AUTHORS

FABRICE BONNEVILLE, MD, PhD
Department of Diagnostic and Therapeutic
Neuroradiology, Toulouse, France

FRANCESCO CARLETTI, PhD
Consultant Neuroradiologist, Lysholm
Department of Neuroradiology, National
Hospital for Neurology and Neurosurgery,
London, United Kingdom

RICCARDO CAU, MD
Department of Radiology, Azienda Ospedaliero
Universitaria (A.O.U.), di Cagliari – Polo di
Monserrato, Monserrato, Cagliari, Italy

JEAN DARCOURT, MD
Department of Diagnostic and Therapeutic
Neuroradiology, Toulouse, France

MYRIAM EDJLALI, MD, PhD
Laboratoire D'imagerie Biomédicale
Multimodale (BioMaps), Université

Paris-Saclay, CEA, CNRS, Inserm, Service
Hospitalier Frédéric Joliot, Orsay, France;
Department of Radiology, APHP, Hôpitaux
Raymond-Poincaré & Ambroise Paré, DMU
Smart Imaging, GH Université Paris-Saclay,
Paris, France

KEIKO A. FUKUDA, MD
Department of Neurology, University of
California, Los Angeles, UCLA Comprehensive
Stroke Center, UCLA Neurovascular Imaging
Research Core, Los Angeles, California, USA

ANDREW J. GAUDEN, MD, PhD
Department of Neurosurgery, Stanford
University School of Medicine, Stanford,
California, USA

AJAY GUPTA, MD
Department of Radiology, Weill Cornell
Medical College, New York, New York,
USA

RAJIV GUPTA, PhD, MD
Department of Radiology, Massachusetts General Hospital, Harvard Medical School, Boston, Massachusetts, USA

ABDERRAHMANE HEDJOUDJE, MD, MSE
Department of Diagnostic and Interventional Neuroradiology, Sion Hospital, CHVR, Sion, Switzerland; Laboratoire D'imagerie Biomédicale Multimodale (BioMaps), Université Paris-Saclay, CEA, CNRS, Inserm, Service Hospitalier Frédéric Joliot, Orsay, France

JEREMY J. HEIT, MD, PhD
Department of Radiology, Stanford University School of Medicine, Stanford, California, USA; Assistant Professor of Radiology and Neurosurgery, Stanford University School of Medicine, Palo Alto, California, USA

SAMUEL S. HUANG, BS
MD Candidate, Albany Medical College, Lexington, Massachusetts, USA

HANS ROLF JÄGER, MD
Professor of Neuroradiology, Consultant Neuroradiologist, Lysholm Department of Neuroradiology, National Hospital for Neurology and Neurosurgery, Neuroradiological Academic Unit, Department of Brain Repair and Rehabilitation, UCL Queen Square Institute of Neurology, London, United Kingdom

MARIANNE ELINE KOOI, MD
Department of Radiology and Nuclear Medicine, CARIM School for Cardiovascular Diseases, Maastricht University Medical Center, Maastricht, the Netherlands

MICHAEL H. LEV, MD
Radiologist, Massachusetts General Hospital, Boston, Massachusetts, USA

SIMON LEVINSON, MD
Department of Neurosurgery, Stanford University School of Medicine, Stanford, California, USA

DAVID S. LIEBESKIND, MD
Department of Neurology, University of California, Los Angeles, UCLA Comprehensive Stroke Center, UCLA Neurovascular Imaging Research Core, Los Angeles, California, USA

JANET YANQING MEI, MD, MPH
Clinical Fellow, Neuroradiology Division, Massachusetts General Hospital, Boston, Massachusetts, USA

MAHMUD MOSSA-BASHA, MD
Professor of Radiology, Vice Chair of Clinical Research, Co-Director of the Research Vascular Imaging Lab, Department of Radiology, Adjunct Professor of Neurology and Electrical Engineering, University of Washington School of Medicine, Director of the Vascular Imaging Lab, University of Washington, Seattle, Washington, USA

JOSHUA P. NICKERSON, MD
Associate Professor, Diagnostic Radiology, School of Medicine, Oregon Health & Science University, Portland, Oregon, USA

LUIS NUNEZ, MD
Department of Diagnostic and Interventional Imaging, Neuroradiology Section, The University of Texas Health Science Center at Houston, Houston, Texas, USA

ARJUN V. PENDHARKAR, MD
Department of Neurosurgery, Stanford University School of Medicine, Stanford, California, USA

CHRISTOPHER A. POTTER, MD
Radiologist, Brigham and Women's Hospital, Boston, Massachusetts, USA

ROBERT W. REGENHARDT, MD, PhD
Neurointerventionalist, Massachusetts General Hospital, Boston, Massachusetts, USA

ROY RIASCOS, MD, FACR
Department of Diagnostic and Interventional Imaging, Neuroradiology Section, The University of Texas Health Science Center at Houston, Houston, Texas, USA

ANDRES RODRIGUEZ, MD
Department of Diagnostic and Interventional Imaging, Neuroradiology Section, The University of Texas Health Science Center at Houston, Houston, Texas, USA

LUISA F. ROJAS-SERRANO, MD
Physician, Candidate for a Master in public health. Residency in Psychiatry. Universidad del Rosario, Bogotá, Colombia

JAVIER M. ROMERO, MD
Associate Professor of Radiology, Harvard
Medical School, Massachusetts General
Hospital, Director, Vascular Ultrasound
Services, Director, RH Ackerman Neurovascular
Lab, Boston, Massachusetts, USA

LUCA SABA, MD
Department of Radiology, Azienda Ospedaliero
Universitaria (A.O.U.), di Cagliari – Polo di
Monserrato, Monserrato, Cagliari, Italy

BHAGYA SANNANANJA, MD
Assistant Professor, Department of Radiology
and Imaging Sciences, Emory University
School of Medicine, Atlanta, Georgia, USA

PAMELA W. SCHAEFER, MD, FACR
Professor of Radiology, Harvard Medical
School, Theresa McLoud Endowed Chair in
Radiology Education, Vice Chair, Education,
MGH and MGB, Neuroradiology Fellowship
Director, Massachusetts General Hospital,
Boston, Massachusetts, USA

ANIWAT SRIYOOK, MD
Department of Radiology, King Chulalongkorn
Memorial Hospital, The Thai Red Cross

Society, Faculty of Medicine, Chulalongkorn
University, Bangkok, Thailand; Department
of Radiology, Massachusetts General
Hospital, Harvard Medical School, Boston,
Massachusetts, USA

LASZLO SZIDONYA, MD, PhD
Radiology Fellow, Diagnostic Radiology,
Oregon Health & Science University, Portland,
Oregon, USA; Assistant Professor, Diagnostic
Radiology, Heart and Vascular Center,
Semmelweis University, Budapest,
Hungary

PEDRO VILELA, MD
Head of Neuroradiology, Hospital da Luz and
Hospital Beatriz Ângelo, Consultant
Neuroradiologist, Neuroradiology Department,
Lisbon Western University Center (Centro
Hospitalar Lisboa Ocidental -CHLO),
PortugalImaging Department, Hospital da Luz,
Lisbon, Portugal

CHENGCHENG ZHU, PhD
Assistant Professor, Department of Radiology,
University of Washington School of Medicine,
Seattle, Washington, USA

Society, Faculty of Medicine, Chulalongkorn
University, Bangkok, Thailand; Department
of Radiology, Massachusetts General
Hospital, Harvard Medical School, Boston,
Massachusetts, USA

LASZLO SZIDONYA, MD, PhD
Radiology Fellow, Diagnostic Radiology,
Oregon Health & Science University, Portland,
Oregon, USA; Assistant Professor, Diagnostic
Radiology, Heart and Vascular Center,
Semmelweis University, Budapest,
Hungary

PEDRO VILELA, MD
Head of Neuroradiology, Hospital da Luz and
Hospital Beatriz Ângelo, Consultant
Neuroradiologist, Neuroradiology Department,
de Carolina Univesity Center (Centro
Hospitalar Lisboa Ocidental—CHLO),
Neuroimaging department, Hospital da Luz,
Lisboa, Portugal

CHENGCHENG ZHU, PhD
Assistant Professor, Department of Radiology,
University of Washington School of Medicine,
Seattle, Washington, USA

JAVIER M. ROMERO, MD
Associate Professor of Radiology, Harvard
Medical School, Massachusetts General
Hospital, Director, Vascular Ultrasound
Section, Director, RH Abbott Neurovascular
Lab, Boston, Massachusetts, USA

LUCA SABA, MD
Department of Radiology, Azienda Ospedaliero
Universitaria (A.O.U.) di Cagliari - Polo di
Monserrato, Monserrato, Cagliari, Italy

SRINIVASAN... , MD
... of Professor, Department of Radiology
and Imaging Sciences, Emory University
School of Medicine, Atlanta, Georgia, USA

FRANKLIN A. ... SCHAFFOUR, MD, FACR
...

... ... PINOOK, MD
Department of Radiology, King Chulalongkorn
Memorial Hospital, Thai Red Cross

Contents

Stroke represents a major cause of morbidity and mortality worldwide with carotid atherosclerosis responsible for a large proportion of ischemic strokes. Given the high burden of the disease, early diagnosis and optimal secondary prevention are essential elements in clinical practice. For a long time, the degree of stenosis had been considered the parameter to judge the severity of carotid atherosclerosis. Over the last 30 years, literature has shifted attention from stenosis to structural characteristics of atherosclerotic lesion, eventually leading to the "vulnerable plaque" model. These "vulnerable plaques" frequently demonstrate high-risk imaging features that can be assessed by various non-invasive imaging modalities.

Ischemic strokes in young adults are increasing in incidence and have emerged as a public health issue. The radiological features are not only diagnostic in identifying ischemic infarctions but also provide important clues in the investigation of the underlying causes or in the identification of risk factors. According to the different imaging patterns associated with ischemic stroke in young adults, the causes can be classified into 5 categories: cardioembolism, large vessel vasculopathy, small vessel vasculopathy, toxic-metabolic, and hypercoagulable disorders. The radiological features of each category and cause are described and summarized in this review.

The cerebral collateral circulation is an increasingly important consideration in the management of acute ischemic stroke and is a key determinant of outcomes. Growing evidence has demonstrated that better collaterals can predict the rate of infarct progression, degree of recanalization, the likelihood of hemorrhagic transformation and various therapeutic opportunities. Collaterals can also identify those unlikely to respond to reperfusion therapies, helping to optimize resources. More randomized trials are needed to evaluate the risks and benefits of endovascular reperfusion with consideration of collateral status. This reviews our current understanding of the pathophysiologic mechanisms, effect on outcomes and strategies for improvement of the collateral system.

There is constant evolution in the diagnosis and treatment of acute ischemic stroke due to advances in treatments, imaging, and outreach. Two major revolutions were the advent of intravenous thrombolysis in the 1990s and endovascular thrombectomy in 2010s. Neuroimaging approaches have also evolved with key goals—detect hemorrhage, augment thrombolysis treatment selection, detect arterial occlusion, estimate infarct core, estimate viable penumbra, and augment thrombectomy treatment selection. The ideal approach to diagnosis and treatment may differ depending on the system of care and available resources. Future directions include expanding indications for these treatments, including a shift from time-based to tissue-based selection.

In this review, we discuss the imaging of aneurysmal subarachnoid hemorrhage (SAH). We discuss emergency brain imaging, aneurysm detection techniques, and the management of CTA-negative SAH. We also review the concepts of cerebral vasospasm and delayed cerebral ischemia that occurs after aneurysm rupture and their impact on patient outcomes. These pathologies are distinct, and the use of multimodal imaging modalities is essential for prompt diagnosis and management to minimize morbidity from these conditions. Lastly, new advances in artificial intelligence and advanced imaging modalities such as PET and MR imaging scans have been shown to improve the detection of aneurysms and potentially predict outcomes early in the course of SAH.

Blunt and penetrating vascular injuries of the head and neck can represent life-threatening emergencies that require accurate detection to prevent devastating and long-lasting consequences. Implementing appropriate screening criteria to indicate imaging studies is crucial as there is a variable latent time before the onset of clinical manifestations. Computed tomography angiography, MR imaging, and digital subtraction angiography represent the imaging modalities of choice to evaluate vascular injuries. The aim of this review is to provide a description of the different types of vascular injuries, describe the importance of each imaging modality, and recognize the imaging appearance of traumatic vessel injury.

Advanced imaging is currently critical in diagnosing, predicting, and managing intracerebral hemorrhage. MD CT angiography has occupied the first line of evaluating patients with a clinical diagnosis of a stroke, given its rapid acquisition time, high resolution of vascular structures, and sensitivity for secondary causes of ICH.

Cryptogenic strokes are symptomatic cerebral ischemic infarcts without a clear etiology identified following standard diagnostic evaluation and currently account for 10% to 40% of stroke cases. Continued research is needed to identify and bridge gaps in knowledge of this stroke grouping. Vessel wall imaging has increasingly shown its utility in the diagnosis and characterization of various vasculopathies. Initial promising evidence suggests rational use of vessel wall imaging in stroke workup may unravel pathologies that otherwise would have been occult and further improve our understanding of underlying disease processes that can translate into improved patient outcomes and secondary stroke prevention.

Cerebral venous thrombosis (CVT) is a rare cerebrovascular disease caused by an occlusion of the cerebral venous sinuses or cortical veins. It has a favorable prognosis if diagnosed and treated early. CVT can be difficult to diagnose on clinical grounds, and imaging plays a key role. We discuss clinical features and provide an overview of current neuroimaging methods and findings in CTV.

Three-dimensional vessel wall MR imaging has gained popularity in the diagnosis and management of patients with cerebrovascular disease in clinical practice. Vessel wall MR imaging is an imaging technique that delivers a fundamentally different viewpoint by emphasizing on the pathology of the vessel wall as opposed to traditional descriptions that focus on the vessel lumen. It shows a crucial power in detecting vessel wall changes in patients with diseases including, but not limited to, central nervous system vasculitis, moyamoya disease, aneurysms, dissections, and intracranial atherosclerotic disease.

Traumatic brain injury is one of the most common causes of morbidity and mortality and significantly impacts the patients' quality of life and socioeconomic status. It can be classified into primary and secondary injuries. Primary injury occurs at the time of the initial head trauma, such as skull fracture, extra-axial hemorrhage, brain contusion, and diffuse axonal injury. Secondary injury develops later as complications such as diffuse cerebral edema, brain herniation, and chronic traumatic encephalopathy. This article describes the indication for imaging, imaging modalities, recommended imaging protocols, and imaging findings of primary and secondary injuries, including pitfalls of each pathology.

Cerebral amyloid angiopathy (CAA) is associated with deposition of amyloid proteins within the intracranial vessels. It is most frequently sporadic and risk increases with advancing age. Amyloid deposition is associated with increased risk of peripheral microhemorrhage, lobar hemorrhage, and/or repetitive subarachnoid hemorrhage. The presence of a peripherally located lobar hemorrhage on computed tomography in an elderly patient should raise concern for underlying CAA, as should multiple foci of peripheral susceptibility artifact or superficial siderosis on susceptibility-weighted imaging, the most sensitive modality for these findings. Newer PET radiotracers are also useful in detecting amyloid deposition.

PROGRAM OBJECTIVE
The objective of the *Radiologic Clinics of North America* is to keep practicing radiologists and radiology residents up to date with current clinical practice in radiology by providing timely articles reviewing the state of the art in patient care.

TARGET AUDIENCE
Practicing radiologists, radiology residents, and other healthcare professionals who provide patient care utilizing radiologic findings.

LEARNING OBJECTIVES
Upon completion of this activity, participants will be able to:
1. Describe cerebrovascular disease.
2. Discuss advances in imaging studies to assist in treatment for acute ischemic stroke.
3. Recognize the signs and symptoms of ischemic strokes in young adults and utilize radiological studies diagnose and help identify underlying causes.

ACCREDITATION
The Elsevier Office of Continuing Medical Education (EOCME) is accredited by the Accreditation Council for Continuing Medical Education (ACCME) to provide continuing medical education for physicians.

The EOCME designates this journal-based CME activity for a maximum of 12 *AMA PRA Category 1 Credit*(s)™. Physicians should claim only the credit commensurate with the extent of their participation in the activity.

All other healthcare professionals requesting continuing education credit for this enduring material will be issued a certificate of participation.

DISCLOSURE OF CONFLICTS OF INTEREST
The EOCME assesses conflict of interest with its instructors, faculty, planners, and other individuals who are in a position to control the content of CME activities. All relevant conflicts of interest that are identified are thoroughly vetted by EOCME for fair balance, scientific objectivity, and patient care recommendations. EOCME is committed to providing its learners with CME activities that promote improvements or quality in healthcare and not a specific proprietary business or a commercial interest.

The planning committee, staff, authors, and editors listed below have identified no financial relationships or relationships to products or devices they or their spouse/life partner have with commercial interest related to the content of this CME activity:
Fabrice Bonneville, MD, PhD; Francesco Carletti, PhD; Riccardo Cau, MD; Jean Darcourt, MD; Myriam Edjlali, MD, PhD; Keiko A. Fukuda, MD; Andrew J. Gauden, MD, PhD; Ajay Gupta, MD, MS; Rajiv Gupta, MD; Abderrahmane Hedjoudje, MDE, MSE; Samuel S. Huang, BS; Hans Rolf Jäger, MD, FRCR; Lynette Jones, MSN, RN-BC; M. Eline Kooi, PhD; Kothainayaki Kulanthaivelu, BCA, MBA; Simon Levinson, MD; David S. Liebeskind, MD; Janet Yanqing Mei, MD, MPH; Mahmud Mossa-Basha, MD; Joshua P. Nickerson, MD; Luis Nunez, MD; Arjun V. Pendharkar, MD; Christopher A. Potter, MD; Roy Riascos, MD; Andres Rodriguez, MD; Luisa F. Rojas-Serrano, MD; Javier M. Romero, MD, FAHA; Luca Saba, MD, PhD; Bhagya Sannananja, MD; Pamela W. Schaefer, MD, FACR; Aniwat Sriyook, MD; Laszlo Szidonya, MD, PhD; Pedro Vilela, MD; Chengcheng Zhu, PhD

The planning committee, staff, authors, and editors listed below have identified financial relationships or relationships to products or devices they or their spouse/life partner have with commercial interest related to the content of this CME activity:
Jeremy J. Heit, MD, PhD: Consultant: Medtronic, MicroVention, Inc., iSchemaView, Inc.

Michael H. Lev, MD: Consultant: GE Healthcare, Takeda Pharmaceuticals, F. Hoffmann-La Roche Ltd, Genentech, Seagen

Robert W. Regenhardt, MD, PhD: Consultant/Advisor: MicroVention, Inc, Penumbra, Inc.

UNAPPROVED/OFF-LABEL USE DISCLOSURE
The EOCME requires CME faculty to disclose to the participants:
1. When products or procedures being discussed are off-label, unlabelled, experimental, and/or investigational (not US Food and Drug Administration [FDA] approved); and
2. Any limitations on the information presented, such as data that are preliminary or that represent ongoing research, interim analyses, and/or unsupported opinions. Faculty may discuss information about pharmaceutical agents that is outside of FDA-approved labelling. This information is intended solely for CME and is not intended to promote off-label use of these medications. If you have any questions, contact the medical affairs department of the manufacturer for the most recent prescribing information.

TO ENROLL
To enroll in the *Radiologic Clinics of North America* Continuing Medical Education program, call customer service at 1-800-654-2452 or sign up online at http://www.theclinics.com/home/cme. The CME program is available to subscribers for an additional annual fee of USD 340.00.

METHOD OF PARTICIPATION

In order to claim credit, participants must complete the following:

1. Complete enrolment as indicated above.
2. Read the activity.
3. Complete the CME Test and Evaluation. Participants must achieve a score of 70% on the test. All CME Tests and Evaluations must be completed online.

CME INQUIRIES/SPECIAL NEEDS

For all CME inquiries or special needs, please contact elsevierCME@elsevier.com.

RADIOLOGIC CLINICS OF NORTH AMERICA

Preface
Imaging Approaches for Cerebrovascular Disease: The Latest and Greatest

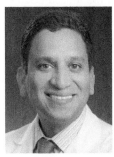 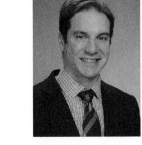

Javier M. Romero, MD   Mahmud Mossa-Basha, MD
Editors

Stroke, including ischemic and hemorrhagic sub-types, is a leading cause of morbidity and mortality worldwide, with a variety of cerebrovascular diseases contributing to its cause. Imaging plays a central role in the diagnosis of stroke and intracranial hemorrhage and the underlying contributing cerebrovascular diseases. Imaging is also key in risk stratification of cerebrovascular lesions, treatment decision making and guidance, primary and secondary stroke prevention, treatment response assessment, and therapeutic interventions. Conventional and advanced imaging applications involving multiple modalities, including computed tomography, MR imaging, ultrasound, digital subtraction angiography, PET, and other nuclear medicine applications, have core clinical applications in neurovascular disease, as well as exciting research promise for further advancing diagnosis, therapy, and risk stratification.

The current *Radiologic Clinics of North America* issue covers major current cerebrovascular disease topics, discussing current imaging, therapeutic paradigms, and cutting-edge research approaches. This issue will highlight the "latest" diagnostic and treatment paradigms, and the "greatest" innovations on the horizon for cerebrovascular disease advanced imaging biomarkers and other biomarkers, including serology and genetic markers. The 12 articles cover carotid atherosclerotic disease, young adult stroke, collateral circulation and its importance in stroke, advanced acute stroke imaging for patient triage, aneurysmal subarachnoid hemorrhage, traumatic cerebrovascular injury, intraparenchymal hemorrhage, vessel wall imaging for cryptogenic stroke, sinus venous thrombosis, central nervous system vasculitis, traumatic brain injury, and cerebral amyloid angiopathy.

The goal of this issue is to provide the reader with a comprehensive understanding of cerebrovascular disease diagnostic algorithms and management in a variety of disease states, introducing them to future directions of imaging, and stimulating their interest in recently breaking research approaches to better diagnose and stratify disease risk, that may potentially ignite researchers and future researchers on a career path in cerebrovascular disease investigation. We hope you

Radiol Clin N Am 61 (2023) xv–xvi
https://doi.org/10.1016/j.rcl.2023.01.013
0033-8389/23/© 2023 Published by Elsevier Inc.

enjoy reading this issue as much as we enjoyed working on it.

Javier M. Romero, MD
Harvard Medical School
Massachusetts General Hospital
Gray/Bigelow
90 Blossom Street
Boston, MA 02114, USA

Mahmud Mossa-Basha, MD
University of Washington
University of Washington Medical Center
1959 NE Pacific Street
Seattle, WA 98195, USA

E-mail addresses:
jmromero@mgh.harvard.edu (J.M. Romero)
mmossab@uw.edu (M. Mossa-Basha)

Pearls and Pitfalls of Carotid Artery Imaging
Ultrasound, Computed Tomography Angiography, and MR Imaging

Riccardo Cau, MD[a], Ajay Gupta, MD[b], Marianne Eline Kooi, MD[c], Luca Saba, MD[a],*

KEYWORDS

• Carotid arteries • Vulnerable plaque • US • CTA • MRA

KEY POINTS

• Non-invasive plaque imaging modalities provide additional information beyond stenosis degree.
• Plaque vulnerability features can be detected with high diagnostic accuracy leveraging various imaging modality strengths.
• Radiologists and other clinicians need to become familiar with pearls and pitfalls of each of the plaque imaging modalities.

INTRODUCTION

Carotid atherosclerosis is a complex and multifactorial disease and a well-established risk factor for ischemic stroke (**Figs. 1** and **2**). The degree of carotid stenosis was considered the sole imaging criterion for stratifying carotid atherosclerosis severity based on prior randomized trials, namely the European Carotid Surgery Trial (ECST), the North American Symptomatic Carotid Endarterectomy Trial (NASCET), and the Asymptomatic Carotid Atherosclerosis Study.[1–3]

Several ex vivo studies reported significant differences in the risk of cardiovascular events given similar degree of luminal stenosis, focusing on "plaque vulnerability" based on plaque composition.[4–7] Vulnerable carotid plaques tend to progress rapidly and are highly associated with cardiovascular complications.[8]

Carotid plaque imaging can identify high-risk imaging markers of future cardiovascular events, directing patient stratification and management.[9,10] Recent years have seen imaging technique advancements, enabling reproducible multi-modality lesion detection and vulnerable feature characterization. Among them, ultrasound (US) represents a widely available imaging modality to evaluate not only the degree of carotid stenosis but also plaque echogenicity as an index of plaque vulnerability.[11,12] Computed tomography angiography (CTA) plays a crucial role in plaque evaluation enabling a more detailed description of plaque composition and morphology.[13–15] Finally, MR imaging is the most specific method for identifying histologically validated vulnerable plaque features, namely intraplaque hemorrhage (IPH), lipid-rich necrotic core (LRNC), and the thickness and integrity of the fibrous cap (FC). The ability to assess high-risk features may also be implemented by adding dedicated sequences to the standard MR imaging examination.[8,16]

In this review, we discuss the role of non-invasive imaging modalities in the landscape of carotid pathology, comparing their strengths, weaknesses, and potentialities.

[a] Department of Radiology, Azienda Ospedaliero Universitaria (A.O.U.), di Cagliari – Polo di Monserrato, s.s. 554, Monserrato, Cagliari 09045, Italy; [b] Department of Radiology Weill Cornell Medical College, New York, NY, USA; [c] Department of Radiology and Nuclear Medicine, CARIM School for Cardiovascular Diseases, Maastricht University Medical Center, Maastricht, the Netherlands
* Corresponding author.
E-mail address: lucasaba@tiscali.it

Radiol Clin N Am 61 (2023) 405–413
https://doi.org/10.1016/j.rcl.2023.01.001

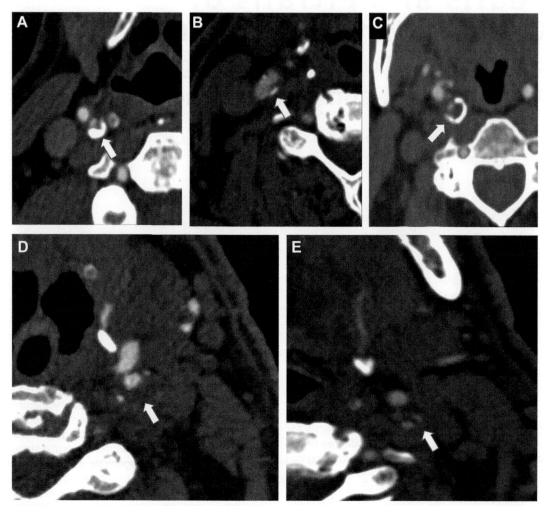

Fig. 1. Examples of different "high-risk" features of carotid plaque using CT. Panel *A–C* demonstrates different carotid plaque calcifications, in particular, heavy calcified plaque (*arrow* in *A*), microcalcification (*arrow* in *B*), and "positive rim" sign, defined as plaque with adventitial calcification (<2 mm thick) and internal soft plaque (>2 mm thickness) (*arrow* in *C*). CTA axial image (*D*) shows a hypodense plaque (HU value = 15) indicating the presence of LRNC (*arrow*). CTA axial image (*E*) demonstrates ulcerated stenosis in the postbulbous left internal carotid artery.

DEGREE OF STENOSIS

Currently, the degree of carotid stenosis was the key point considered in deciding management approaches, based on the NASCET and ECST trial results.[17,18] According to the current European Society of Cardiology (ESC) guidelines, US is the first-line examination.[19] The degree of carotid stenosis is estimated through different hemodynamic criteria on Doppler US, including peak systolic velocity, end-diastolic velocity, and carotid index allowing direct measurement of flow velocity,[19] with B-mode a supplementary method to evaluate carotid stenosis.[19]

The diagnostic accuracy of Duplex US demonstrated a sensitivity of 98% (95% CI, 97%–100%) and specificity of 88% (95% CI, 76%–100%) for

detecting 50% to 70% stenosis and sensitivity of 90% (95% CI, 84%–94%) and specificity of 94% (95% CI, 88%–97%) for ≥70% stenosis.[20] US, despite its wide availability, ease, and low cost, is limited by intrinsic and extrinsic weaknesses. First, unfavorable patient anatomy (vessel tortuosity, short thick neck, high carotid bifurcation, external devices), calcified carotid plaque obscuring assessment, limited windows, and overestimation due to a contralateral carotid occlusion are limitations. Second, the US is operator-dependent and image quality often directly correlates to operator experience.[21]

The ESC guidelines recommend CTA and magnetic resonance angiography (MRA) as a complement to the US for carotid stenosis evaluation.[22,23]

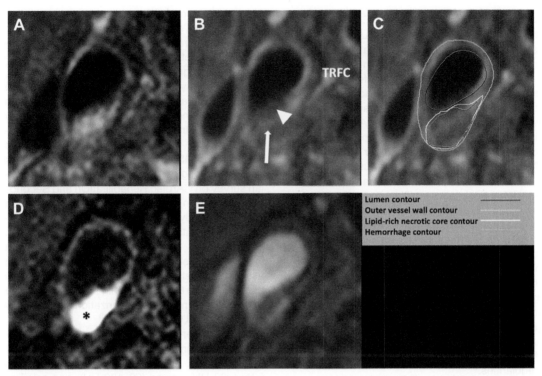

Fig. 2. Multi-sequence carotid MR imaging at the same cross-sectional level. The following MR images are acquired in the transverse plane: (A) pre-contrast T1-weighted (T1w) quadruple inversion recovery (QIR) turbo spin echo (TSE), (B) pre-contrast and (C) post-contrast T1w QIR TSE, (D) T1w inversion recovery (IR) turbo field echo (TFE), and (E) time of flight (TOF). LRNC was identified as an intraplaque region that does not show contrast enhancement (arrow). A hyperintense signal in the bulk of the plaque can be clearly observed in the IR-TFE image, indicating the presence of intraplaque hemorrhage (asterisk). The fibrous cap was scored as thin or ruptured (TRFC) because there was no signal enhancement in the region between the LRNC and the lumen (arrowhead).

CT demonstrates excellent diagnostic accuracy with sensitivity and specificity of 95% and 98% for the detection of >70% stenosis, respectively. Conversely, CT is limited by heavy calcified plaque.[21] Finally, contrast-enhanced (CE)-MRA represents the most sensitive tool for carotid stenosis.[24]

CAROTID PLAQUE

High-risk carotid plaque features, including IPH, thinning or rupture of FC, maximum wall thickness or plaque volume, plaque morphology, LRNC, plaque inflammation, plaque neovascularization, and calcifications may be investigated by different non-invasive modalities with lesser or greater capacity to provide insight into plaque composition and morphology. In the following section, features related to plaque vulnerability are presented with a particular focus on the pearls and pitfalls of the various modalities.

Maximum Wall Thickness

Maximum wall thickness is the maximum thickness of the plaque,[25] and correlates with plaque

volume, a feature of plaque vulnerability. Plaque thickness is relatively easily assessed by US, CTA, or MRA.[8] In daily clinical practice, US, due to its availability and feasibility, is the first-line modality to assess carotid plaque thickness.[26,27] A prospective cohort study of 43 patients from the ORION trial with 16% to 79% carotid stenosis who underwent carotid MRA and US demonstrated significant inter-modality plaque thickness measurement agreement (Pearson correlation coefficient r = 0.93; $P < 0.001$).[28] However, when US imaging is limited,[29] CTA or MRA can appropriately evaluate plaque characteristics.[16]

The carotid plaque area and volume are highly reproducible parameters associated with plaque size.[30,31] In the Plaque At RISK (PARISK) study, carotid plaque volume and area were independently associated with recurrent ipsilateral cerebrovascular ischemic events (HR: 1.07 per 100 mL increase for plaque volume; 95% CI 1.00–1.22).[31] Plaque area and volume are more accurate than plaque thickness in measuring plaque progression/regression because plaque grows in all directions.[32]

Plaque Surface Morphology and Ulcerations

The luminal surface of carotid plaque can be categorized as smooth (regular luminal morphology), irregular (small luminal alteration from 0.3 to 0.9 mm), and ulcerated (intimal defect causing an extension of the lumen into the plaque measuring at least 1 mm).[13,16] The plaque surface can be evaluated using US, CTA, and MRA, with variable diagnostic accuracy.[8,10] US is specifically suboptimal compared with CTA or MRA unless ultrasound-enhancing agents are used.[16]

Carotid contrast-enhanced ultrasound (CEUS) can enhance image quality, improving luminal and plaque anatomy evaluation including plaque surface irregularities and ulcerations.[25] Widespread utilization of CEUS for plaque imaging, however, is off-label and is not addressed in the most recent American Society of Echocardiography guidelines.[33] 3D US methods have also shown promise in the assessment of carotid plaque irregularities.[34,35] The main strength of 3D quantification of carotid plaque is its multiplanar capacity, enabling a comprehensive assessment of plaque morphology, geometry, and surface irregularities.[25]

Time of flight-MRA (TOF-MRA) is limited in ulceration detection due to signal dephasing and saturation in focal areas of complex flow such as an ulcer crater.[36] It can also overestimate the degree of stenosis.[27] Contrast-enhanced (CE) MRA can overcome these limitations because it is not dependent on blood flow. Etesami et al. reported that 37.5% of ulcerated plaques detected with CE-MRA images were not visualized with TOF-MRA.[37] In addition, CE-MRA can identify ulcerations in calcified plaque.[27]

CT is the reference standard non-invasive imaging modality to evaluate plaque ulcerations. A cross-sectional study of 237 patients reported a higher sensitivity and specificity for CT in comparison with the US (sensitivity of 93.75% vs 37.5% and specificity of 98.59% vs 91.3%, respectively)[38] in comparison to surgical specimens for ulcerated plaque. The primary limitation of CT for carotid plaque assessment is beam hardening from extensive calcification. This limitation can be overcome with dual-source CT, which uses low- and high-peak kilovoltage acquisitions allowing the removal of calcified plaque components from the lumen, permitting a more accurate assessment of plaque and lumen.[27,39]

Plaque Composition

Carotid plaque consists of several components and the proportion of subcomponents can correlate with future ischemic events.[16,40] The characterization of different tissue types, including carotid plaque, was initially qualitatively evaluated using US via grayscale values according to echogenicity and heterogeneity; however, this information can be augmented with quantitative analyses, specifically grayscale median (GSM).[25] GSM is the median gray value of the US pixel and has been evaluated in the Imaging in Carotid Angioplasty and Risk of Stroke study, an international multicenter registry that investigated the relationship between the GSM of carotid plaque and the risk of stroke during carotid artery stenting.[41] The Italian survey on CArdiac RehabilitatiOn and Secondary prevention after cardiac revascularization (ICARIOS) study reported that the rate of cerebrovascular events was higher in patients with GSM<25 in comparison to patients with GSM>25.[41] Histological studies also reported an association between less calcification, unstable plaque, a large lipid core, a thin FC, and increased inflammation and neovascularization histologically and low GSM US values.[30,42,43]

Carotid atherosclerotic plaque component differentiation using CT is based on Hounsfield unit (HU) densities. Carotid plaques are classified as fatty (<60 HU), mixed (60–130 HU), and calcified (>130 HU) on CT.[44] Dual-energy CT (DECT) facilitates better tissue characterization, with higher spatial resolution, lower contrast agent utilization, lower radiation dose, and reduced artifacts.[45] In addition, the introduction of spectral CT with photon counting brings the promise of improved plaque characterization through the generation of contrast agent concentration and photon attenuation maps.[46] Histological validation and longitudinal studies are warranted to evaluate the impact and predictive value of spectral photon counting CT on carotid plaque vulnerability for stroke assessment. Specifically, using data from randomized prospective trials (eg, Comparison of Spectral Photon Counting CT with Dual-Energy CT and MR Imaging for Plaque and Lumen Carotid Arteries Evaluation (CAPL) [NCT04466787]) may contribute to better understanding the role of spectral photon counting CT.

Different plaque components can be identified using high-resolution, multiparametric MRA, including pre- and post-contrast high-resolution 2D or 3D T1-weighted, magnetization-prepared rapid gradient-echo (MPRAGE), T2-weighted, and TOF-MRA sequences. Fat suppression and blood suppression are valuable for optimal lesion contrast from surrounding tissues, and to avoid artifacts that may mimic pathological lesions.[47,48]

LRNC consists of heterogeneous collections of cholesterol crystals and cellular debris. MR imaging is the gold standard for LRNC visualization due to superior soft tissue contrast.[8,10] LRNC presents as a focal hypointense area on T2-weight images and is best appreciated on CE-MRA as a focal non-enhancing area.[8]

LRNC can be also visualized using CT due to lipid attenuation properties with HU values < 60. A histological study by Walker and colleagues[49] reported a trend toward lower attenuation measurements with increased intraplaque lipid, but with a high standard deviation of HU values. These results highlighted an important limitation to the application of CT for the characterization of LRNC, namely the significant overlap of HU values between LRNC, fibrous tissue, and IPH.[49] Another potential limitation of intraplaque lipid assessment on CT is obscuration from heavily calcified plaque.[6] De Weert and colleagues[50] reported that LRNC can be detected with good correlation with the histological specimen ($R^2 = 0.77$) only in mildly calcified plaques.

US can detect LRNC as a hypoechogenic area, also known as a juxta-luminal black area. Plaques with juxtaluminal LRNC on histology demonstrated significantly lower GSM values, reflecting a hypoechoic region at the plaque surface ($P = 0.009$).[51] Nonetheless, US is not useful for discriminating between IPH and LRNC, thus limiting US value in carotid plaque characterization.[8,13]

FC is a connective tissue layer that divides the plaque from the lumen. FC ulceration and/or rupture exposes the LRNC to platelets and coagulation factors leading to a thromboembolic cascade.

Currently, MRA is the best non-invasive imaging modality to investigate FC status. On MRA, a normal FC appears as a juxtaluminal band of low signal on TOF-MRA.[52] The absence of the dark juxtaluminal band or presence of focal juxtaluminal hyperintensity is indicative of "vulnerable plaque".[8,52] Contrast agents can help discriminate between FC and LRNC. The contrast increases the signal intensity of fibrous tissue in comparison with LRNC and, therefore, contrast-enhanced MR imaging has good reproducibility of FC status assessment.[53,54]

On US, FC appears as an echogenic structure with stronger echoes compared to plaque and blood.[55] The evaluation of FC status and thickness has a 73% sensitivity and 67% specificity using stratified GSM parameters.[51] Conversely, CT is not suitable for FC assessment due to edge-blur and halo effect artifacts.[13] Some studies, however, suggest that fissured FC can be detected using CT. Saba and colleagues[56] demonstrated that plaques with histologically confirmed fissured FC showed higher enhancement on CT compared to non-fissured plaques.

IPH is considered one of the most important features associated with plaque instability. MR imaging is the best modality for the detection of IPH, due to its ability to characterize the hemoglobin oxidative state.[13,57] Several studies suggested the use of fat-suppressed T1-weighted sequences in clinical practice to identify IPH. This sequence, thanks to an inversion pulse for blood suppression, identifies IPH as a focal intraplaque hyperintense signal with intensity >150% of that of adjacent muscles.[4,8]

A number of recent studies have suggested that CT can also detect IPH,[36,58,59] including studies that showed a good correlation between IPH detected by CT and the corresponding histologic section ($\kappa = 0.712$; $P = 0.102$),[60] with limitations in smaller plaques and heavily calcified plaques.[60] The sensitivity and specificity of CT to detect IPH was 100% and 64%, respectively.[61,62]

Plaque inflammation and neovascularization: Plaque inflammation, another vulnerable plaque feature, remains predominantly investigative. MRA using ultrasmall superparamagnetic iron oxide nanoparticles as a surrogate marker of macrophage accumulation and activity has shown promising results.[63,64] Alternatively, fluorodeoxyglucose positron emission tomography (18-FDG PET) can identify areas of inflammation.[65] Another indirect approach to assess plaque inflammation is to evaluate the perivascular adipose tissue for stranding using CTA.[66]

Plaque imaging can also detect plaque neovascularization using US, CTA, or MRA.[13] In particular, dynamic contrast-enhanced (DCE)-MRA is well-suited to evaluate intraplaque neovessels.[13,67] CEUS can also be used to detect plaque neovascularization, defined as the movement of microbubbles from the adventitia to the plaque core.[68,69] A meta-analysis including 20 studies demonstrated the association between plaque enhancement on CEUS and intraplaque neo-vessels.[70] Finally, some studies suggested that the amount of plaque enhancement on CTA is associated with the extent of intraplaque neovascularization.[56,71]

Calcifications: Controversial results have emerged regarding the role of calcium in atherosclerosis and its relationship with plaque vulnerability.[14] The size and location of carotid calcifications are related to the variable risk of cerebrovascular events. Studies have suggested that microcalcifications were significantly associated with unstable plaques,[72,73] whereas large calcifications are protective.[14]

Recently, Saba and colleagues[73] investigated the relationship between calcium configuration and the prevalence of cerebrovascular events using CT, highlighting the potential role of calcium in plaque vulnerability. CTA is considered the reference standard in the detection of calcification. Nevertheless, plaque calcification can be detected with US (as a hyperechogenic area) and MR imaging (as a hypointense region on all contrast sequences) with lower sensitivity and specificity compared to CTA.[55]

GENERAL TECHNIQUE LIMITATIONS

Beyond the limitations of each modality in identifying high-risk plaque, it is necessary to know the general technique limitations. In particular, the US application is limited by the operator's skill, composition (calcifications), anatomy, and a limited anatomic window.[21]

The CTA disadvantages include ionizing radiation exposure and adverse reactions to iodinated contrast media. Another CTA limitation is limited differentiation of the outer carotid wall in the absence of the surrounding adipose tissue.[57]

The limitations of MR imaging include its long acquisition time, the need for specialized hardware (carotid coils) for high-resolution images to detect FC status, the complexity of interpretation, and limited access.[74] If only IPH is scored on carotid MR imaging, a short MR image examination with a standard neurovascular coil is sufficient and image interpretation is straightforward.

SUMMARY

Various non-invasive plaque imaging modalities can provide detailed information on the carotid plaque with supplementary and complementary roles in identifying high-risk features. Further evidence is necessary to incorporate each of these imaging modalities with their advantages and limitations into a standardized diagnostic flowchart with the purpose to offer a significant contribution to risk stratification and patient management.

CLINICS CARE POINTS

- Carotid artery atherosclerosis is associated with an increased risk of cardiovascular events.
- IPH, thinning or rupture of FC, maximum wall thickness or plaque volume, plaque morphology, LRNC, plaque inflammation, plaque neovascularization, and calcifications are markers of plaque vulnerability and predictors of future events.

- Non-invasive plaque imaging techniques complement each other in their ability to identify features of plaque instability.

REFERENCES

1. North American Symptomatic Carotid Endarterectomy Trial. Methods, patient characteristics, and progress. Stroke 1991;22(6):711–20.
2. Randomised trial of endarterectomy for recently symptomatic carotid stenosis: final results of the MRC European Carotid Surgery Trial (ECST). Lancet (London, England) 1998;351(9113):1379–87.
3. Abbott AL. Medical (nonsurgical) intervention alone is now best for prevention of stroke associated with asymptomatic severe carotid stenosis: results of a systematic review and analysis. Stroke 2009; 40(10):e573–83.
4. Saba L, Brinjikji W, Spence JD, et al. Roadmap consensus on carotid artery plaque imaging and impact on therapy strategies and guidelines: an international, multispecialty, expert review and position statement. AJNR Am J Neuroradiol 2021;42(9): 1566–75.
5. Saba L, Sanfilippo R, Sannia S, et al. Association between carotid artery plaque volume, composition, and ulceration: a retrospective assessment with MDCT. AJR Am J Roentgenol 2012;199(1):151–6.
6. Zhu G, Hom J, Li Y, et al. Carotid plaque imaging and the risk of atherosclerotic cardiovascular disease. Cardiovasc Diagn Ther 2020;10(4):1048–67.
7. Schindler A, Schinner R, Altaf N, et al. Prediction of stroke risk by detection of hemorrhage in carotid plaques: meta-analysis of individual patient data. JACC Cardiovasc Imaging 2020;13(2 Pt 1):395–406.
8. Saba L, Moody AR, Saam T, et al. Vessel wall–imaging biomarkers of carotid plaque vulnerability in stroke prevention trials. JACC Cardiovasc Imaging 2020;13(11):2445–56.
9. Singh N, Marko M, Ospel JM, et al. The risk of stroke and TIA in nonstenotic carotid plaques: a systematic review and meta-analysis. AJNR Am J Neuroradiol 2020;41(8):1453–9.
10. Saba L, Yuan C, Hatsukami TS, et al. Carotid Artery Wall Imaging: Perspective and Guidelines from the ASNR Vessel Wall Imaging Study Group and Expert Consensus Recommendations of the American Society of Neuroradiology. Am J Neuroradiol 2018; 39(2). https://doi.org/10.3174/ajnr.A5488.
11. Picano E, Paterni M. Ultrasound tissue characterization of vulnerable atherosclerotic plaque. Int J Mol Sci 2015;16(5):10121–33.
12. Jashari F, Ibrahimi P, Bajraktari G, et al. Carotid plaque echogenicity predicts cerebrovascular symptoms: a systematic review and meta-analysis. Eur J Neurol 2016;23(7):1241–7.

13. Saba L, Agarwal N, Cau R, et al. Review of imaging biomarkers for the vulnerable carotid plaque. JVS Vasc Sci 2021. https://doi.org/10.1016/j.jvssci.2021.03.001.

14. Saba L, Nardi V, Cau R, et al. Carotid artery plaque calcifications: lessons from histopathology to diagnostic imaging. Stroke 2022;53(1):290–7.

15. Cademartiri F, Balestrieri A, Cau R, et al. Insight from imaging on plaque vulnerability: similarities and differences between coronary and carotid arteries—implications for systemic therapies. Cardiovasc Diagn Ther 2020;10(4):1150–62.

16. Saba L, Saam T, Jäger HR, et al. Imaging biomarkers of vulnerable carotid plaques for stroke risk prediction and their potential clinical implications. Lancet Neurol 2019;4422(19):1–14.

17. Endarterectomy for asymptomatic carotid artery stenosis. Executive Committee for the Asymptomatic Carotid Atherosclerosis Study. JAMA 1995;273(18):1421–8.

18. Barnett HJ, Taylor DW, Eliasziw M, et al. Benefit of carotid endarterectomy in patients with symptomatic moderate or severe stenosis. North American Symptomatic Carotid Endarterectomy Trial Collaborators. N Engl J Med 1998;339(20):1415–25.

19. Messas E, Goudot G, Halliday A, et al. Management of carotid stenosis for primary and secondary prevention of stroke: state-of-the-art 2020: a critical review. Eur Heart J Suppl 2020;22(Suppl M):M35–42.

20. Jahromi AS, Cinà CS, Liu Y, et al. Sensitivity and specificity of color duplex ultrasound measurement in the estimation of internal carotid artery stenosis: a systematic review and meta-analysis. J Vasc Surg 2005;41(6):962–72.

21. Adla T, Adlova R. Multimodality imaging of carotid stenosis. Int J Angiol 2015;24(3):179–84.

22. Aboyans V, Ricco J-B, Bartelink M-LEL, et al. 2017 ESC Guidelines on the Diagnosis and Treatment of Peripheral Arterial Diseases, in collaboration with the European Society for Vascular Surgery (ESVS): Document covering atherosclerotic disease of extracranial carotid and vertebral, mesenteric, renal. Eur Heart J 2018;39(9):763–816.

23. Prokop M, Waaijer A, Kreuzer S. CT angiography of the carotid arteries. JBR-BTR 2004;87(1):23–9.

24. Yang CW, Carr JC, Futterer SF, et al. Contrast-enhanced MR angiography of the carotid and vertebrobasilar circulations. AJNR Am J Neuroradiol 2005;26(8):2095–101.

25. Johri AM, Nambi V, Naqvi TZ, et al. Recommendations for the assessment of carotid arterial plaque by ultrasound for the characterization of atherosclerosis and evaluation of cardiovascular risk: from the american society of echocardiography. J Am Soc Echocardiogr 2020;33(8):917–33.

26. Landry A, Spence JD, Fenster A. Measurement of carotid plaque volume by 3-dimensional ultrasound. Stroke 2004;35(4):864–9.

27. Zhao X, Hippe DS, Li R, et al. Prevalence and characteristics of carotid artery high-risk atherosclerotic plaques in chinese patients with cerebrovascular symptoms: a chinese atherosclerosis risk evaluation II study. J Am Heart Assoc 2017;6(8):e005831.

28. Underhill HR, Kerwin WS, Hatsukami TS, et al. Automated measurement of mean wall thickness in the common carotid artery by MRI: a comparison to intima-media thickness by B-mode ultrasound. J Magn Reson Imaging 2006;24(2):379–87.

29. Yuan J, Usman A, Das T, et al. Imaging carotid atherosclerosis plaque ulceration: comparison of advanced imaging modalities and recent developments. AJNR Am J Neuroradiol 2017;38(4):664–71.

30. Mitchell CC, Stein JH, Cook TD, et al. Histopathologic validation of grayscale carotid plaque characteristics related to plaque vulnerability. Ultrasound Med Biol 2017;43(1):129–37.

31. van D-ND HK, TM TB, van der KA G, et al. Carotid plaque characteristics predict recurrent ischemic stroke and TIA. JACC Cardiovasc Imaging 2022;0(0). https://doi.org/10.1016/j.jcmg.2022.04.003.

32. Spence JD. Carotid plaque measurement is superior to IMT Invited editorial comment on: carotid plaque, compared with carotid intima-media thickness, more accurately predicts coronary artery disease events: a meta-analysis-Yoichi Inaba, M.D., Jennifer A. Chen M.D. Atherosclerosis 2012;220(1):34–5.

33. Porter TR, Mulvagh SL, Abdelmoneim SS, et al. Clinical applications of ultrasonic enhancing agents in echocardiography: 2018 american society of echocardiography guidelines update. J Am Soc Echocardiogr 2018;31(3):241–74.

34. Rafailidis V, Sidhu PS. Vascular ultrasound, the potential of integration of multiparametric ultrasound into routine clinical practice. Ultrasound 2018;26(3):136–44.

35. Rafailidis V, Huang DY, Yusuf GT, et al. General principles and overview of vascular contrast-enhanced ultrasonography. Ultrason (Seoul, Korea) 2020;39(1):22–42.

36. Saba L, Saam T, Jäger HR, et al. Imaging biomarkers of vulnerable carotid plaques for stroke risk prediction and their potential clinical implications. Lancet Neurol 2019;18(6):559–72.

37. Etesami M, Hoi Y, Steinman DA, et al. Comparison of carotid plaque ulcer detection using contrast-enhanced and time-of-flight MRA techniques. AJNR Am J Neuroradiol 2013;34(1):177–84.

38. Saba L, Caddeo G, Sanfilippo R, et al. CT and ultrasound in the study of ulcerated carotid plaque compared with surgical results: potentialities and

advantages of multidetector row CT angiography. AJNR Am J Neuroradiol 2007;28(6):1061–6.

39. Vlahos I, Chung R, Nair A, et al. Dual-energy CT: vascular applications. AJR Am J Roentgenol 2012; 199(5 Suppl):S87–97.

40. Cau R, Flanders A, Mannelli L, et al. Artificial intelligence in computed tomography plaque characterization: a review. Eur J Radiol 2021;109767. https://doi.org/10.1016/j.ejrad.2021.109767.

41. Biasi GM, Froio A, Diethrich EB, et al. Carotid plaque echolucency increases the risk of stroke in carotid stenting. Circulation 2004;110(6):756–62.

42. Salem MK, Bown MJ, Sayers RD, et al. Identification of patients with a histologically unstable carotid plaque using ultrasonic plaque image analysis. Eur J Vasc Endovasc Surg 2014;48(2):118–25.

43. Spanos K, Tzorbatzoglou I, Lazari P, et al. Carotid artery plaque echomorphology and its association with histopathologic characteristics. J Vasc Surg 2018;68(6):1772–80.

44. Saba L, Anzidei M, Marincola BC, et al. Imaging of the carotid artery vulnerable plaque. Cardiovasc Intervent Radiol 2014;37(3):572–85.

45. Opincariu D, Benedek T, Chitu M, et al. From CT to artificial intelligence for complex assessment of plaque-associated risk. Int J Cardiovasc Imaging 2020;(50). https://doi.org/10.1007/s10554-020-01926-1.

46. Boussel L, Coulon P, Thran A, et al. Photon counting spectral CT component analysis of coronary artery atherosclerotic plaque samples. Br J Radiol 2014; 87(1040):20130798.

47. Kassem M, Florea A, Mottaghy FM, et al. Magnetic resonance imaging of carotid plaques: current status and clinical perspectives. Ann Transl Med 2020;8(19):1266.

48. Mazzacane F, Mazzoleni V, Scola E, et al. Vessel wall magnetic resonance imaging in cerebrovascular diseases. Diagnostics 2022;12(2):1–20.

49. Walker LJ, Ismail A, McMeekin W, et al. Computed tomography angiography for the evaluation of carotid atherosclerotic plaque. Stroke 2002;33(4): 977–81.

50. de Weert TT, Ouhlous M, Meijering E, et al. In vivo characterization and quantification of atherosclerotic carotid plaque components with multidetector computed tomography and histopathological correlation. Arterioscler Thromb Vasc Biol 2006;26(10): 2366–72.

51. Sztajzel R, Momjian S, Momjian-Mayor I, et al. Stratified Gray-Scale Median Analysis and Color Mapping of the Carotid Plaque. Stroke 2005;36(4):741–5.

52. Yuan C, Zhang S, Polissar NL, et al. Identification of fibrous cap rupture with magnetic resonance imaging is highly associated with recent transient ischemic attack or stroke. Circulation 2002;105(2): 181–5.

53. Dong L, Kerwin WS, Ferguson MS, et al. Cardiovascular magnetic resonance in carotid atherosclerotic disease. J Cardiovasc Magn Reson 2009;11(1):53.

54. Kwee RM, van Engelshoven JMA, Mess WH, et al. Reproducibility of fibrous cap status assessment of carotid artery plaques by contrast-enhanced MRI. Stroke 2009;40(9):3017–21.

55. Huibers A, De Borst GJ, Wan S, et al. Non-invasive carotid artery imaging to identify the vulnerable plaque: current status and future goals. Eur J Vasc Endovasc Surg 2015;50(5):563–72.

56. Saba L, Tamponi E, Raz E, et al. Correlation between fissured fibrous cap and contrast enhancement: preliminary results with the use of CTA and histologic validation. AJNR Am J Neuroradiol 2014;35(4): 754–9.

57. Murgia A, Erta M, Suri JS, et al. CT imaging features of carotid artery plaque vulnerability. Ann Transl Med 2020;8(19):1261.

58. Saba L, Lanzino G, Lucatelli P, et al. Carotid Plaque CTA Analysis in Symptomatic Subjects with Bilateral Intraparenchymal Hemorrhage: A Preliminary Analysis. AJNR Am J Neuroradiol 2019;40(9):1538–45.

59. Saba L, Francone M, Bassareo PP, et al. CT Attenuation Analysis of Carotid Intraplaque Hemorrhage. AJNR Am J Neuroradiol 2018;39(1):131–7.

60. Wintermark M, Jawadi SS, Rapp JH, et al. High-resolution CT imaging of carotid artery atherosclerotic plaques. AJNR Am J Neuroradiol 2008;29(5): 875–82.

61. Ajduk M, Pavić L, Bulimbašić S, et al. Multidetector-row computed tomography in evaluation of atherosclerotic carotid plaques complicated with intraplaque hemorrhage. Ann Vasc Surg 2009; 23(2):186–93.

62. Ajduk M, Bulimbašić S, Pavić L, et al. Comparison of multidetector-row computed tomography and duplex Doppler ultrasonography in detecting atherosclerotic carotid plaques complicated with intraplaque hemorrhage. Coll Antropol 2013;37(1): 213–9.

63. Andelovic K, Winter P, Jakob PM, et al. Evaluation of Plaque Characteristics and Inflammation Using Magnetic Resonance Imaging. Biomedicines 2021; 9(2). https://doi.org/10.3390/biomedicines9020185.

64. Kooi ME, Cappendijk VC, Cleutjens KBJM, et al. Accumulation of Ultrasmall Superparamagnetic Particles of Iron Oxide in Human Atherosclerotic Plaques Can Be Detected by In Vivo Magnetic Resonance Imaging. Circulation 2003;107(19): 2453–8.

65. Poredos P, Gregoric ID, Jezovnik MK. Inflammation of carotid plaques and risk of cerebrovascular events. Ann Transl Med 2020;8(19):1281.

66. Baradaran H, Myneni PK, Patel P, et al. Association between carotid artery perivascular fat density and

cerebrovascular ischemic events. J Am Heart Assoc 2018;7(24):e010383.

67. van Hoof RHM, Heeneman S, Wildberger JE, et al. Dynamic contrast-enhanced MRI to study atherosclerotic plaque microvasculature. Curr Atheroscler Rep 2016;18(6):33.

68. Coli S, Magnoni M, Sangiorgi G, et al. Contrast-enhanced ultrasound imaging of intraplaque neovascularization in carotid arteries: correlation with histology and plaque echogenicity. J Am Coll Cardiol 2008;52(3):223–30.

69. Hoogi A, Adam D, Hoffman A, et al. Carotid plaque vulnerability: quantification of neovascularization on contrast-enhanced ultrasound with histopathologic correlation. AJR Am J Roentgenol 2011;196(2):431–6.

70. Huang R, Abdelmoneim SS, Ball CA, et al. Detection of carotid atherosclerotic plaque neovascularization using contrast enhanced ultrasound: a systematic review and meta-analysis of diagnostic accuracy studies. J Am Soc Echocardiogr 2016;29(6):491–502.

71. Saba L, Lai ML, Montisci R, et al. Association between carotid plaque enhancement shown by multidetector CT angiography and histologically validated microvessel density. Eur Radiol 2012;22(10):2237–45.

72. Montanaro M, Scimeca M, Anemona L, et al. The paradox effect of calcification in carotid atherosclerosis: microcalcification is correlated with plaque instability. Int J Mol Sci 2021;22(1). https://doi.org/10.3390/ijms22010395.

73. Saba L, Chen H, Cau R, et al. Impact analysis of different CT configurations of carotid artery plaque calcifications on cerebrovascular events. AJNR Am J Neuroradiol 2022;43(2):272–9.

74. Cau R, Bassareo PP, Mannelli L, et al. Imaging in COVID-19-related myocardial injury. Int J Cardiovasc Imaging 2020. https://doi.org/10.1007/s10554-020-02089-9.

Ischemic Infarction in Young Adults

Janet Yanqing Mei, MD, MPH[a], Pamela W. Schaefer, MD[b],*

KEYWORDS

- Ischemic infarction • Stroke • Vasculopathy • Young adults • Radiology • MR imaging • CT
- Angiography

KEY POINTS

- Compared with older patients, young individuals more often have ischemic stroke secondary to cardioembolism, extracranial artery dissection, reversible cerebral vasoconstriction syndrome (RCVS), monogenic disorders, illicit and recreational drug use, hypercoagulable disorders, and pregnancy.
- Cardioembolic stroke, the most common subtype of ischemic stroke in young adults, typically demonstrates multifocal small infarcts in multiple arterial territories from showering of emboli. However, a single arterial territorial infarct can also occur because of a single vessel occlusion from a solitary embolus.
- Large artery vasculopathies (atherosclerosis, extracranial and intracranial dissection, radiation-induced arteriopathy, Takayasu arteritis, fibromuscular dysplasia, carotid web, and vascular Ehlers-Danlos syndrome) and small vessel vasculopathies (central nervous system vasculitis, RCVS, moyamoya disease, cerebral autosomal dominant arteriopathy with subcortical infarcts and leukoencephalopathy, Susac syndrome, and infectious causes exemplified by tuberculous meningitis, varicella zoster virus vasculopathy, and SARS-CoV2 infection) comprise a wide variety of causes demonstrating various imaging features.
- Toxic-metabolic causes including mitochondrial encephalopathy with lactic acidosis and strokelike episodes and illicit and recreational drug use are another important group of stroke causes in young adults.
- Hypercoagulable disorders can lead to arterial or venous infarction in young adults. Venous infarction typically shows more vasogenic edema than cytotoxic edema and intracranial hemorrhage, with evidence of cerebral venous thrombosis on vascular imaging.

INTRODUCTION

More than 2 million young adults (15–55 years old) have an ischemic stroke yearly worldwide,[1] and the incidence is increasing.[2] Modifiable risk factors account for almost 80% of all ischemic strokes in young individuals.[3] Although atherosclerosis remains an important risk factor (15%–25% of cases),[4] cardioembolic stroke is more common (15%–47% of cases).[5] Other frequent causes include cervical artery dissection (2%–25% of cases),[6] reversible cerebral vasoconstriction syndrome, monogenic disorders, illicit and recreational drug use, hypercoagulable disorders, and pregnancy (**Table 1**).

Neuroimaging features are diagnostic in identifying ischemic infarctions and provide important clues in determining underlying causes. According to the different imaging patterns, the causes are classified into 5 categories: cardioembolism, large vessel vasculopathy, small vessel vasculopathy, toxic-metabolic conditions, and hypercoagulable disorders.

a Neuroradiology Division, Massachusetts General Hospital, 55 Fruit Street, Gray 241G, Boston, MA 02114, USA; b Harvard Medical School, Massachusetts General Hospital, 55 Fruit Street, Gray 241 G, Boston, MA 02114, USA
* Corresponding author. 55 Fruit Street, Gray 241G, Boston, MA 02114.
E-mail address: pschaefer@partners.org

Radiol Clin N Am 61 (2023) 415–434
https://doi.org/10.1016/j.rcl.2023.01.010

Table 1
Ischemic infarction causes in young adults

Cardioembolism	Clinical Features	Radiological Features
Atrial myxoma (see **Fig. 1**)	Intracardiac obstruction, embolic infarcts, constitutional symptoms	• Cardioembolic infarction: multifocal small infarcts in multiple arterial territories • Myxomatous intracranial aneurysms: multiple, distal MCA branches, hyperdense from myxoid matrix or calcification • Cerebral myxomatous metastases: multiple, hemorrhagic frontoparietal masses
Bland emboli	A-fib, dilated cardiomyopathy	Multifocal small infarcts in multiple arterial territories
Septic emboli (see **Fig. 2**)	Aortic or mitral valve endocarditis	Abscesses, parenchymal and subarachnoid hemorrhage, mycotic aneurysms
Fat emboli (see **Fig. 3**)	Long bone or pelvic fractures; acute respiratory failure, skin petechiae, ischemic stroke	Punctate foci of restricted diffusion throughout the brain in acute phase (1–4 d), confluent restricted diffusion in subcortical and deep white matter in subacute phase (5–14 d), innumerable microhemorrhages
Air emboli	Invasive procedures	• Arterial: punctate parenchymal foci of air • Venous: serpiginous air in cortical veins with adjacent gyriform infarction

Large Vessel Vasculopathy	Clinical Features	Radiological Features
Atherosclerosis	Cardiovascular disease; classic risk factors: smoking, obesity, hypercholesterolemia, hypertension, and diabetes	• MRA/CTA: atheromatous plaques with stenosis at ICA origins, carotid siphons, M1 and M2 MCA segments, and intracranial vertebral arteries. • MR imaging/CT: territorial and/or border zone infarctions
Dissection		
Cervical artery (see **Fig. 4**)	Neck/facial pain, headache, Horner syndrome, cranial nerve palsy, tinnitus	Irregular filiform stenosis (string of pearls), tapering of true lumen to a point (flame sign), intramural hematoma, intimal flap, pseudoaneurysm (subacute phase)
Intracranial	Headache, vertigo, focal neurological deficit	Infarction and/or subarachnoid hemorrhage, VW-MR imaging helps differentiate from other intracranial arterial narrowing
Radiation-related arteriopathy (see **Fig. 5**)	Radiotherapy to head and neck cancer or brain tumor	• Neck: accelerated atherosclerosis • Head: large vessel stenosis at terminal ICAs and proximal circle of Willis branches with a moyamoya pattern, cavernous malformations, intracranial aneurysms, capillary telangiectasias

(continued on next page)

Table 1
(continued)

Large Vessel Vasculopathy	Clinical Features	Radiological Features
Takayasu arteritis (see Fig. 6A–D)	Inflammatory vasculopathy predominantly affecting aorta and major branches in young women	Vessel wall thickening and enhancement, luminal narrowing, occlusion, aneurysmal dilation, pseudoaneurysms
FMD (see Fig. 6E, F)	Noninflammatory, nonatherosclerotic angiopathy of small- and medium-sized arteries	Alternating stenoses and dilatations in extracranial carotid and vertebral arteries, vascular loops, fusiform vascular ectasia, arterial dissection, aneurysm, subarachnoid hemorrhage
Carotid web (see Fig. 6G–I)	Ischemic stroke in the ipsilateral anterior circulation	Thin, linear membrane from posterior carotid bulb
Vascular EDS (see Fig. 7)	Autosomal dominant disorder, fragility of medium and large arteries from type III procollagen deficiency	Intracranial aneurysms, subarachnoid hemorrhage, cervical and intracranial arterial ectasias and dissections, carotid-cavernous fistula

Small Vessel Vasculopathy	Clinical Features	Radiological Features
CNS vasculitis (see Fig. 8)	• PACNS: idiopathic inflammatory disease of medium-small cerebral arteries. • Secondary CNS vasculitis: systemic vasculitis involving multiple organs secondary to connective tissue disorders, infection, malignancy, drug use, radiation therapy	Multiterritorial infarcts, hemorrhage, white matter edema Beaded appearance, concentric wall thickening, and enhancement of cerebral arteries
RCVS (see Fig. 9)	Recurrent thunderclap headache, focal neurologic deficits	Border zone infarcts, cerebral convexity subarachnoid hemorrhage Tapered narrowing of medium-sized arteries followed by dilatation. No or mild contrast enhancement on vessel-wall MR imaging
Moyamoya disease (see Fig. 10)	Idiopathic, noninflammatory, nonatherosclerotic progressive steno-occlusive disease	Tapered narrowing or occlusion at terminal ICAs and proximal MCAs/ACAs, compensatory collaterals (puff of smoke). Ischemic infarctions secondary to arterial occlusion and hemorrhages secondary to arterial rupture
CADASIL (see Fig. 11)	Inherited small vessel disease, early cerebrovascular events, functional disability	White matter hyperintensities (periventricular, anterior temporal, external capsule, frontal, parietal), subcortical infarcts, cerebral microhemorrhages
Susac syndrome (see Fig. 12).	Autoimmune encephalopathy, branch retinal artery occlusions, neurosensorial hearing loss	Multifocal small T2/FLAIR hyperintense white matter lesions with predilection for the central and superior aspect of the corpus callosum

Selected Infections	Clinical Features	Radiological Features
Tuberculous meningitis (see Fig. 13)	Headache, fever, neck stiffness, vomiting, mental status changes	• Florid basilar meningitis with thick leptomeningeal enhancement • Multifocal infarcts in caudate head, anteromedial thalamus, internal capsule anterior limb/genu • Cortical and border zone infarcts secondary to involvement of terminal ICAs, COW, basilar artery
VZV vasculopathy (see Fig. 14)	Primary infection with VZV or viral reactivation, immunocompromised	Ischemic infarcts involving cortex, deep white matter, and gray matter Segmental stenosis and dilatation, concentric vessel wall enhancement
SARS-CoV2 infection	Ischemic stroke, intracerebral hemorrhage, cerebral venous sinus thrombosis	Large vessel occlusion with multiterritorial involvement, PRES, vasculitis, arterial dissection

Toxic-Metabolic	Clinical Features	Radiological Features
MELAS (see Fig. 15)	Strokelike episodes, seizures, lactic acidosis	Multifocal strokelike lesions in different stages of evolution crossing vascular territories, predilection to the parietal, temporal, and occipital lobes; elevated lactate peaks throughout brain
Illicit drug use	History of drug abuse	• Cocaine and amphetamines: MCA territory white matter, intracranial hemorrhage • MDMA: globus pallidus, occipital cortex • Heroin: border zones, globus pallidus, hippocampus, cerebellum • Other complications: PRES, diffuse edema, toxic leukoencephalopathy (see Fig. 16), cerebral atrophy, and CNS infection

Hypercoagulable Disorders	Clinical Features	Radiological Features
APS (see Fig. 18)	Autoimmune disorder with circulating APLAs, arterial or venous thrombosis, thrombocytopenia, frequent miscarriages	Infarcts of various ages, focal T2/FLAIR hyperintense white matter lesions
Pregnancy and peripartum	From third trimester to 6 wk postpartum	• Arterial: cortical/subcortical infarcts • Venous sinus thrombosis (see Fig. 17): MR imaging: vasogenic more than cytotoxic edema, hemorrhage; absence of flow voids with blooming on SWI NCCT: hyperdense veins/sinuses CTV/MRV/postcontrast MR imaging: Absent dural sinus or cortical vein flow/enhancement

Cardioembolism

Cardioembolic stroke is the most common subtype of ischemic stroke in young adults. Imaging findings typically demonstrate multifocal small infarcts in multiple arterial territories from the showering of emboli. A single arterial territorial infarct can also occur because of a single vessel occlusion from a solitary embolus.

Atrial myxoma

Atrial myxoma is the most common primary cardiac tumor in adults. Cerebral embolization results from surface thrombus surrounding the myxoma or from tumor fragmentation, which leads to infarction, aneurysm formation, and metastases.[7]

Both myxomatous intracranial aneurysms and cerebral myxomatous metastases are rare. Myxomatous intracranial aneurysms are usually multiple and have a predilection for distal branches of the middle cerebral arteries (MCA) (**Fig. 1**). They are hyperdense on noncontrast head computed tomography (NCCT) due to the accumulation of myxoid matrix or calcification in the aneurysmal wall. Cerebral myxomatous metastases are typically multiple and hemorrhagic and are most common in the frontoparietal region.[8]

Bland emboli

Bland emboli result from blood stasis in cardiac chambers and thrombus formation, commonly seen with atrial fibrillation and dilated cardiomyopathy. Patent foramen ovale (PFO) may place a patient at an increased risk of paradoxical thromboembolism. However, the prevalence of PFO in a stroke-free population is as high as 25%, and other causes of stroke should be excluded before designating PFO as the cause.

Septic emboli

Septic emboli are mostly caused by aortic and mitral valve endocarditis. Septic embolism can

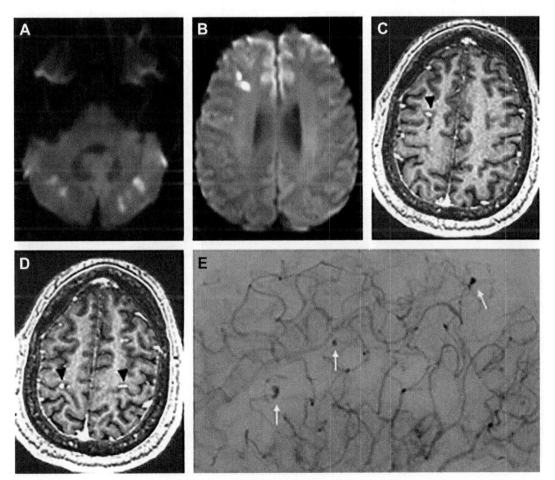

Fig. 1. Atrial myxoma. Multifocal embolic acute to subacute infarctions involving cerebellum and right frontal lobe on DWI (*A, B*). Two years later, multiple enhancing foci within frontal sulci bilaterally (*arrowheads on C, D*), representing myxomatous aneurysms on angiogram (*arrows on E*).

lead to brain abscesses, parenchymal and sub-arachnoid hemorrhage, and mycotic aneurysms, in addition to small, scattered infarcts throughout the brain parenchyma (**Fig. 2**).

Fat emboli

Cerebral fat embolism is classically seen in patients with long bone fractures or pelvic trauma with a triad of acute respiratory failure, skin petechiae, and ischemic stroke. A right-to-left cardiac shunt is not a precondition, as the marrow fat droplets can deform and travel through pulmonary capillaries.

In the acute phase (1–4 days), MR imaging shows numerous scattered punctate foci of restricted diffusion, particularly in the white matter, corpus callosum, basal ganglia, thalami, brainstem, and cerebellum (**Fig. 3**). In the subacute phase (5–14 days), there is confluent restricted diffusion in subcortical and deep white matter. Innumerable punctate foci of susceptibility, representing microhemorrhages, can occur in the same regions as the cytotoxic edema or seem more extensive.[9]

Air emboli

Cerebral air embolism is rare but can occur during invasive procedures and may involve veins or arteries. The venous pattern seems as serpiginous air in cortical veins with adjacent gyriform infarctions. The arterial pattern presents as infarctions with parenchymal punctate or curvilinear foci of air, often in a watershed distribution.[10]

Large Vessel Vasculopathy

Atherosclerosis

Large-artery atherosclerosis accounts for 2% to 8% of ischemic strokes in young adults and mostly occurs in patients older than 40 years.[5] It is associated with cardiovascular atherosclerosis and risk factors, including hypertension, hyperlipidemia, hypercholesterolemia, diabetes mellitus, obesity, and smoking. The stroke mechanism includes thromboembolic stroke, hypoperfusion from high-grade stenosis or occlusion, and a mixed mechanism.

On CT angiogram (CTA) or MR angiogram (MRA), atheromatous calcified and/or noncalcified

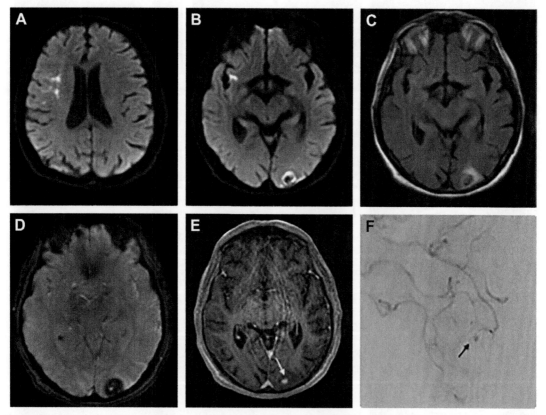

Fig. 2. Septic emboli. DWI (*A, B*) shows multifocal supratentorial acute to subacute infarctions. A dominant left occipital lesion on FLAIR (*C*) has associated hemorrhage on SWI (*D*). Internal punctate enhancement on the post-contrast T1-weighted image (*white arrow* on *E*) represents a mycotic aneurysm on cerebral angiography (*black arrow* on *F*).

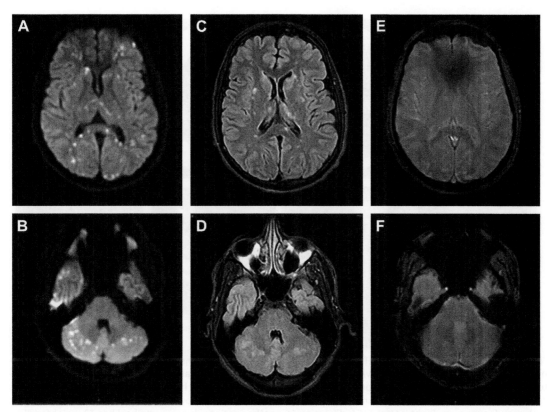

Fig. 3. Fat emboli. Numerous punctate acute to subacute infarctions throughout the cerebrum and cerebellum with involvement of deep gray nuclei and the corpus callosum splenium on DWI (*A* and *B*) and FLAIR (*C* and *D*) and innumerable microhemorrhages on SWI (*E* and *F*).

plaques with resultant stenosis are evident, most commonly occurring at the common carotid artery bifurcations and internal carotid artery (ICA) origins, carotid siphons, MCA M1 and M2 branches and intracranial vertebral arteries as well as the aortic arch and great vessel origins. Plaque size, content, and integrity are important indicators for vulnerable plaques at risk for thromboembolic strokes and can be assessed using CTA, MRA, or carotid ultrasound. Vessel wall-MR imaging (VW-MR imaging) typically demonstrates eccentric arterial wall enhancement.[11]

Dissection

Cervical artery dissection Cervical carotid or vertebral artery dissection cause approximately 20% of strokes in young adults.[12] Patients can present with neck and facial pain, headache, Horner syndrome, cranial nerve palsy, and tinnitus, with or without identifiable preceding trauma.

CTA and MRA can demonstrate a long thin irregular stenosis (string of pearls sign), tapering of the true lumen to a point (flame sign), mural thickening from the intramural hematoma, or an intimal flap. On MR imaging, the intramural hematoma is

typically T1 hyperintense in the subacute stage, and the narrowed residual lumen is present as a flow void. In the subacute phase, pseudoaneurysms can form (**Fig. 4**).

Intracranial dissection Intracranial dissection is much less common compared with extracranial dissection. However, subsequent aneurysm formation and extravascular bleeding are more likely because the medial and adventitial layers of intradural arteries are thin.[13]

VW-MR imaging can help differentiate dissection from intracranial atherosclerotic plaque, vasculitis, and reversible cerebral vasoconstriction syndrome. The imaging features include a curvilinear hyperintensity on T2-weighted images (intimal flap) separating the true lumen from the false lumen, eccentric arterial wall thickening with the signal characteristic of blood (intramural hematoma),[11] and layered enhancement of the luminal boundary and outer margin of the vessel on postcontrast T1-weighted images.[14]

Radiation-induced arteriopathy

Carotid arteries receive significant doses of radiation in the management of head and neck cancer.

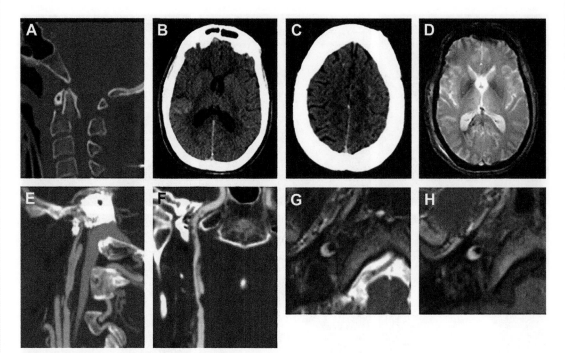

Fig. 4. Cervical artery dissection. NCCT (*A–C*) shows right anterior frontal hemorrhagic contusion and subarachnoid hemorrhage within the right Sylvian fissure and bilateral frontoparietal sulci following acute odontoid fracture. SWI (*D*) shows right occipital horn intraventricular hemorrhage and hemorrhagic foci at the right corpus callosum splenium, suggestive of traumatic axonal injury. CTA (*E* and *F*) shows distal right cervical ICA dissection with pseudoaneurysm. Right petrous ICA dissection in another patient shows a small caliber T2-weighted flow void (*G*) and adjacent intramural hematoma with crescent intrinsic T1 hyperintensity (*H*).

Radiation can result in morphological features such as those seen in spontaneous atherosclerosis. Differentiating factors are accelerated progression, a longer segment of involvement, and a higher incidence of complications after carotid endarterectomy and carotid stenting. Vascular injury after radiotherapy may result in severe carotid artery stenosis (**Fig. 5**) and stroke/transient ischemic attack (TIA) related to thromboembolism and/or hypoperfusion.[15]

Intracranially, steno-occlusive vasculopathy of the large cerebral arteries may evolve slowly after radiation, often accompanied by cavernous malformations, intracranial aneurysms, and capillary telangiectasias. At imaging, there is wall thickening and enhancement of the large cerebral arteries, resulting in a stenotic or occlusive state. Furthermore, moyamoya-like collateral circulation and transdural anastomoses may be observed as the terminal ICA, and the major branches of the circle of Willis are especially vulnerable.[16]

Takayasu arteritis
Takayasu arteritis (TA) is a rare inflammatory vasculopathy that predominantly affects the aorta and major branches. Young women account for 80% to 90% of TA cases, with an onset age range of 10 to 40 years.

In the acute phase, the aorta and pulmonary arteries may demonstrate vessel wall thickening and enhancement, suggestive of active inflammation. As the disease progresses, inflammation can lead to narrowing, occlusion, aneurysmal dilation, or pseudoaneurysm formation of large vessels[17] (**Fig. 6**A–D).

Approximately 10% to 20% of patients with TA exhibit neurological manifestations. Nearly 48% with vertebral artery involvement experience visual disturbance, whereas 80% with carotid and vertebral artery involvement exhibit TIA or stroke, mostly secondary to hypoperfusion.[18] Brain imaging usually shows small- to medium-sized infarctions in multiple vascular territories and at arterial border zones.

Fibromuscular dysplasia
Fibromuscular dysplasia (FMD) is a heterogeneous group of vascular lesions characterized by an idiopathic, noninflammatory, and nonatherosclerotic angiopathy of small- and medium-sized arteries. After renal arteries, extracranial internal carotid arteries and vertebral arteries are the most common locations.[19]

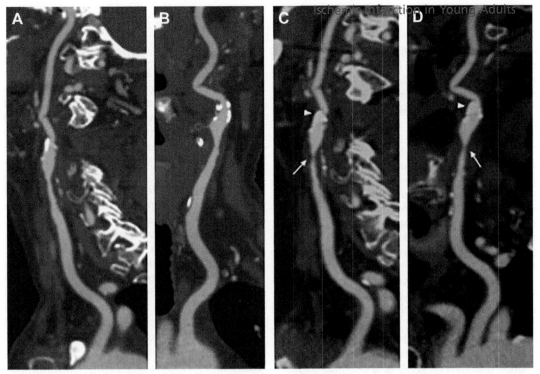

Fig. 5. Radiation vasculitis. CTAs in a patient 5 years after radiation therapy for tongue SCC demonstrate progressive narrowing in the distal left CCA (*arrows* on *C* and *D* compared with *A* and *B*) and more prominent calcified plaques in the proximal left ICA (*arrowheads* on *C* and *D* compared with *A* and *B*).

FMD is characterized by alternating stenoses and dilatations, causing a string of beads appearance (**Fig. 6**E, F). Less common imaging findings include vascular loops, fusiform vascular ectasia, arterial dissection, and aneurysm. TIA and stroke occur due to arterial stenosis, extracranial arterial dissection, or, less commonly, intracranial dissection.

FMD can also lead to subarachnoid hemorrhage secondary to intracranial dissection or rupture of intracranial aneurysms.[19,20]

Carotid web
A carotid web is a thin, linear membrane extending from the posterior aspect of the carotid bulb

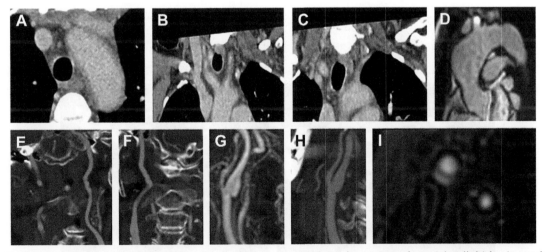

Fig. 6. Large vessel vasculopathy. CTA of the chest in a patient with TA shows circumferential wall thickening and enhancement of the aorta and great vessels (*A–C*). In another patient, MRA of the chest (*D*) shows aneurysmal dilatation of the ascending aorta without prominent wall thickening or enhancement. Neck CTA in a patient with FMD shows the characteristic "string of beads" appearance in the distal ICAs bilaterally (*E* and *F*). A carotid web is a thin, linear membrane from the posterior aspect of the carotid bulb on MRA (*G*) and CTA (*H*). The web appears like a dissection on the axial view (*I*).

into the lumen (**Fig. 6**G–I). Carotid web has a confirmed association with ischemic stroke of undetermined cause, especially in the ipsilateral anterior circulation. It is important to differentiate it from dissection using the sagittal view of CTA or MRA.[21]

Vascular Ehlers-Danlos syndrome

Vascular Ehlers-Danlos syndrome (vEDS) is an autosomal dominant disorder characterized by the fragility of medium and large arteries due to type III procollagen deficiency. The most common general vascular findings are aneurysms, dissections, ectasias, and fistula formation, with complications of hemorrhagic events and end-organ infarcts (**Fig. 7**).[22]

Most neurovascular disease reports include intracranial aneurysms (typically developing in the cavernous ICA or along the carotid siphon), subarachnoid hemorrhage, cervical or intracranial arterial dissection, cervical vertebral and carotid artery ectasias, and carotid-cavernous fistula.[23] Although uncommon, vEDS is a potential cause of stroke in young people and should be suspected in young patients presenting with unusual or extensive vascular findings.

Small Vessel Vasculopathy

Central nervous system vasculitis

Central nervous system (CNS) vasculitis is a heterogeneous group of disorders with diverse clinical manifestations. Primary angiitis of the CNS (**Fig. 8**) is an idiopathic inflammatory disease of small- to medium-sized arteries affecting the CNS or peripheral nervous system, with no evidence of generalized inflammation. It is most often observed in the fifth and sixth decades of life.[24] Secondary CNS vasculitis comprises systemic vasculitis involving multiple organs and vasculitis secondary to systemic connective tissue disorders, infection, malignancy, drug use, or radiation therapy.

The imaging findings are highly variable and include multiple territorial infarctions, parenchymal and subarachnoid hemorrhage, leptomeningeal enhancement, white matter edema, a beaded appearance of multiple arteries, and vessel wall thickening with concentric enhancement.[11]

Reversible cerebral vasoconstriction syndrome

Reversible cerebral vasoconstriction syndrome (RCVS) is characterized by recurrent thunderclap headaches and reversible segmental, multifocal

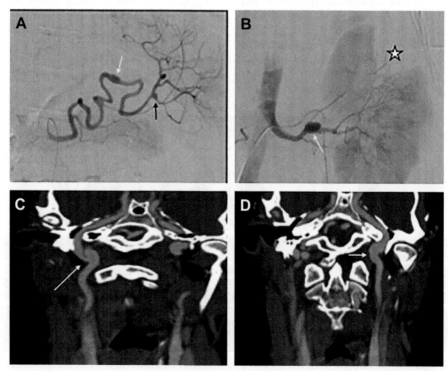

Fig. 7. Vascular Ehlers-Danlos syndrome. A 5-mm splenic artery aneurysm (*A, black arrow*) and fusiform dilatation in the proximal splenic artery (*A, white arrow*) are noted. On renal arteriogram, a left renal artery focal outpouching (*B, white arrow*) was present with distal filling defect and infarct of the upper pole (*star*), suggestive of dissection. Head and neck CTA demonstrates a pseudoaneurysm in the right distal cervical ICA (*C, arrow*) and fusiform dilatation on the left (*D, arrow*).

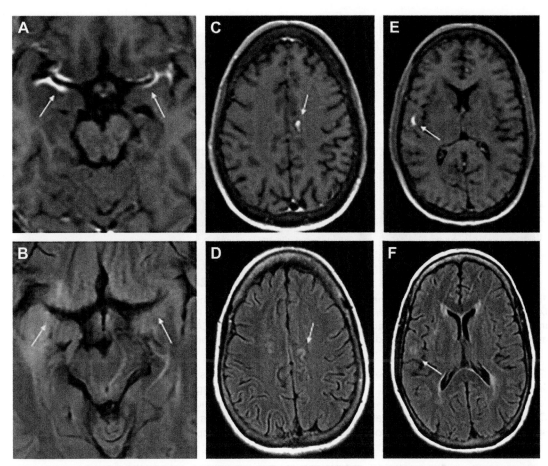

Fig. 8. PACNS. VW-MR imaging shows concentric vessel wall enhancement along M1 and proximal M2 segments (*A, arrows*) with adjacent parenchymal edema (*B, arrows*). There are additional multifocal vessel wall enhancements with adjacent parenchymal edema involving a left ACA distal branch in the left parasagittal frontal lobe (*C and D, arrows*) and a right MCA distal branch at the right frontal operculum (*E and F, arrows*).

vasoconstriction of the cerebral arteries (**Fig. 9**). Hemorrhage, seizures, and associated posterior reversible encephalopathy syndrome (PRES) usually occur within the first week, whereas ischemic sequelae occur during the second and third weeks after the symptom onset.[25]

Imaging findings include border zone infarctions, cerebral convexity subarachnoid hemorrhage, and intraparenchymal hemorrhage. The most characteristic vascular finding is diffuse, bilateral tapered narrowing of medium-sized arteries followed by abnormally dilated segments of second- and third-order branches.[26] Normalization of the vascular findings is usually seen within 8 to 12 weeks.[25] VW-MR imaging demonstrates either no or mild vessel wall enhancement.[27]

Moyamoya disease

Moyamoya disease is an idiopathic, noninflammatory, nonatherosclerotic progressive steno-occlusive disease involving the terminal ICA and proximal anterior cerebral artery (ACA) and MCA (**Fig. 10**), with relative sparing of the posterior cerebral artery. These steno-occlusive changes stimulate the compensatory development of collateral vessels at the base of the brain and create the "puff of smoke" appearance on cerebral angiography. Clinical manifestations include acute neurologic deficits from intracranial artery occlusion or intraparenchymal hemorrhage (caused by rupture of fragile collateral vessels), epilepsy (frequently seen in children), and migraines.[28]

Cerebral angiography represents the gold-standard technique for evaluating the intracranial arteries, although both MRA and CTA usually lead to the diagnosis. The MR imaging and CT are used to evaluate associated ischemic or hemorrhagic changes (see **Fig. 10**). Quantitative analysis of cerebral blood flow and cerebrovascular reserve can evaluate the risk of surgical complications.[29]

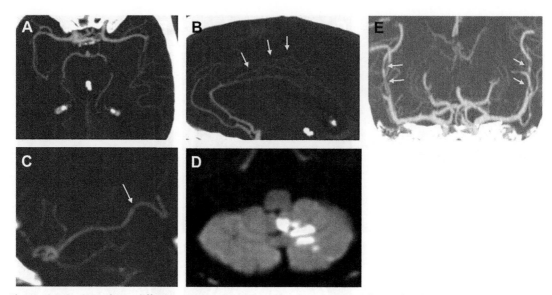

Fig. 9. RCVS. CTAs show diffuse narrowing and multifocal stenosis involving distal ACAs (*B, arrows*), MCAs (*A* and *C, arrow*), and PCAs (*A*), as well as severe stenosis at the left PCA P2 segment. DWI shows acute infarction in the left PICA territory (*D*). A beaded appearance of the bilateral MCA M2 segments (*E, arrows*) is present in another patient with RCVS who did not have an acute or subacute infarction.

Cerebral autosomal dominant arteriopathy with subcortical infarcts and leukoencephalopathy

Cerebral autosomal dominant arteriopathy with subcortical infarcts and leukoencephalopathy (CADASIL) is the most common single-gene disorder leading to stroke and vascular dementia, caused by mutations in the NOTCH3 gene. CADASIL presents with various neurological and psychiatric symptoms, including migraine, transient

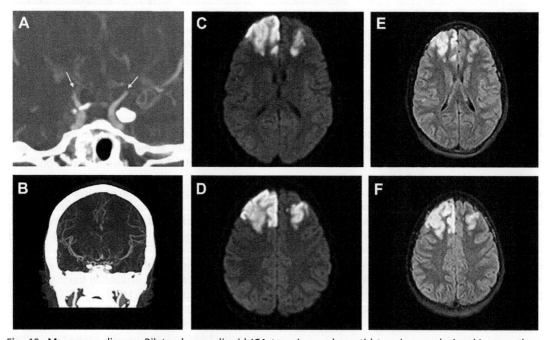

Fig. 10. Moyamoya disease. Bilateral supraclinoid ICA tapering and carotid terminus occlusion (*A, arrows*) are shown on CTA. The prominent lenticulostriate collaterals surrounding the occluded bilateral MCA M1 segments give the typical puff of smoke appearance (*B*). Subacute bilateral MCA and ACA territorial and MCA/ACA border zone infarcts are present on DWI (*C* and *D*) and FLAIR (*E* and *F*).

ischemic attack, acute stroke, cognitive impairment, gait abnormality, and mood disturbance, with a mean onset age of 35 to 40 years.[30]

MR imaging abnormalities include symmetric white matter hyperintensities (predominantly in the periventricular region, anterior temporal poles, external capsules, and frontal and parietal lobes with sparing of the subcortical U-fibers), subcortical infarcts, and cerebral microbleeds (**Fig. 11**).[31]

Susac syndrome

Susac syndrome is an autoimmune microangiopathy characterized by the clinical triad of encephalopathy, branch retinal artery occlusions, and sensorineural hearing loss. The estimated mean onset age is 31.6 years, and the male-to-female ratio is 1: 3.5.[32]

MR imaging shows multifocal small T2/fluid attenuated inversion recovery (FLAIR) hyperintense white matter lesions, including characteristic snowball-like, rounded lesions in the central corpus callosum and icicle-like wedge-shaped lesions along the roof of the corpus callosum (**Fig. 12**).[33] The deep gray matter, cerebellum, cerebellar peduncles, and brain stem are occasionally involved. Because these lesions are secondary to arteriolar infarction, they show restricted diffusion in the acute and subacute phases, enhancement in the subacute phase, and cavitation in the chronic phase. Leptomeningeal enhancement is also present in approximately 33% of cases.[34]

Infection

The infectious causes of stroke are extensive, including bacterial (syphilis and tuberculosis), fungal (cryptococcus, aspergillus, and mucormycosis are common in immunocompromised patients), parasitic (most commonly neurocysticercosis), and viral infections (varicella). The underlying mechanisms include vasculitis, meningitis, cardioembolism, arachnoiditis, arterial compression, and arterial occlusion.[35] The imaging findings vary depending on the mechanism and areas of involvement. Examples of tuberculous meningitis and varicella-zoster virus vasculitis are included in this article to show how intracranial infection contributes to ischemic infarction. The authors have also included COVID-19–related strokes, an emerging topic.

Tuberculous meningitis Tuberculosis has a predilection for the basal meninges and typically results in multiple, bilateral infarctions located in the "tubercular zone," comprising the caudate nucleus head, anteromedial thalamus, and anterior limb and genu of the internal capsule due to the involvement of the medial striate, thalamotuberal, and thalamoperforating arteries that are embedded in exudates and likely to be stretched by coexistent hydrocephalus (**Fig. 13**). Cortical

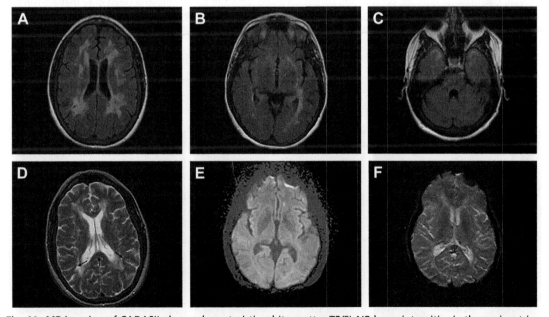

Fig. 11. MR imaging of CADASIL shows characteristic white matter T2/FLAIR hyperintensities in the periventricular region, anterior temporal juxtacortical white matter, and left external capsule on FLAIR (*A–C*) with subcortical U-fiber sparing on T2-weighted imaging (*D, arrows*). A punctate subacute infarct is noted in the inferior left frontal lobe on DWI (*E*), and a left thalamic microbleed is noted on SWI (*F*).

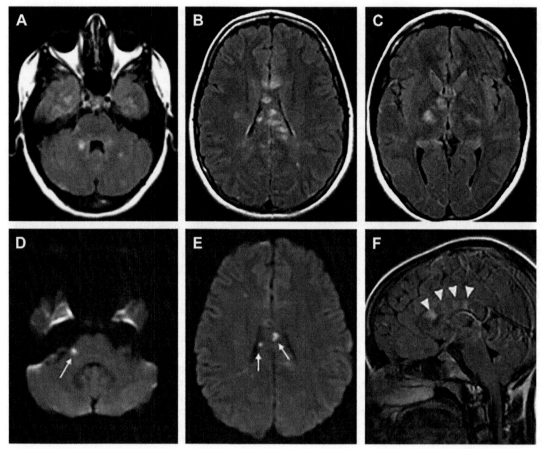

Fig. 12. Susac syndrome. FLAIR images (*A–C* and *F*) demonstrate multifocal small T2/FLAIR hyperintense lesions involving cerebellar peduncles, cerebellum, corpus callosum, centrum semiovale, and deep gray matter. The lesions at right cerebellar peduncle and corpus callosum demonstrate restricted diffusion (*arrows* on *D* and *E*), suggestive of acute to subacute infarctions. Snowball-like lesions (*arrowheads* on *F*) have a rounded morphology and span the whole corpus callosum width.

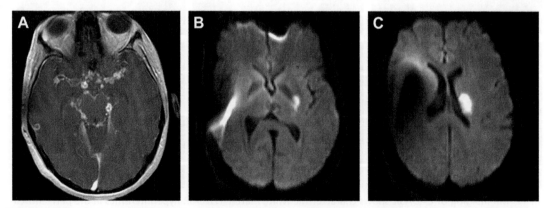

Fig. 13. Tuberculous meningitis. Basilar predominant thick nodular leptomeningeal enhancement is present on postcontrast T1-weighted imaging (*A*). There are acute infarcts involving left basal ganglia, internal capsule, and corona radiata on DWI (*B* and *C*).

and border zone infarcts can also occur due to involvement of the proximal major intracranial arteries at the skull base.[36,37]

Varicella zoster virus vasculopathy Varicella zoster virus (VZV) vasculopathy occurs after either primary infection with VZV (varicella; chickenpox) or viral reactivation (zoster; shingles), typically in immunocompromised patients.[38] It presents with TIA and ischemic strokes and less frequently with intracranial hemorrhage secondary to a ruptured aneurysm.[39]

CT or MR imaging often reveals single or multiple ischemic infarcts involving both cortex and deep white and gray matter. Vascular imaging shows segmental stenosis with poststenotic dilatation (**Fig. 14**). Concentric vessel wall enhancement and diffuse vessel wall irregularity have also been reported.[40]

SARS-CoV2 infection Cerebrovascular disease, including ischemic stroke, intracerebral hemorrhage, and cerebral venous sinus thrombosis, has been reported in patients with COVID-19.[41] Although most patients were older than 60 years and the stroke mechanism was associated with preexisting vascular risk factors, strokes in young adults, associated with thrombus in the aorta, deep vein thrombosis, and pulmonary embolism have also occurred.[42]

Typical neuroimaging features include large vessel occlusion and multiterritorial involvement. Atypical presentations include PRES, vasculitis, and arterial dissection.[43] Both arterial and venous vascular imaging are essential, given the high risk of coagulopathy.

Toxic-Metabolic

Mitochondrial encephalopathy with lactic acidosis and strokelike episodes

Mitochondrial encephalopathy with lactic acidosis and strokelike episodes (MELAS) is a mitochondrial disorder characterized by strokelike episodes, seizures, and lactic acidosis. The disease usually manifests between 2 and 10 years of age, and 90% present before age 40 years.[44]

Typical neuroimaging findings include strokelike lesions, basal ganglia calcifications, and brain atrophy. The strokelike cortical lesions are multifocal, in different stages of evolution, cross cerebral arterial territories, and show a predilection for the parietal, temporal, and occipital lobes (**Fig. 15**).[45] Head and neck arteries are typically normal, and MR spectroscopy may demonstrate elevated lactate peaks.

Illicit and recreational drug use

Illicit drug use is an important cause of ischemic stroke in young adults. The underlying mechanisms include severe acute hypertension, cardiac

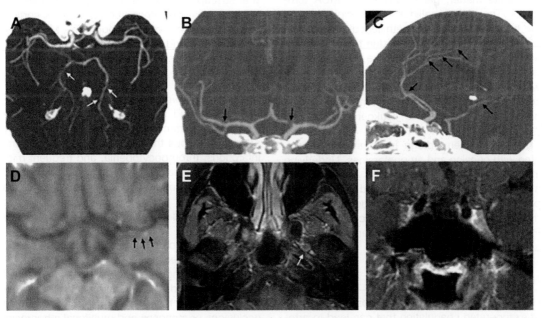

Fig. 14. VZV vasculopathy. Diffuse multifocal stenoses of the major intracranial arteries are present on head CTA (*A–C, arrows*). Short-segmental concentric wall thickening and enhancement of the left MCA M1 segment is shown VW-MR imaging (*D, black arrows*). On postcontrast T1-weighted sequences, thickening of left cranial nerve V2 at foramen ovale is present (*E, white arrow*) and thickening and enhancement of left cranial nerve III, IV V1, and V2 are demonstrated within the prominent left cavernous sinus (*F*).

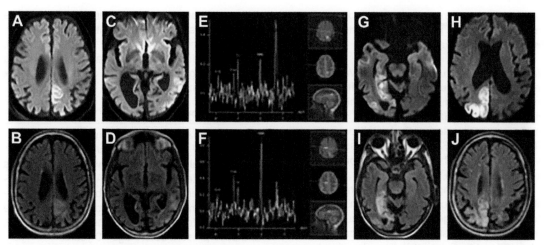

Fig. 15. MELAS. Large areas of restricted diffusion representing cytotoxic edema (*A, C*) with associated FLAIR hyperintensity (*B, D*) are present in the left temporal, parietal, and occipital lobes. On MRS, there is a prominent lactate peak in a region with cytotoxic edema in the left parietal lobe (*E*) and a small lactate peak in the normal-appearing right posterior frontal lobe (*F*). Later, new FLAIR hyperintense lesions with restricted diffusion are seen in the right parietal, occipital, and temporal lobes (*G–J*).

arrhythmias, cerebral vasospasm, vasculitis, venous and arterial thrombosis, cardioembolism secondary to infective endocarditis or dilated cardiomyopathy, and embolization due to injected foreign material.[46]

The location of drug-induced ischemic infarcts varies with different agents. Infarcts related to cocaine and amphetamines often involve the cerebral white matter, particularly in the MCA territory.[47] The globus pallidus and occipital cortex are most susceptible to methylenedioxymethamphetamine-induced ischemia due to the distribution of serotonin receptors.[48] The globus pallidus is also most involved in infarcts caused by heroin with frequent involvement of bilateral border zones, cerebellum, and hippocampus.[49] Inhaled heroin can cause toxic leukoencephalopathy ("Chasing the dragon" in **Fig. 16**).

Intracranial hemorrhage is commonly associated with cocaine and amphetamines. Underlying intracranial aneurysms and/or arteriovenous malformations have been reported in one-half of patients with cocaine-related intracranial hemorrhage.[50] Other neurologic complications include PRES, diffuse cerebral edema, cerebral atrophy, and CNS infection.[51]

Hypercoagulable Disorders

Hypercoagulability describes the pathologic state of exaggerated coagulation that can lead to arterial infarcts due to thromboembolism, paradoxical infarcts frequently secondary to an intracardiac shunt such as PFO, or venous infarcts secondary to venous sinus thrombosis.[52]

The clinical symptoms of venous infarcts are vague, including headache, seizures, and other neurologic deficits.[53] MR imaging typically shows vasogenic edema more than cytotoxic edema and intracranial hemorrhage (**Fig. 17**). The dural venous thrombosis is evident as hyperdensity of the major dural sinuses and/or cortical veins on NCCT, absence of the T2-hypointense flow voids with susceptibility weighted imaging blooming on MR imaging, or absence of dural sinus or cortical vein enhancement on CT venography, MR venography (MRV), and certain postcontrast 3-dimensional T1-weighted MR sequences.[54]

Antiphospholipid antibody syndrome

Antiphospholipid antibody syndrome (APS) is a systemic autoimmune disorder characterized by arterial or venous thrombosis leading to cerebral infarctions, thrombocytopenia, and frequent miscarriages, caused by circulating antiphospholipid antibodies. Secondary APS is found in up to 30% to 50% of patients with SLE and in up to 30% of patients with human immunodeficiency virus.[24]

APS has also been implicated in cardioembolic infarcts associated with left cardiac valvular abnormalities, including irregular leaflets, nonbacterial vegetations, and valve dysfunction.[55] Vascular imaging studies have shown extracranial arterial occlusions or stenoses and multifocal intracranial arterial narrowing and dilatation, suggestive of vasculopathy.[56] MR imaging usually shows infarcts of various sizes and ages and focal T2/FLAIR hyperintense white matter lesions (**Fig. 18**).[57]

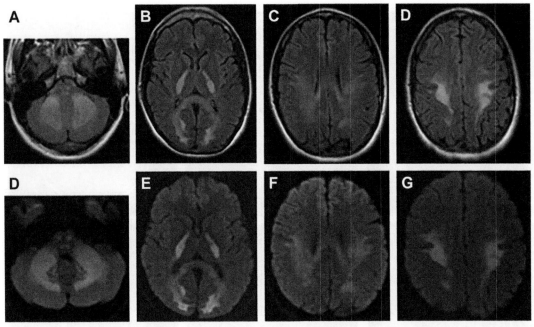

Fig. 16. Heroin leukoencephalopathy. Symmetric white matter T2/FLAIR hyperintensities and restricted diffusion involving cerebellum (*A, E*), posterior limb of the internal capsules (*B, F*), and parietal and occipital lobes (*C, D, F, G*).

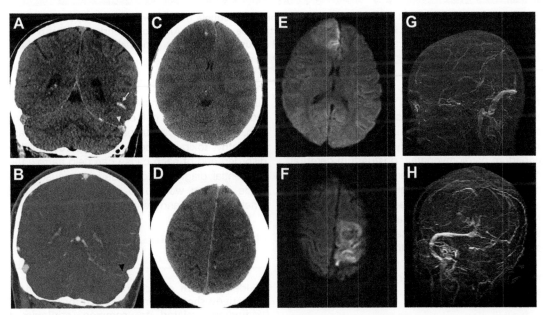

Fig. 17. Cerebral venous sinus thrombosis. NCCT shows a left temporal intraparenchymal hemorrhage with surrounding edema (*A, arrow*). Hyperdensity within the left transverse sinus (*A, white arrowhead*) suggests cerebral venous thrombosis, confirmed by CTV (*B, black arrowhead*). Another patient has subacute infarcts involving the right anterior frontal lobe and left posterior frontal and parietal lobes on NCCT (*C* and *D*) and DWI (*E* and *F*) not confined within arterial territories, with small intraparenchymal and subarachnoid hemorrhages. MRV (*G, H*) shows absence of flow within the superior sagittal sinus and partial thrombosis of the left transverse and sigmoid sinuses.

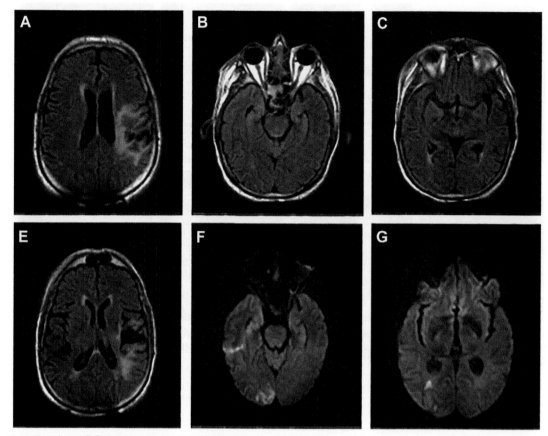

Fig. 18. A large left MCA territory encephalomalacia represents sequela from a remote infarct (A, D). Cortical/subcortical restricted diffusion involving the right occipital lobe with T2 FLAIR hyperintensity represents acute to subacute infarct (B, E). A triangular area of restricted diffusion in the right periatrial white matter without T2 FLAIR hyperintensity represents an acute infarct (C, F).

Pregnancy and peripartum

Pregnancy and puerperium, especially from the third trimester to 6 weeks postpartum, are associated with an increased risk of ischemic and hemorrhagic stroke.[58] The underlying causes include peripartum cardiomyopathy, postpartum cerebral angiopathy, amniotic fluid embolism, eclampsia, and physiological hypercoagulable state.[59]

MR imaging is the preferred image modality for pregnant and lactating patients. Gadolinium-based contrast agents are category-C drugs that cause adverse effects on the fetus in animals. Therefore, phase-contrast or time-of-flight MRV techniques are preferred for evaluating cerebral venous thrombosis.

SUMMARY

Compared with older patients, young individuals more often have ischemic stroke secondary to cardioembolism, extracranial artery dissection, reversible cerebral vasoconstriction syndrome, monogenic disorders, illicit drug use, hypercoagulable disorders, pregnancy, and puerperium. The radiological features of 5 categories (cardioembolism, large vessel vasculopathy, small vessel vasculopathy, toxic-metabolic, and hypercoagulable disorder) and of each cause can help narrow the differential diagnoses of underlying causes and guide imaging workup to ensure accurate and timely diagnosis and treatment.

CLINICS CARE POINTS.

- Identification of ischemic infarcts in young patients should prompt a search for imaging findings related to common etiologies, including cardioembolism, extracranial artery dissection, RCVS, monogenic disorders, illicit and recreational drug use, infection, hypercoagulable disorders, and pregnancy.

- According to the different imaging patterns, the underlying causes can be classified into five categories: cardioembolism, large vessel vasculopathy, small vessel vasculopathy, toxic-metabolic conditions, and hypercoagulable disorders.

- Vascular imaging, vessel-wall MRI, and MR spectroscopy are frequently used in addition to CT and conventional MRI for investigating underlying diseases and should be applied according to the imaging features of the suspected causes

DISCLOSURE

The authors disclose no commercial or financial conflicts of interest and no funding sources for this article.

REFERENCES

1. Béjot Y, Bailly H, Durier J, et al. Epidemiology of stroke in Europe and trends for the 21st century. Presse Med 2016;45(12 Pt 2):e391–8.

2. Madsen TE, Khoury JC, Leppert M, et al. Temporal trends in stroke incidence over time by sex and age in the GCNKSS. Stroke 2020;51(4):1070–6.

3. Griffiths D, Sturm J. Epidemiology and etiology of young stroke. Stroke research and treatment. 2011.

4. Lee T-H, Hsu W-C, Chen C-J, et al. Etiologic study of young ischemic stroke in Taiwan. Stroke 2002;33(8): 1950–5.

5. Ji R, Schwamm LH, Pervez MA, et al. Ischemic stroke and transient ischemic attack in young adults: risk factors, diagnostic yield, neuroimaging, and thrombolysis. JAMA Neurol 2013;70(1):51–7.

6. Putaala J, Metso AJ, Metso TM, et al. Analysis of 1008 consecutive patients aged 15 to 49 with first-ever ischemic stroke. Stroke 2009;40(4):1195–203.

7. Lee VH, Connolly HM, Brown RD Jr. Central nervous system manifestations of cardiac myxoma. Arch Neurol 2007;64(8):1115–20.

8. Niño AO, Ramirez LAC, Leal JCA, et al. Brain manifestations secondary to auricular myxoma. Radiol Case Rep 2020;15(11):2371–4.

9. Yeap P, Kanodia AK, Main G, et al. Role of susceptibility-weighted imaging in demonstration of cerebral fat embolism. BMJ Case Rep 2015.

10. Kang SR, Choi SS, Jeon SJ. Cerebral air embolism: a case report with an emphasis of its pathophysiology and MRI findings. Investig Magn Reson Imaging 2019;23(1):70–4.

11. Mandell DM, Mossa-Basha M, Qiao Y, et al. Intracranial vessel wall MRI: principles and expert consensus recommendations of the American Society of Neuroradiology. AJNR Am J Neuroradiol 2017; 38(2):218–29.

12. Debette S. Pathophysiology and risk factors of cervical artery dissection: what have we learnt from large hospital-based cohorts? Curr Opin Neurol 2014; 27(1):20–8.

13. Mehdi E, Aralasmak A, Toprak H, et al. Craniocervical dissections: radiologic findings, pitfalls, mimicking diseases: a pictorial review. Curr Med Imag Rev 2018;14(2):207–22.

14. Wang Y, Lou X, Li Y, et al. Imaging investigation of intracranial arterial dissecting aneurysms by using 3 T high-resolution MRI and DSA: from the interventional neuroradiologists' view. Acta Neurochir 2014; 156(3):515–25.

15. Leboucher A, Sotton S, Gambin Flandrin I, et al. Head and neck radiotherapy-induced carotid toxicity: pathophysiological concepts and clinical syndromes. Oral Oncol 2022;129:105868.

16. Katsura M, Sato J, Akahane M, et al. Recognizing radiation-induced changes in the central nervous system: where to look and what to look for. Radiographics 2020;41(1):224–48.

17. Gao P, Dmytriw AA, Wang T, et al. Contemporary challenges of acute ischemic stroke in takayasu arteritis. Stroke 2020;51(10):e280–4.

18. Hershberger R, Cho JS. Neurologic complications of aortic diseases and aortic surgery. Handb Clin Neurol 2014;119:223–38.

19. Varennes L, Tahon F, Kastler A, et al. Fibromuscular dysplasia: what the radiologist should know: a pictorial review. Insights Imaging 2015;6(3):295–307.

20. Furie D, Tien RD. Fibromuscular dysplasia of arteries of the head and neck: imaging findings. AJR Am J Roentgenol 1994;162(5):1205–9.

21. Kim SJ, Allen JW, Bouslama M, et al. Carotid webs in cryptogenic ischemic strokes: a matched case-control study. J Stroke Cerebrovasc Dis 2019;28(12): 1–7.

22. Zilocchi M, Macedo TA, Oderich GS, et al. Vascular ehlers-danlos syndrome: imaging findings. Am J Roentgenol 2007;189(3):712–9.

23. Castori M, Voermans NC. Neurological manifestations of Ehlers-Danlos syndrome(s): a review. Iran J Neurol 2014;13(4):190–208.

24. Abdel Razek AAK, Alvarez H, Bagg S, et al. Imaging spectrum of CNS vasculitis. Radiographics 2014;34: 873–94.

25. Arrigan MT, Heran MKS, Shewchuk JR. Reversible cerebral vasoconstriction syndrome: an important and common cause of thunderclap and recurrent headaches. Clin Radiol 2018;73(5):417–27.

26. Miller T, Shivashankar R, Mossa-Basha M, et al. Reversible cerebral vasoconstriction syndrome, part 2: diagnostic work-up, imaging evaluation, and differential diagnosis. Am J Neuroradiol 2015;36(9):1580–8.

27. Mossa-Basha M, Hwang WD, De Havenon A, et al. Multicontrast high-resolution vessel wall magnetic resonance imaging and its value in differentiating

intracranial vasculopathic processes. Stroke 2015; 46(6):1567–73.

28. Ihara M, Yamamoto Y, Hattori Y, et al. Moyamoya disease: diagnosis and interventions. Lancet Neurol 2022.

29. Velo M, Grasso G, Fujimura M, et al. Moyamoya vasculopathy: cause, clinical manifestations, neuroradiologic features, and surgical management. World Neurosurg 2022;159:409–25.

30. Dichgans M, Markus HS, Salloway S, et al. Donepezil in patients with subcortical vascular cognitive impairment: a randomised double-blind trial in CADASIL. Lancet Neurol 2008;7(4):310–8.

31. Mahammedi A, Wang L, Williamson B, et al. Small vessel disease, a marker of brain health: what the radiologist needs to know. Am J Neuroradiol 2022; 43(5):650–60.

32. Dörr J, Krautwald S, Wildemann B, et al. Characteristics of Susac syndrome: a review of all reported cases. Nat Rev Neurol 2013;9(6):307–16.

33. Sveinsson O, Kolloch J, Träisk F, et al. Susac syndrome-an unusual syndrome which can be mistaken for multiple sclerosis. Lakartidningen 2020;117:1–7.

34. Bagaglia SA, Passani F, Oliverio GW, et al. Multimodal Imaging in Susac Syndrome: a case report and literature review. Int J Environ Res Publ Health 2021;18(7):3435.

35. Li W, Kim J, Zhang J, et al. Infectious causes of acute ischemic stroke: pathomechanisms and distribution of brain infarct. Precis Future Med 2020;4(3): 114–8.

36. Misra UK, Kalita J, Maurya PK. Stroke in tuberculous meningitis. J Neurol Sci 2011;303(1):22–30.

37. Synmon B, Das M, Kayal AK, et al. Clinical and radiological spectrum of intracranial tuberculosis: a hospital based study in Northeast India. Indian J Tubercul 2017;64(2):109–18.

38. Gilden D, Cohrs RJ, Mahalingam R, et al. Varicella zoster virus vasculopathies: diverse clinical manifestations, laboratory features, pathogenesis, and treatment. Lancet Neurol 2009;8(8):731–40.

39. Amlie-Lefond C, Gilden D. Varicella Zoster Virus: a common cause of stroke in children and adults. J Stroke Cerebrovasc Dis 2016;25(7):1561–9.

40. Cheng-Ching E, Jones S, Hui FK, et al. High-resolution MRI vessel wall imaging in varicella zoster virus vasculopathy. J Neurol Sci 2015;351(1–2):168–73.

41. Ellul MA, Benjamin L, Singh B, et al. Neurological associations of COVID-19. Lancet Neurol 2020;19(9): 767–83.

42. Beyrouti R, Adams ME, Benjamin L, et al. Characteristics of ischaemic stroke associated with COVID-19. J Neurol Neurosurg Psychiatr 2020;91(8): 889–91.

43. Nannoni S, de Groot R, Bell S, et al. Stroke in COVID-19: a systematic review and meta-analysis. Int J Stroke 2020;16(2):137–49.

44. Gonçalves FG, Pinheiro CA, Alves F, et al. Primary mitochondrial disorders of the pediatric central nervous system: neuroimaging findings. Radiographics 2020;40(7):2042–67.

45. Goodfellow JA, Dani K, Stewart W, et al. Mitochondrial myopathy, encephalopathy, lactic acidosis and stroke-like episodes: an important cause of stroke in young people. Postgrad Med 2012; 88(1040):326–34.

46. Ramot Y, Nyska A, Spectre G. Drug-induced thrombosis: an update. Drug Saf 2013;36(8):585–603.

47. Jacobs IG, Roszler M, Kelly J, et al. Cocaine abuse: neurovascular complications. Radiology 1989; 170(1):223–7.

48. Squier M, Jalloh S, Hilton-Jones D, et al. Death after ecstasy ingestion: neuropathological findings. J Neurol Neurosurg Psychiatry 1995;58(6):756.

49. Niehaus L, Meyer B-U. Bilateral borderzone brain infarctions in association with heroin abuse. J Neurol Sci 1998;160(2):180–2.

50. Brown E, Prager J, Lee H, et al. CNS complications of cocaine abuse: prevalence, pathophysiology, and neuroradiology. AJR American journal of roentgenology 1992;159(1):137–47.

51. Hagan IG, Burney K. Radiology of recreational drug abuse. Radiographics 2007;27(4):919–40.

52. Senst B, Tadi P, Goyal A, et al. Hypercoagulability. StatPearls. StatPearls publishing copyright © 2022. StatPearls Publishing LLC.; 2022.

53. van den Bergh WM, van der Schaaf I, van Gijn J. The spectrum of presentations of venous infarction caused by deep cerebral vein thrombosis. Neurology 2005;65(2):192–6.

54. Connor S, Jarosz J. Magnetic resonance imaging of cerebral venous sinus thrombosis. Clin Radiol 2002; 57(6):449–61.

55. Grimes K, Klein AP, Lalla R, et al. Antiphospholipid syndrome and stroke. Antiphospholipid syndrome: recent advances in clinical and basic aspects. Cardiovascular Research 2022;cvac115.

56. Saidi S, Mahjoub T, Almawi W. Lupus anticoagulants and anti-phospholipid antibodies as risk factors for a first episode of ischemic stroke. J Thromb Haemostasis 2009;7(7):1075–80.

57. Rodrigues CE, Carvalho JF, Shoenfeld Y. Neurological manifestations of antiphospholipid syndrome. Eur J Clin Invest 2010;40(4):350–9.

58. Van Alebeek ME, De Heus R, Tuladhar AM, et al. Pregnancy and ischemic stroke: a practical guide to management. Curr Opin Neurol 2018;31(1): 44–51.

59. Ekker MS, Boot EM, Singhal AB, et al. Epidemiology, aetiology, and management of ischaemic stroke in young adults. Lancet Neurol 2018;17(9):790–801.

Evaluation of Collateral Circulation in Patients with Acute Ischemic Stroke

Check for updates

Keiko A. Fukuda, MD, David S. Liebeskind, MD*

KEYWORDS

- Collaterals • Acute ischemic stroke • Extended time window • Endovascular reperfusion
- Leptomeningeal anastomoses • Cerebral blood flow • Vasodilation

KEY POINTS

- Collateral status has been shown to affect the therapeutic time window for revascularization, infarct growth, recanalization success, hemorrhagic transformation, and long-term functional status.
- Augmentations to improve collateral status include induced hypertension, external counter pulsation, vasodilation, sphenopalatine ganglion stimulation, and partial aortic obstruction.
- The development of empiric and novel collateral therapeutic interventions will likely require clinical trials using refined diagnostic imaging to select therapeutic candidates based on collateral status.
- More attention should be paid to collateral status to help guide treatment decisions in acute ischemic stroke moving forward.

INTRODUCTION

Collaterals have moved from the periphery to an essential consideration for acute ischemic stroke (AIS) treatment. As advancing technologies and techniques have broadened the criteria for acute reperfusion therapies in recent years, leveraging cerebral collateral circulation remains the next frontier. Here, we review our current understanding of the pathophysiologic mechanisms, effect on outcomes, and strategies for improvement of the collateral system.

Collateral circulation refers to the subsidiary cerebral vessels that redistribute blood flow when the primary network fails.[1] It may be thought of as the brain's adaptability and reserve when the neurovascular system is under ischemic threat. Growing evidence has demonstrated that better collateral grade can predict the rate of infarct progression, degree of recanalization, the likelihood of hemorrhagic transformation, and various therapeutic opportunities.[2]

Collateral status differs markedly among patients with AIS (Table 1). In the IMS-III trial, 65% had poor collaterals (grade 0–2) and 35% had good collaterals (grade 3 or 4) per the American Society of Interventional and Therapeutic Neuroradiology/ Society of Interventional Radiology (ASITN/SIR) scale.[3] In the SWIFT trial cohort, 67% had poor collateral grades and 32% had good collateral grades on the ASITN/SIR scale.[4] However, pretreatment collateral status in patients treated in the extended time windows skewed toward favorable collateral status. A recent multicenter retrospective registry study of 554 patients presenting within 10 hours of anterior circulation large vessel occlusion (LVO) with successful recanalization indicated 84.5% were classified into good collaterals and 15.5% into poor collaterals based on single-phase computed tomography angiography (CTA).[5] In the DAWN trial, 74.5% had good or fair collaterals and 17.7% had poor collaterals.[6] This suggests a high level of collateral status variability among those

Department of Neurology, University of California, Los Angeles, UCLA Comprehensive Stroke Center, UCLA Neurovascular Imaging Research Core, 635 Charles East Young Drive South, Suite 225, Los Angeles, CA 90095-7334, USA
* Corresponding author.
E-mail address: davidliebeskind@yahoo.com

Radiol Clin N Am 61 (2023) 435–443
https://doi.org/10.1016/j.rcl.2023.01.002
0033-8389/23/

Table 1
Collateral status and outcomes with endovascular therapy

Trial	Patient Selection Criteria	Proportion of Good Vs. Bad Collaterals	Collateral Flow Grading System	Effect of Collaterals on Outcomes
DEFUSE-2 (2012)[57]	<12 h, AC LVO	Good-48% Bad-52%	DSA ASITN/SIR scale	Greater infarct growth in poor collateral group. No significant difference in good functional outcomes between good and poor collateral groups with perfusion.
SWIFT (2012)[58]	<8h, NIHSS≥8, AC LVO	Good-67% Bad-33%	DSA ASITN/SIR scale	Better collaterals associated with better mRS 0–2 at 3 mo (P < .001).
IMS-III (2013)[59]	<5h, IV tPA given, NIHSS≥10	Good-65% Bad-35%	DSA ASITN/SIR scale	Higher proportion of mRS 0–2 at 3 mo in those with good collaterals (P < .004).
MR CLEAN (2014)[60]	<6 h, NIHSS≥2, AC LVO	Good-67% Bad-33%	Single-phase CTA Tan scale	Ordinal odds ratio for favorable shift in mRS: good = 3.2, moderate = 1.6, poor = 1.2, absent = 1.0. Also better effect of EVT with higher collateral grades. Good collaterals = 86.8 mL reduction in infarct growth. Bad collaterals = 88.6 mL increase in infarct volume.
ENDOSTROKE registry (2015)[61]	MCA occlusion	Good-48.8% Bad-51.3%	DSA ASITN/SIR	Collateral status is independent predictor of mRS at 3 months–good with 46% and poor with 51%.
DAWN (2017)[62]	6–24 h, NIHSS>5, ASPECTS>5, AC LVO, clinical-core mismatch	Good-44.4% Fair-31.3% Poor-24.3%	CTA, DSA Tan	Those with the most favorable baseline NIHSS score, ASPECTS, infarct core volume and mRS 0–2 at 3 mo was 43.7% in good, 30.8% in fair, and 17.7% in poor.
Triple-S (2018)[63]	<8 h AC LVO	Good-35% Bad-65%	DSA ASITN/SIR	Collateral status as independent predictor of mRS 0–2 at 3 mo.
ETIS registry [64]2021)	AC LVO	Good-47.5% Poor-52.5%	DSA ASITN/SIR	Drop in probability of good outcome in both good and poor collateral groups in extended time window.

Good collaterals are defined as grades 3–4 and bad collaterals are defined as grades 0–2 on the ASITN/SIR scale.
Abbreviation: AC, anterior circulation.

with large vessel occlusions and its role in determining the rate of stroke progression.

The optimal imaging modalities available to assess pretreatment collateral status include multiphase CTA and CT perfusion (CTP). These correspond well with a leptomeningeal collateral grade on conventional angiography and have been used to predict final infarct volume, growth, and clinical response after thrombolysis. CTP provides information on collateral status, core, and penumbra.[7] Conventional MRI and magnetic resonance angiography (MRA), susceptibility contrast perfusion, and arterial spin labeling are other MRI techniques available that also demonstrate a good correlation with conventional angiography collateral grades.[7]

Although collateral status is known as a significant contributor to stroke pathophysiology, it is not commonly used as selection criteria for clinical trials. Trials have, however, suggested the importance of assessing collaterals when weighing the risks and benefits of endovascular therapy (EVT) in acute ischemic stroke (AIS). More attention should be paid to collateral status to help guide treatment decisions moving forward.

Pathophysiology and Collateral Failure in Stroke

Our understanding of the collateral circulation has evolved over time with several advances in our mechanistic understanding and therapeutic options (Table 2). Currently, we understand that leptomeningeal anastomoses (LMAs) are a specialized vascular niche that respond differently to aberrant hemodynamic changes. Aging causes LMAs to undergo pruning, decreased numbers as brain size and vessel diameters increase. Aging correlates with collateral rarefaction. Rodent studies show that collateral reduction occurs in an age-dependent manner with older animals having significantly fewer LMAs than younger animals.[8] Cardiovascular risk factors including hypertension, diabetes, and obesity can further exacerbate collateral rarefaction.[9] Other markers of oxidative stress and endothelial inflammation are associated with diminished collateral supply.[10] Patients with a poor collateral grade, such as elderly patients, have larger infarct volumes particularly if there is incomplete recanalization.[8,11]

Unlike angiogenesis, arteriogenesis in the LMAs is triggered by an increase in the mechanical forces on the collateral vessel wall and not hypoxemia.[12] Arterial occlusions lead to pressure gradient changes with accelerated retrograde flow from the non-occluded artery through nascent collateral vessels, causing increased fluid shear stress (FSS).[13] Since FSS is inversely related to vessel diameter, as the collateral vessel wall undergoes outward expansion, FSS decreases. Because of this, the collateral vessels are limited in growth to restore up to 40% of the original blood flow, and growth factors and cytokines (fibroblast growth factor [FGF]-1, FGF-2, vascular endothelial growth factor [VEGF], and MCP-1) can further restore up to 50% of original flow.[14,15] To date, increasing FSS on the collateral vessel wall by using an arteriovenous (AV) shunt has been the only effective way to fully restore and surpass the maximum conductance of the occluded parent vessel. This inherent shortfall highlights the need to fully elucidate the mechanisms governing LMA arteriogenesis to maximize their therapeutic potential and to overcome additional challenges that may exist due to age and chronic inflammatory conditions.[8]

A role for nitric oxide (NO), a potent vasodilatory agent, in enhancing cerebral blood flow (CBF) is also debated. When activated by shear stress, endothelial cells increase the expression of endothelial NO synthase, elevating NO release. However, as collateral vessels vasodilate and increase in

Table 2
Experimental techniques and therapeutics aimed at increasing cerebral blood flow

Technique	Mechanism
Vasodilators (nitric oxide, prostaglandins, leptins, PDE-5 inhibitors, erythropoietin/trophic factors)	Complements ongoing arteriogenesis; promotes angiogenesis/vasculogenesis
Induced hypertension	Increases CBF
Sphenopalatine ganglion stimulation	Increases CBF via vasodilation and arteriogenesis
Partial aortic occlusion	Increases CBF via vasodilation and arteriogenesis
External compression devices	Theoretic increased CBF, not fully established
NO, VE-Cadherin, VEGF	Increased vascular permeability; promotes angiogenesis

diameter, FSS is reduced, potentially serving to negatively regulate arteriogenesis. This implies NO is indispensable for initial vasodilation of collateral vessels, possibly through dilation of upstream feeding arteries, but does not significantly affect arteriogenesis. Inhaled NO is being investigated for clinical applications to reduce ischemic brain damage and increase collateral flow through vasodilation. To combat an increase in oxidative stress that accompanies inducible NO synthase, prostaglandins are considered for improving acute vasodilation due to their delayed and moderate effect on vasodilation. Leptin is another agent that may support collateral flow, but it does not impact cellular proliferation or collateral conductance when maximally dilated. Initial studies have shown the importance of taking advantage of collateral vessels for acute vasodilation and subsequent arteriogenesis to improve blood flow restoration in ischemic stroke. Pharmacologic collateral vasodilatation could improve tissue perfusion in the short-term before recanalization. It could also complement ongoing arteriogenesis, which may take additional time for maximum vessel growth.

Certain medical comorbidities also affect intracranial collateral development. In a recent analysis of the MR CLEAN registry, poor collateral status was associated with old age and male sex, high glucose levels and history of peripheral arterial disease, and internal carotid artery terminus occlusion.[16] In the SWIFT trial, a history of hypertension, smoking, and higher blood glucose levels predicted worse collaterals and worse outcomes.[4] In animal models, hypertension weakens the development of collaterals and significantly constricts the anastomoses leading to reduced collateral capacity.[4] Chronic hypertension impairs endothelial function and stiffens myogenic vessel tone, leading to reduced vasodilator capacity of arterioles, capillaries, and leptomeningeal collaterals. Chronic hypertension may also downregulate cerebral autoregulation, leading to collateral development.

In contrast, chronic hypoperfusion due to flow restrictions such as extracranial or intracranial stenosis and use of statins promote collateral development mediated by an increase in endothelial progenitor cell growth.[17] It is also possible that acute hyperglycemia and hypertension in AIS may be indirect markers of poor collaterals, causing more extensive ischemia and worse outcomes post-intervention. A graded association between lower blood glucose and blood pressure was noted with better collateral flow.[4] In patients in the extended window of the DAWN trial, a history of diabetes and higher glucose levels on presentation were also significantly associated with poor collaterals and larger core infarcts. Likewise, good collaterals were associated with lower baseline glucose levels, lack of diabetes history, and higher likelihood of angiographic reperfusion following endovascular therapy.[18] The pathophysiology of the association between collaterals and glycemia may correspond with larger core infarcts, yet requires further study.

A likely contributor to collateral status is the presence of small vessel disease (SVD) as this is almost certainly related to a long history of hypertension and diabetes. In a study evaluating patients with a high burden of chronic SVD concurrently undergoing mechanical thrombectomy for large vessel occlusions, there were double the odds of poor collateral status compared with patients with LVOs without SVD. A dose-dependent relationship was seen between higher burden of SVD and poor collaterals. Significant chronic microvascular ischemic changes may be a marker for impaired cerebrovascular reserve, manifesting as limited recruitment and poor perfusion of ischemic tissue during LVO. Hypoperfusion may also impair collateral recruitment as either a consequence of or cause of increased SVD.[19]

The mechanisms of SVD include chronically reduced blood flow due to arteriolosclerosis, lipohyalinosis, and small artery and arteriole fibrinoid changes leading to leukoaraiosis. As the leptomeningeal collateral system is also composed of small arteries and arterioles, it is possible that the mechanisms causing leukoaraiosis might also affect the leptomeningeal collateral system. In several analyses of acute embolic LVOs treated with thrombectomy, good collateral flow was found to be associated with reduced leukoaraiosis in both cardiac and noncardiac embolism mechanisms, particularly thrombi with shorter lengths. Age and vascular risk factors have not been univariately associated with poor leptomeningeal collateral flow though the severity of leukoaraiosis has been associated with several of these parameters including older age, hypertension, diabetes, smoking, and obesity. Studies have indicated that leukoaraiosis, as an individual's cumulative burden of SVD from multiple risk factors, more strongly correlates with leptomeningeal impairment. In a study of white matter hyperintensities (WMH) and functional outcome, those with higher WMH volumes (>9 mL) were less likely to be functionally independent at 90 days.[19] This is thought to be due to disturbance in vasodilation of leptomeningeal collaterals and blood flow resulting in faster infarct growth, and thus, poorer outcomes.[20] As such, leukoaraiosis may serve as an imaging marker of global cerebrovascular dysfunction and a determinant of differences in leptomeningeal collaterals.[21]

Better Collaterals Improve Outcomes

Good collateral status predicts infarct growth, recanalization success, hemorrhagic transformation after EVT, and the therapeutic time window for revascularization.[19] Studies further indicate that pretreatment collateral circulation is associated with both clinical and imaging outcomes after EVT in patients with AIS due to LVO despite most patients' selection by other imaging or clinical criteria.[6,22] Numerous trials have shown that patients with high collateral grade in AIS have a better response to IV alteplase and EVT, slower stroke progression, and better neurologic outcomes.[3,4,23] In a collateral analysis in patients with LVOs treated with EVT in the extended window, good collaterals were associated with smaller core infarcts at presentation, slower infarct evolution, less hemorrhagic transformation, and higher rates of 90-day functional independence.[4,18,24]

The IMS-III trial authors speculated that strong collaterals may be associated with a stronger degree of recanalization due to a greater volume of systemic thrombolytics delivered to the clot surface, enhancing thrombolysis and facilitating thrombectomy. Reperfusion of the downstream territory may be more complete after occluded large vessel recanalization if such regions receive more robust collateral perfusion. In both IMS-III and SWIFT, the degree of final reperfusion with a modified TICI score$\geq$2 was related to collateral extent.[3] However, recanalization was still possible even when baseline collateral flow was poor.[4]

Retrograde collateral filling allows thrombolytic and neuroprotective molecules (extrinsic, intrinsic, or both) greater access to the distal clot segments. Robust collaterals may facilitate fragmented thrombi dissolution, thrombus retrieval, and device pass efficacy.[25] Robust retrograde flow may place distal force on the thrombus and facilitate retrieval in more proximal locations. Collateral circulation may also determine thrombus characteristics. MR CLEAN investigators showed that patients with good collaterals had both a lower burden of thrombus and higher perviousness.[26] Another single-center study of 626 patients found that those with excellent collaterals were more likely to achieve first-pass effect for successful reperfusion (eTICI 2b–3) and complete reperfusion (eTICI 2c–3) than in the other groups.[25] Lastly, collateral circulation may protect blood vessels by minimizing ischemic vascular injury.

Infarct Growth

The association between pretreatment collateral circulation with post-EVT infarct growth was demonstrated in an early study.[2] In a later study,

the hyperacute infarct growth rate (ischemic core volume divided by time from symptom onset) in patients with good, intermediate, and poor collaterals was 0.17, 0.26, and 0.41 mL/min, respectively.[27] Similarly, another study found the median infarct progression rate was 2.2 mL/h with wide variability in the first 6 hours after onset. Faster infarct progression was associated with poor collaterals, whereas slower infarct progression was associated with reduced disability levels at discharge, increased reperfusion by EVT, and reduced hemorrhagic transformation.[28]

Rapid infarct progression is relatively common. The control arm of the ESCAPE trial saw faster infarct progression, defined as ASPECTS decay$\geq$3 from baseline to 2 to 8 hours of follow-up imaging, occurring in 34.9% of patients. Faster progressors had worse collaterals and more frequent carotid T or L occlusions at baseline causing impaired collateral flow via the anterior and posterior cerebral arteries.[29] Recently, a prospective multicenter cohort study showed that fast progressors had worse outcomes when receiving EVT beyond 6 hours of stroke onset. The early infarct growth rate strongly correlated with both collateral grade and clinical outcome after EVT in this study.[6] These results suggest that collateral status may help support decisions on patients who are fast progressors in the extended window.[30]

Extended Time Window

Identification of good collaterals can help physicians when considering recanalization in the late time window. Several studies have shown that patients with good baseline collaterals are significantly more likely to have better functional outcomes from EVT beyond 6 and up to 24 hours from the last known well.[18,31] Similarly, another study showed that EVT after 5 hours from onset-to-puncture led to significantly reduced functional independence at 3 months in the poor collateral group. This was not significantly influenced by time in the good collateral group.[32] Of note, LVOs due to progressive intracranial atherosclerosis allow robust collaterals to develop. These studies emphasize how important assessing collaterals in patients presenting in the late window is and its strong predictive capability of response to treatment and long-term neurologic outcomes.[33]

Hemorrhagic Transformation

Poor collaterals predict the progression of malignant cerebral edema after EVT. Although most studies show an elevated risk of hemorrhagic transformation after EVT in patients with poor collaterals, there is inconsistency especially in those with CTA to assess collateral status.[34,35] One possible explanation is that poor collaterals are associated with larger infarcts, which confer a greater risk of hemorrhage post-revascularization. Thus, the risk of symptomatic hemorrhagic conversion may be lower in patients with good collaterals in whom infarct volume at presentation is smaller and the infarct growth rate is lower.

Strategies to Enhance Collateral Circulation

Outside of the ultimate enhancement to collateral circulation (reperfusion), there are several old and newly emerging collateral enhancements with potential value as interventional adjuncts. Relevant hemodynamic augmentation includes induced hypertension, lowering the head of the bed, vasodilation, expanded volume status, external counterpulsation, partial aortic obstruction routing splanchnic blood to the upper body and brain, and sphenopalatine ganglion stimulation.[7,36]

Most work observing changes in blood flow with intrinsic-innervation stimulation has been done in animals. Although the precise mechanisms underlying cerebral autoregulation are not fully understood, experts believe they are mediated at the levels of the neurons, neuropil, and cerebral blood vessels.[37] Extrinsic and intrinsic innervations to the vessels regulate blood flow.[38,39] The intrinsic nerves originate mainly in the brainstem and are distributed predominantly on the parenchymal vessels compared with the extrinsic nerves, which supply vessels on the brain surface.[40] Sympathetic nerve stimulation, especially around the locus coeruleus and parabrachial nucleus, causes reduced CBF and brain water permeability.[41,42] Stimulation of several other structures throughout the brainstem and cerebellum including the dorsal medullary reticular formation, rostral ventrolateral medulla, dorsal raphe nuclei, and fastigial nucleus of the cerebellum can result in vasodilation of cortical vessels.[39] Unfortunately, due to the invasive approach, these techniques would be impractical in acute stroke.[43]

Studies in small numbers of patients with SPECT imaging have shown that elevating blood pressure may decrease the penumbra. A retrospective assessment of 30 patients reported that a third of patients with phenylephrine-induced hypertension showed neurologic improvement. Phenylephrine was used within 12 hours of symptom onset and continued for between 24 hours and 6 days.[44] The American Heart Association's guidelines recommend that induced hypertension can be used in "exceptional cases" and that

cardiac and neurologic status should be closely monitored during its use.[45]

In animal models, the application of nitric oxide, albumin, and tumor necrosis factor-alpha inhibitor has been shown to increase arteriogenesis (collateral formation from pre-existing channels) in animal stroke models. Preclinical and clinical studies have also shown that various pharmacologic therapies may enhance angiogenesis (capillary formation from pre-existing vessels) and vasculogenesis (de novo capillary formation), which include sildenafil and phosphodiesterase-type 5 inhibitors, erythropoietin/trophic factors, and statins with or without cell therapy.[7,46–49] Large randomized trials in patients with acute stroke have however failed to show results. Possible reasons for these failures include inadequate patient selection and lack of assessment of effects such as interventions on collateral blood vessels and flow. More studies are needed with optimized patient selection and rigorous consideration of the available collateral-enhancing strategies via advanced imaging techniques.

A considerable amount of preclinical and clinical data supporting parasympathetic fibers of the facial nerve as a potential therapeutic option for rapid AIS treatment exist. The parasympathetic nerves arise from the superior salivatory nucleus and pass along cranial nerve VII to the sphenopalatine and otic ganglia. Several neurotransmitters such as acetylcholine, vasoactive intestinal polypeptide, peptide histidine isoleucine, and nitrous oxide are involved in vasodilation.[50,51] Stimulation of the sphenopalatine ganglion in rats, cats, and human beings results in an almost immediate vasodilatory response in the ipsilateral cerebral vessels, which lasts as long as the stimulus is applied. The effect can be quite profound, with an increase in blood flow of more than 40% in the ipsilateral cortex.[52] Various human trials have investigated electrical stimulation of the sphenopalatine ganglion transorally but have suffered from operational limitations and non-significant clinical findings. In the future, optimal use for facial nerve stimulation will likely be to augment and improve gold-standard treatments such as thrombolytic and mechanical thrombectomy.[53]

Another possible method is restricting abdominal aortic blood flow by temporary occlusion. This has been shown to reduce infarction volume when used alone and in combination with alteplase in rodents with embolic stroke.[54] The Neuro-Flo catheter, which restricts the aortic lumen by up to 80% at the suprarenal and infrarenal levels, has been developed for use in acute stroke and is safe in patients up to 24 hours after symptom onset. It has also been tested on patients who received alteplase without increased risk of hemorrhagic transformation.[55] However, the SENTIS trial, which included 515 patients enrolled within 14 hours of symptom onset, did not show clinical benefit from the device compared with standard medical therapy. The study likely was not powered to show a clear clinical benefit in unselected patients treated far after symptom onset. A subgroup of patients greater than 70 years with moderate deficits may have shown an improvement in outcomes. It is still possible this approach is effective in patients with pretreatment penumbral tissue.[56]

SUMMARY

In the current era of acute stroke treatment, collaterals have emerged as one of the most important considerations in decision-making. Despite the mechanisms of remodeling remaining under continued investigation, collaterals are a key determinant of stroke outcomes. At present, collaterals can identify those unlikely to respond to reperfusion therapies due to poor collaterals and thus allow for more efficient triage and resource utilization. Proven measures of collaterals should be taken into consideration in predicting stroke outcomes. More randomized trials are needed to evaluate the risks and benefits of EVT in consideration of collateral status.

CLINICS CARE POINTS

- The rate of penumbral loss in untreated stroke is not directly related to the duration of symptoms but primarily depends on the quality and maintenance of collateral flow. In the presence of a large vessel occlusion, infarct core growth and penumbral loss progresses more rapidly with malignant collateral patterns (i.e., fast progressors) and more slowly in patients with good collateral patterns (i.e., slow progressors).

- A malignant collateral pattern on delayed-phase CT can be characterized by a lack of contrast filling at least 50% of the intracranial vessels in the at-risk territory. Unless recanalization occurs soon after the onset of a stroke, poor collateral flow is associated with a low probability of penumbral salvage and significant clinical benefit from EVT.

- A good collateral pattern has symmetric or nearly symmetric leptomeningeal flow when comparing the affected to the unaffected hemisphere. Good collateral flow is an essential indicator of the potential efficacy of EVT.

DISCLOSURE

The authors have nothing to disclose.

REFERENCES

1. Liebeskind DS. Collateral circulation. Stroke 2003; 34(9):2279–84.
2. Bang OY, Saver JL, Buck BH, et al. Impact of collateral flow on tissue fate in acute ischaemic stroke. J Neurol Neurosurg Psychiatry 2008;79(6):625–9.
3. Liebeskind DS, Tomsick TA, Foster LD, et al. Collaterals at angiography and outcomes in the Interventional Management of Stroke (IMS) III trial. Stroke 2014;45(3):759–64.
4. Liebeskind DS, Jahan R, Nogueira RG, et al. Impact of collaterals on successful revascularization in Solitaire FR with the intention for thrombectomy. Stroke 2014;45(7):2036–40.
5. Kim BM, Baek JH, Heo JH, et al. Collateral status affects the onset-to-reperfusion time window for good outcome. J Neurol Neurosurg Psychiatry 2018;89(9): 903–9.
6. Lee JS, Bang OY. Collateral Status and Outcomes after Thrombectomy. Transl Stroke Res 2022. https://doi.org/10.1007/s12975-022-01046-z.
7. Bang OY, Goyal M, Liebeskind DS. Collateral Circulation in Ischemic Stroke: Assessment Tools and Therapeutic Strategies. Stroke 2015;46(11):3302–9.
8. Kaloss AM, Theus MH. Leptomeningeal anastomoses: Mechanisms of pial collateral remodeling in ischemic stroke. WIREs Mech Dis 2022;3:e1553.
9. Moore SM, Zhang H, Maeda N, et al. Cardiovascular risk factors cause premature rarefaction of the collateral circulation and greater ischemic tissue injury. Angiogenesis 2015;18(3):265–81.
10. Zhang H, Jin B, Faber JE. Mouse models of Alzheimer's disease cause rarefaction of pial collaterals and increased severity of ischemic stroke. Angiogenesis 2019;22(2):263–79.
11. Seker F, Pereira-Zimmermann B, Pfaff J, et al. Collateral Scores in Acute Ischemic Stroke : A retrospective study assessing the suitability of collateral scores as standalone predictors of clinical outcome. Clin Neuroradiol 2020;30(4):789–93.
12. Heil M, Schaper W. Influence of mechanical, cellular, and molecular factors on collateral artery growth (arteriogenesis). Circ Res 2004;95(5):449–58.
13. Roux E, Bougaran P, Dufourcq P, et al. Fluid Shear Stress Sensing by the Endothelial Layer. Front Physiol 2020;11:861.
14. Hoefer IE, van Royen N, Buschmann IR, et al. Time course of arteriogenesis following femoral artery occlusion in the rabbit. Cardiovasc Res 2001;49(3): 609–17.
15. Schaper W, Flameng W, Winkler B, et al. Quantification of collateral resistance in acute and chronic

experimental coronary occlusion in the dog. Circ Res 1976;39(3):371–7.

16. Wiegers EJA, Mulder M, Jansen IGH, et al. Clinical and Imaging Determinants of Collateral Status in Patients With Acute Ischemic Stroke in MR CLEAN Trial and Registry. Stroke 2020;51(5):1493–502.

17. Ovbiagele B, Saver JL, Starkman S, et al. Statin enhancement of collateralization in acute stroke. Neurology 2007;68(24):2129–31.

18. Liebeskind DS, Saber H, Xiang B, et al. Collateral Circulation in Thrombectomy for Stroke After 6 to 24 Hours in the DAWN Trial. Stroke 2022;53(3):742–8.

19. Lin MP, Brott TG, Liebeskind DS, et al. Collateral Recruitment Is Impaired by Cerebral Small Vessel Disease. Stroke 2020;51(5):1404–10.

20. Boulouis G, Bricout N, Benhassen W, et al. White matter hyperintensity burden in patients with ischemic stroke treated with thrombectomy. Neurology 2019;93(16):e1498–506.

21. Hashimoto T, Kunieda T, Honda T, et al. Reduced Leukoaraiosis, Noncardiac Embolic Stroke Etiology, and Shorter Thrombus Length Indicate Good Leptomeningeal Collateral Flow in Embolic Large-Vessel Occlusion. AJNR Am J Neuroradiol 2022;43(1):63–9.

22. Leng X, Fang H, Leung TW, et al. Impact of Collateral Status on Successful Revascularization in Endovascular Treatment: A Systematic Review and Meta-Analysis. Cerebrovasc Dis 2016;41(1–2):27–34.

23. Liebeskind DS, Flint AC, Budzik RF, et al. Carotid I's, L's and T's: collaterals shape the outcome of intracranial carotid occlusion in acute ischemic stroke. J Neurointerv Surg 2015;7(6):402–7.

24. Bang OY, Saver JL, Kim SJ, et al. Collateral flow averts hemorrhagic transformation after endovascular therapy for acute ischemic stroke. Stroke 2011;42(8):2235–9.

25. Garcia-Tornel A, Ciolli L, Rubiera M, et al. Leptomeningeal Collateral Flow Modifies Endovascular Treatment Efficacy on Large-Vessel Occlusion Strokes. Stroke 2021;52(1):299–303.

26. Alves HC, Treurniet KM, Dutra BG, et al. Associations Between Collateral Status and Thrombus Characteristics and Their Impact in Anterior Circulation Stroke. Stroke 2018;49(2):391–6.

27. Puhr-Westerheide D, Tiedt S, Rotkopf LT, et al. Clinical and Imaging Parameters Associated With Hyperacute Infarction Growth in Large Vessel Occlusion Stroke. Stroke 2019;50(10):2799–804.

28. Seo WK, Liebeskind DS, Yoo B, et al. Predictors and Functional Outcomes of Fast, Intermediate, and Slow Progression Among Patients With Acute Ischemic Stroke. Stroke 2020;51(8):2553–7.

29. Ospel JM, Hill MD, Kappelhof M, et al. Which Acute Ischemic Stroke Patients Are Fast Progressors?: Results From the ESCAPE Trial Control Arm. Stroke 2021;52(5):1847–50.

30. Sarraj A, Hassan AE, Grotta J, et al. Early Infarct Growth Rate Correlation With Endovascular Thrombectomy Clinical Outcomes: Analysis From the SELECT Study. Stroke 2021;52(1):57–69.

31. Ribo M, Flores A, Rubiera M, et al. Extending the time window for endovascular procedures according to collateral pial circulation. Stroke 2011;42(12):3465–9.

32. Hwang YH, Kang DH, Kim YW, et al. Impact of time-to-reperfusion on outcome in patients with poor collaterals. AJNR Am J Neuroradiol 2015;36(3):495–500.

33. Lee JS, Hong JM, Kim JS. Diagnostic and Therapeutic Strategies for Acute Intracranial Atherosclerosis-related Occlusions. J Stroke 2017;19(2):143–51.

34. de Havenon A, Mlynash M, Kim-Tenser MA, et al. Results From DEFUSE 3: Good Collaterals Are Associated With Reduced Ischemic Core Growth but Not Neurologic Outcome. Stroke 2019;50(3):632–8.

35. Renu A, Laredo C, Montejo C, et al. Greater infarct growth limiting effect of mechanical thrombectomy in stroke patients with poor collaterals. J Neurointerv Surg 2019;11(10):989–93.

36. Shuaib A, Bornstein NM, Diener HC, et al. Partial aortic occlusion for cerebral perfusion augmentation: safety and efficacy of NeuroFlo in Acute Ischemic Stroke trial. Stroke 2011;42(6):1680–90.

37. Attwell D, Buchan AM, Charpak S, et al. Glial and neuronal control of brain blood flow. Nature 2010;468(7321):232–43.

38. Ainslie PN, Ogoh S. Regulation of cerebral blood flow in mammals during chronic hypoxia: a matter of balance. Exp Physiol 2010;95(2):251–62.

39. Goadsby PJ. Neurovascular headache and a midbrain vascular malformation: evidence for a role of the brainstem in chronic migraine. Cephalalgia 2002;22(2):107–11.

40. Hamel E. Perivascular nerves and the regulation of cerebrovascular tone. J Appl Physiol(1985) 2006;100(3):1059–64.

41. Mraovitch S, Iadecola C, Ruggiero DA, et al. Widespread reductions in cerebral blood flow and metabolism elicited by electrical stimulation of the parabrachial nucleus in rat. Brain Res 1985;341(2):283–96.

42. de la Torre JC, Surgeon JW, Walker RH. Effects of locus coeruleus stimulation on cerebral blood flow in selected brain regions. Acta Neurol Scand Suppl 1977;64:104–5.

43. Shuaib A, Butcher K, Mohammad AA, et al. Collateral blood vessels in acute ischaemic stroke: a potential therapeutic target. Lancet Neurol 2011;10(10):909–21.

44. Rordorf G, Cramer SC, Efird JT, et al. Pharmacological elevation of blood pressure in acute stroke. Clinical effects and safety. Stroke 1997;28(11):2133–8.

45. Adams HP Jr, del Zoppo G, Alberts MJ, et al. Guidelines for the early management of adults with

ischemic stroke: a guideline from the American Heart Association/American Stroke Association Stroke Council, Clinical Cardiology Council, Cardiovascular Radiology and Intervention Council, and the Atherosclerotic Peripheral Vascular Disease and Quality of Care Outcomes in Research Interdisciplinary Working Groups: The American Academy of Neurology affirms the value of this guideline as an educational tool for neurologists. Circulation 2007;115(20):e478–534.

46. Ding G, Jiang Q, Li L, et al. Angiogenesis detected after embolic stroke in rat brain using magnetic resonance T2*WI. *Stroke*. May 2008;39(5):1563–8.

47. Silver B, McCarthy S, Lu M, et al. Sildenafil treatment of subacute ischemic stroke: a safety study at 25-mg daily for 2 weeks. J Stroke Cerebrovasc Dis 2009;18(5):381–3.

48. Tongers J, Roncalli JG, Losordo DW. Role of endothelial progenitor cells during ischemia-induced vasculogenesis and collateral formation. Microvasc Res 2010;79(3):200–6.

49. Todo K, Kitagawa K, Sasaki T, et al. Granulocyte-macrophage colony-stimulating factor enhances leptomeningeal collateral growth induced by common carotid artery occlusion. Stroke 2008;39(6):1875–82.

50. Gonzalez C, Barroso C, Martin C, et al. Neuronal nitric oxide synthase activation by vasoactive intestinal peptide in bovine cerebral arteries. J Cereb Blood Flow Metab 1997;17(9):977–84.

51. Uddman R, Tajti J, Moller S, et al. Neuronal messengers and peptide receptors in the human sphenopalatine and otic ganglia. Brain Res 1999;826(2):193–9.

52. Seylaz J, Hara H, Pinard E, et al. Effect of stimulation of the sphenopalatine ganglion on cortical blood flow in the rat. J Cereb Blood Flow Metab 1988;8(6):875–8.

53. Baker TS, Robeny J, Cruz D, et al. Stimulating the Facial Nerve to Treat Ischemic Stroke: A Systematic Review. Front Neurol 2021;12:753182.

54. Noor R, Wang CX, Todd K, et al. Partial intra-aortic occlusion improves perfusion deficits and infarct size following focal cerebral ischemia. J Neuroimaging 2010;20(3):272–6.

55. Emery DJ, Schellinger PD, Selchen D, et al. Safety and feasibility of collateral blood flow augmentation after intravenous thrombolysis. Stroke 2011;42(4):1135–7.

56. Hammer MD, Schwamm L, Starkman S, et al. Safety and feasibility of NeuroFlo use in eight- to 24-hour ischemic stroke patients. Int J Stroke 2012;7(8):655–61.

57. Lansberg MG, Straka M, Kemp S, et al. MRI profile and response to endovascular reperfusion after stroke (DEFUSE 2): a prospective cohort study. Lancet Neurol 2012;11(10):860–7.

58. Saver JL, Jahan R, Levy EI, et al. Solitaire flow restoration device versus the Merci Retriever in patients with acute ischaemic stroke (SWIFT): a randomised, parallel-group, non-inferiority trial. Lancet 2012;380(9849):1241–9.

59. Broderick JP, Palesch YY, Demchuk AM, et al. Endovascular therapy after intravenous t-PA versus t-PA alone for stroke. N Engl J Med 2013;368(10):893–903.

60. Berkhemer OA, Fransen PS, Beumer D, et al. A randomized trial of intraarterial treatment for acute ischemic stroke. N Engl J Med 2015;372(1):11–20.

61. Singer OC, Berkefeld J, Nolte CH, et al. Collateral vessels in proximal middle cerebral artery occlusion: the ENDOSTROKE study. Radiology 2015;274(3):851–8.

62. Nogueira RG, Jadhav AP, Haussen DC, et al. Thrombectomy 6 to 24 Hours after Stroke with a Mismatch between Deficit and Infarct. N Engl J Med 2018;378(1):11–21.

63. Kim JT, Liebeskind DS, Jahan R, et al. Impact of Hyperglycemia According to the Collateral Status on Outcomes in Mechanical Thrombectomy. Stroke 2018;49(11):2706–14.

64. Anadani M, Januel AC, Finitsis S, et al. Effect of intravenous thrombolysis before endovascular therapy on outcome according to collateral status: insight from the ETIS Registry. J Neurointerv Surg 2022. https://doi.org/10.1136/neurintsurg-2021-018170.

Advanced Imaging for Acute Stroke Treatment Selection
CT, CTA, CT Perfusion, and MR Imaging

Robert W. Regenhardt, MD, PhD[a,1], Christopher A. Potter, MD[b,1,*],
Samuel S. Huang, BS[c], Michael H. Lev, MD[a]

KEYWORDS

- Neuroimaging • MR imaging • Computed tomography • Acute ischemic stroke
- Large vessel occlusion • Intravenous thrombolysis • Endovascular thrombectomy
- Systems of care

KEY POINTS

- The diagnosis and treatment of acute ischemic stroke (AIS) is complex with large differences in systems of care and resources across different geographies.
- Intravenous thrombolysis was introduced in the 1990s and involves the peripheral administration of a tissue plasminogen activator to eliminate thrombus.
- Endovascular thrombectomy was introduced in the 2010s and involves the intra-arterial catheter-based retrieval of thrombus.
- The neuroimaging approach is crucial to diagnose and treat AIS; candidacy for both thrombolysis and thrombectomy hinges on imaging data in addition to clinical data.
- Expanding indications for these treatments is the focus of future ongoing research, much of which revolves around imaging data.

INTRODUCTION

The diagnosis and treatment of acute ischemic stroke (AIS) have been changing rapidly in the last several decades due to advances in treatment technology, imaging development and stroke outreach. In this article, we will review diagnostic imaging, treatment approaches, and stroke emergency medical systems (EMS) systems, focusing on the most recent updates.

AIS is a clinical syndrome caused by arterial occlusion/stenosis and can occur in all age groups but occurs most commonly in adults. The most common causes in adults include atherosclerotic disease and atrial fibrillation, whereas in younger patients, causes such as cardiac and hematologic diseases predominate. The human and financial cost of AIS is large, with stroke-related care costing up to US$53 billion from 2017 to 2018.[1]

Both computed tomography (CT) and MR imaging can achieve the goals of imaging triage for AIS—exclusion of hemorrhage, detection of vessel occlusion, and candidacy for endovascular therapy (EVT)—although each approach has its strengths and weaknesses in the evaluation of early and late window patients.[2,3]

Intravenous thrombolysis for AIS was first approved in the mid 1990s and was revolutionary.

[a] Massachusetts General Hospital, 55 Fruit Street, WAC 7-745, Boston, MA 02114, USA; [b] Brigham and Women's Hospital, 45 Francis Street, Boston, MA 02115, USA; [c] Albany Medical College, 438 Waltham Street, Lexington, MA 02421, USA
[1] The authors contributed equally.
* Corresponding-author.
E-mail address: cpotter3@bwh.harvard.edu
Twitter: @rwregen (R.W.R.)

Radiol Clin N Am 61 (2023) 445–456
https://doi.org/10.1016/j.rcl.2023.01.003
0033-8389/23/© 2023 Elsevier Inc. All rights reserved.

The initial intravenous thrombolysis treatment window of 3 hours was subsequently extended to 4.5 hours in the late 2000s. More recently, diffusion weighted imaging (DWI) and fluid attenuated inversion recovery (FLAIR) mismatch has been introduced as a biomarker for the identification of patients with unknown time of symptom onset that may be safely treated with intravenous thrombolysis.[4,5] In addition, extension of the intravenous treatment time beyond 4.5 hours has been explored in the recent EXTEND trial in patients after up to 9 hours last known well (LKW).[6]

EVT was the second revolutionary step in stroke treatment and continues to rapidly advance. Multiple concurrent studies demonstrated the efficacy of thrombectomy in the anterior circulation in 2015 within 6 hours LKW. This was followed by studies showing efficacy up to 24 hours from LKW in patients selected with advanced imaging such as perfusion imaging or DWI,[7,8] although the need for advanced imaging in this extended window patient group has recently been questioned.[9] Studies and experience have shown that each patient has their own tissue clock that is dependent on the robustness of their collateral flow and other factors. Estimating an individual patient's infarct progression has become a focus in advanced imaging, such as collateral imaging.

This article will review the current guidelines, recent changes, and future directions in diagnosis and treatment of AIS.

IMAGING APPROACH

The goals of imaging triage for AIS are 4-fold: (1) detection of hemorrhage to exclude patients who cannot be safely treated with intravenous thrombolysis, (2) detection of a treatable arterial occlusion, (3) estimation of infarct core volume or tissue that cannot be saved DESPITE reperfusion, and (4) estimation of penumbra, which is tissue at risk that may be salvaged with reperfusion.[2,3,10] In the era on EVT, vascular imaging in AIS is now an established part of imaging triage. Either CT, MR imaging, or a combination of the 2 imaging modalities may be used for AIS triage, depending on local resources and expertise.

Noncontrast Computed Tomography and CTA Head/Neck

Noncontrast CT (NCCT) and computed tomography angiography (CTA) head and neck has the advantage of being widely available, rapid, and free of the safety concerns of MR imaging, with radiation dose the main and relatively minor concern. Intravenous contrast can be safely administered to most patients, with contrast-induced nephropathy

thought to be much less frequent than initially reported.[11,12] NCCT has a high sensitivity and specificity for intracranial hemorrhage. CTA can rapidly characterize the intracranial and cervical vasculature to evaluate for large vessel occlusion and candidacy for EVT. Thick maximum intensity projection (MIP) reconstructions can increase sensitivity for vessel occlusion and can be rapidly performed and made available at the CT console or on picture archiving and communication system (PACS).[10] NCCT is limited for the evaluation of infarct core and penumbra, although recent studies suggest that NCCT and CTA may be sufficient for patient selection in the extended time window[9] because they found similar rates in functional disability in patients selected with advanced imaging (CT and MR perfusion imaging, DWI) versus selection using NCCT and CTA alone.

Computed Tomography Perfusion

CT perfusion imaging (CTP) has become a widely available method for characterizing core infarct volume and penumbra for patient selection in the late treatment window, with the current criteria established by the DAWN and DEFUSE3 trials.[7,8] Following the DAWN and DEFUSE3 trials, cerebral blood flow (CBF) and time to maximum enhancement (Tmax) have become the key reference values for automated estimation of infarct core and penumbra, respectively. However, there is limited reliability of infarct core size on CTP compared with DWI,[13] and CBF and Tmax values can vary depending on the postprocessing algorithm.[14]

Although CTP can be performed rapidly, it is of equivocal benefit in early window patients because the added imaging may increase door to needle time.[11] Because CTP may not be helpful for early window evaluation, many centers currently do not routinely perform CTP in early window candidates. Stroke mimics, such as seizure, may also be visible on CTP and always important to consider on interpretation of CTP data.[10] CTP can also be helpful in identifying small infarcts and distal vessel occlusions in some patients without large vessel occlusion.

Collaterals

It is well established that patients with LVO and robust pial collaterals, known as slow progressors, tend to preserve penumbra longer and infarct core increases less rapidly compared with patients with poor pial collaterals, known as fast progressors.[15,16] These slow progressors are often better candidates for EVT depending on the time from LKW. Collateral imaging can be used to identify a benign or malignant collateral pattern and the likelihood of a favorable core to penumbra ratio for

EVT.[15] CTA can be used to evaluate collateral flow to estimate the penumbral size for EVT candidacy.[11] Whether multiphase or single phase imaging is superior has not yet been established. Collateral status has also been assessed using MR angiography and CT or MR imaging perfusion.

MR Imaging

MR imaging has strengths and weaknesses compared with CT in AIS imaging triage. Image acquisition is longer than CT, safety screening is necessary before imaging, and patient preparation and transportation can potentially increase door to needle time. Because of these obstacles, MR imaging should be used where comparable door to needle times with CT can be achieved using rapid MR imaging protocols, and efficient screening and workflow. The availability of MR imaging is another drawback because many institutions do not have 24-hour MR imaging access.

The main advantage of MR imaging is the accuracy of DWI in the determination of core infarct volume; indeed, MR imaging is the imaging standard. Although DWI can slightly overestimate the core infarct volume in patients who have been successfully reperfused, this tends to be less than 10% of the total core volume and during the early time window.[2,17] For patients transferred to a comprehensive stroke center with LVO identified on recent NCCT/CTA imaging at a spoke hospital, it is reasonable to forego repeat imaging on arrival with the exception of DWI or CTP for extended window patients.[2,18,19] Because the eligibility criteria of the early trials demonstrating the efficacy of EVT were necessarily restrictive, more inclusive criteria are being studied, particularly in groups with lower NIHSS scores and those with larger infarct core volumes. This demands accurate assessment of infarct core and penumbra. Improving infarct core volume measurement using DWI can potentially expand treatment criteria.

In addition to utility in EVT selection, the DWI-FLAIR mismatch imaging biomarker has been recently shown to reliably identify patients with unknown LKW, such as wake up strokes, who can be safely treated with intravenous thrombolysis by identifying low diffusivity on DWI without corresponding elevated FLAIR signal[4,5] (Fig. 1). The Massachusetts General Hospital (MGH) imaging triage strategy has evolved over time to encompass the latest changes in imaging and therapy and reflects local resources (Fig. 2).

INTRAVENOUS THROMBOLYSIS

IVT involves the peripheral intravenous administration of a tissue plasminogen activator, such as alteplase or tenecteplase. There are several criteria for treatment selection, based largely on inclusion and exclusion criteria for the trials demonstrating the efficacy of IVT.[20,21] IVT should be considered for all patients aged 18 years and older who are diagnosed with likely AIS causing a measurable neurologic deficit after undergoing noncontrast head CT that shows neither hemorrhage nor significant established infarct. Earlier IVT was only considered within 4.5 hours from LKW.[21] However, if certain imaging criteria are met, it can be considered outside of this window.[6,22]

There are several contraindications for IVT[20,21]: significant head trauma or earlier stroke within 3 months, arterial puncture at a noncompressible site within 7 days, history of intracranial hemorrhage, malignant intracranial tumor, arteriovenous malformation, large aneurysm, recent cranial or spinal surgery, elevated blood pressure (>185/110 mm Hg; treatable before administration), blood glucose less than 50 mg/dL (treatable before administration), active internal hemorrhage, platelets less than 100k, anticoagulation within 48 hours (heparin and aPTT > upper limit of normal, warfarin and INR > 1.7, NOAC), and other active bleeding diatheses. Although not absolute contraindications, there are several other situations where the risks versus benefits should be carefully weighed.[21]

The time from LKW is an important factor when evaluating a patient's candidacy for IVT. Initially, the early time window was considered within 3 hours, and the late between 3 to 4.5 hours. These windows were derived from the clinical trials that demonstrated the efficacy and safety of IVT.[20,21] However, recent evidence aims to redefine "late" as beyond 4.5 hours from LKW. Indeed, through advanced imaging we are transitioning from a time-based assessment to a tissue-based assessment of IVT treatment candidacy.[6,22] Importantly, there is a difference in outcomes when patients are selected for reperfusion based on tissue viability rather than the time from onset of stroke.[6] The EXTEND trial showed that patients with favorable perfusion imaging stand to benefit from IVT between 4.5 and 9 hours after stroke onset or awakening with stroke symptoms.[6] In addition, the WAKEUP and WITNESS trials showed that patients with reduced FLAIR hyperintensity in DWI-defined lesions, that is, DWI-FLAIR mismatch, stand to benefit from IVT without higher hemorrhage risks when the stroke onset time is unknown.[4,5,23]

In addition to alteplase, tenecteplase is another form of IVT that is gaining in popularity because it offers several advantages. Evidence supports that tenecteplase is more effective at achieving recanalization and has been associated with improved

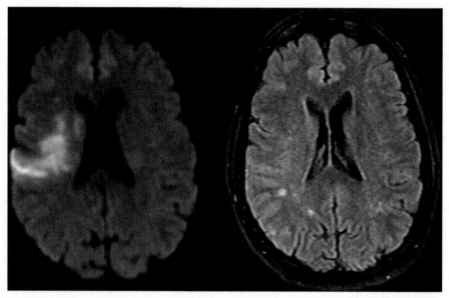

Fig. 1. DWI-FLAIR mismatch: A 60-year-old woman with chronic obstructive pulmonary disease (COPD) and remote right carotid endarterectomy (CEA) presented with left sided weakness and NIHSS 11. She was LKW 17 hours and 30 min before presentation. Given this late window, an MR imaging was performed revealing a 40-mL infarct core on DWI with nondetectable FLAIR hyperintensity, suggesting that (1) IV-tPA was appropriate based on the WAKE-UP trial results, and that (2) endovascular thrombectomy was appropriate based on the DAWN trial results (DWI core volume <50 mL). In this case, thrombectomy was performed; the patient had mRS 2 at 90 days.

outcomes.[24] For severe stroke, data support the lower dose of 0.25 mg/kg is safer than higher doses.[25] This has led to 0.25 mg/kg becoming the most common dose used in clinical practice because it leads to improved long-term outcomes without additional hemorrhage risks.[24] Furthermore, it can be administered as an intravenous push injection and does not require a drip. This allows for faster administration and makes the transfer and transport of patients more straightforward. Tenecteplase 0.25 mg/kg has even shown promise when administered in mobile stroke units.[26] Currently, the TIMELESS trial is testing the utility of tenecteplase between 4.5 and 24 hours in patients with LVO.

Imaging has substantially improved our ability to estimate the long-term efficacy and risks after treatment with IVT. For example, clot burden is an important marker that predicts recanalization after IVT. Furthermore, leptomeningeal collaterals help predict who is likely to benefit and who may have additional risks. Indeed, different imaging modalities have contributed substantially to outcome prognostication, and new approaches are being used in different time windows.

ENDOVASCULAR THROMBECTOMY

EVT involves intra-arterial mechanical thrombus retrieval through either transfemoral, transradial, or direct carotid access.[27] Catheters are used to navigate to the site of occlusion under fluoroscopic guidance. Options for thrombus retrieval include aspiration alone, the use of a stent retriever, or a combination of techniques.[28] There are several criteria for treatment selection; similar to IVT, criteria are based largely on inclusion and exclusion criteria for the trials that demonstrated efficacy and safety.[27] Importantly, these criteria are evolving, and they continue to be challenged. Initially, EVT was limited to those patients presenting within 6 hours from LKW.[27] However, there is now overwhelming evidence supporting treatment of patients who present within 24 hours from LKW, particularly if there is a small DWI core or substantial mismatch on CTP.[7,8] There is proven benefit for patients meeting the following criteria: age 18 to 90 years, baseline modified Rankin Score (mRS) 2 or less, life expectancy greater than 12 months, NIHSS 6 or greater, occlusion of the intracranial internal carotid artery (ICA) or middle cerebral artery (MCA) M1 division, ASPECTS 7 or greater, DWI core 70 cc or less, and nonmalignant collateral pattern. There is potential benefit for patients meeting the following criteria: NIHSS 4 or greater; age greater than 90 years; mRS 3 or less; adequate life expectancy; basilar occlusion with 70% or less infarction of the pons, midbrain, thalamus; M2 occlusion; ASPECTS 3 or greater; and DWI core 120 cc or less. Indeed, the

MGH Acute Stroke Imaging Algorithm 2021

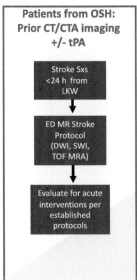

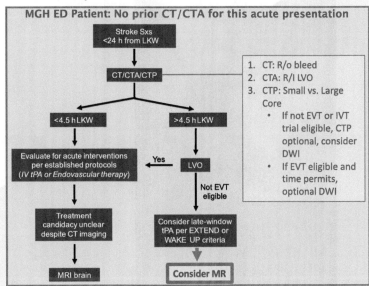

Fig. 2. The current MGH acute stroke imaging triage algorithm reflects the latest advances in imaging and treatment, as well as the optimal use of local resources and system of care. (*Courtesy of* R Gupta, MD PhD, Boston, MA.)

ASPECTS threshold is currently undergoing much study.[29] Finally, there is unlikely benefit for patients with the following: nondisabling stroke symptoms; more than 24 hours from LKW; mRS of 4 or greater; limited life expectancy; distal occlusions (M3, M4, anterior cerebral artery (ACA), posterior cerebral artery (PCA)), especially those not associated with disabling symptoms; basilar occlusion with greater than 70% infarction of the pons, midbrain, thalamus; ASPECTS less than 3; malignant collateral pattern; and DWI greater than 120 cc (**Fig. 3**).

Because the EVT trials were designed differently for patients presenting with LKW less than 6 hours versus those with LKW 6 to 24 hours, there are important imaging and clinical considerations for both groups of patients. The first trials excluded patients with LKW greater than 6 hours to select for patients most likely to benefit in order to prove the efficacy of EVT.[27] Indeed, data support there are differences in outcomes comparing patients who present in these time windows.[30] There are also differences in outcomes comparing different imaging modalities for patient selection.[9,13,31] It is important to note that there are several biomarkers, particularly in neuroimaging, which enhance our ability to predict outcomes and have implications

for patient selection.[18] For example, collateral patterns have been associated with both infarct growth and long-term outcomes.[32] There are also growing data supporting the importance of infarct topography, perhaps more important than the overall total volume.[33] One study emphasized the importance of white matter infarct volume as a key determinant for long-term outcome after EVT.[34] Although advanced imaging yields more data, some advocate for keeping imaging fast and simple. A recent study supports that when used for patient selection for EVT, an NCCT may be all that is needed even in the extended window.[35–37] However, at centers with resources, such as the ability to perform CTP and MR imaging quickly, a patient-centered approach also offers advantages.[31]

In the early window, there is substantial benefit from EVT across a wide range of clinical subgroups.[38,39] Indeed, 90-day outcomes are dramatically improved after EVT compared with medical management; EVT has among the lowest number needed to treat (NNT) in modern medicine.[6] As such, the role of IVT for patients who ultimately undergo EVT has recently been questioned.[40] After several recent trials, guidelines still advocate for the administration of IVT for all eligible patients.[41]

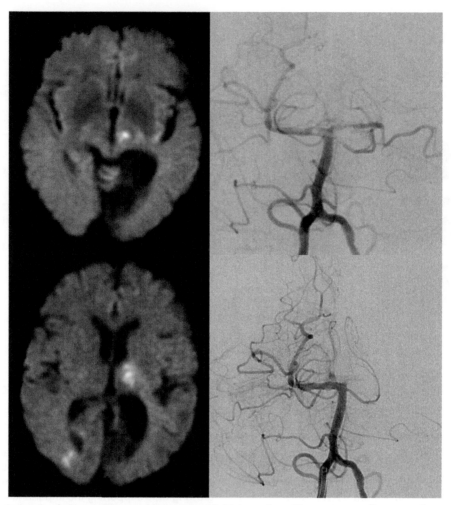

Fig. 3. Posterior circulation: A 62-year-old woman with history of smoking, coronary disease, and a remote PCA stroke who presented with right-sided weakness, CTA revealed left M2 occlusion, which migrated to a distal M4 segment at the time of angiography, so thrombectomy was not performed. The following morning, she was drowsy so a repeat head CT/CTA was obtained, which identified a basilar tip thrombus. MR imaging was without extensive brainstem infarction, so a decision was made to proceed with thrombectomy. The basilar tip was cleared of thrombus for a thrombolysis in cerebral infarction (TICI) 2b result, although there was persistent left P1 thrombus despite multiple passes. Unfortunately, the patient did not significantly improve, given multiple infarcts in both the anterior and posterior circulations.

Perhaps, not surprisingly, bypassing IVT was associated with a lower percentage of successful reperfusion before EVT.[40] This is an especially important point for patients who require transfer from a hospital that can administer IVT but not offer EVT.[42,43] As discussed above, a shorter time to EVT is significantly associated with better outcomes.[30] This likely relates to the prevention of infarct growth and preservation of ischemic penumbra.[44] Interestingly, there is substantial variability of DWI reversal in the early window, especially between 1 and 3 hours. However, the volume that undergoes DWI reversal is no more than 10% the total volume beyond 0.5 hours.[2,17]

The late window encompasses an active area of ongoing study to determine the ideal imaging and clinical assessments for patient treatment selection and optimizing 90-day outcomes. Indeed, there is much debate about the appropriate imaging triage approach.[9] Advanced imaging was used in both the late window trials.[7,8] The DAWN trial enrolled patients with LKW 6 to 24 hours before EVT; it required patients have a mismatch between the severity of the clinical deficit and the infarct volume for inclusion. Patients were divided into 3 groups: group A had patients aged 80 years and older, NIHSS 10 or greater, and infarct volume less than 21 cc; group B had patients aged younger

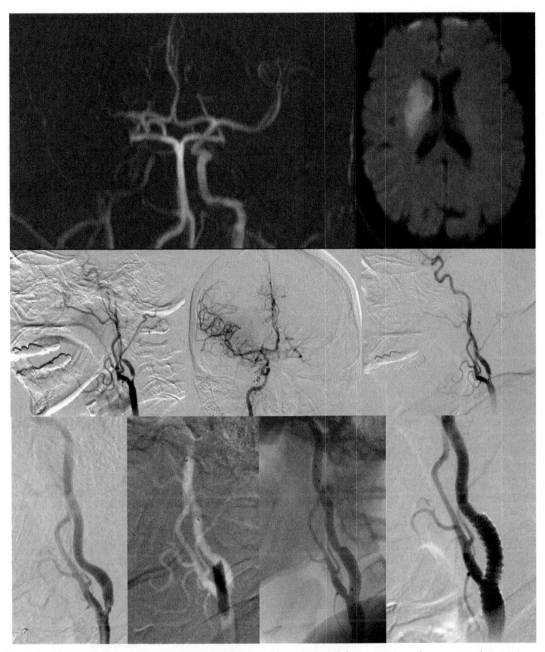

Fig. 4. Tandem lesions in a transfer patient: A 58-year-old woman with hypertension who presented to a primary stroke center community hospital with left-sided weakness and NIHSS score 15. CT revealed an ASPECTS of 10; CTA showed tandem lesions, critical stenosis of the right cervical ICA and occlusion of the M1. She was evaluated by Telestroke assessment and administered intravenous alteplase. She was then transferred to the tertiary comprehensive stroke center for thrombectomy. Transfer was delayed, and she arrived 6 hours from her LKW. MR imaging showed persistent right M1 occlusion, limited filling of the ICA, and <50 mL infarct core. Thrombectomy was performed by first navigating the cervical lesion and advancing a guide catheter into the ICA. Intracranially, the M1 thrombus was retrieved for a TICI 3 result after a single pass. Reevaluation of the cervical lesion showed moderate stenosis. She underwent carotid artery stenting 4 weeks later.

than 80 years, NIHSS 10 or greater, and infarct volume less than 31 cc; and group C had patients aged younger than 80 years, NIHSS 20 or greater, and infarct volume 31 to 50 cc. Infarct volume could be assessed by DWI or CTP. There was a robust treatment effect using this approach.[7] Similarly, the DEFUSE 3 trial enrolled patients with LKW 6 to 16 hours before EVT. However, patient selection was determined by a ratio of penumbra to infarct core as determined by perfusion imaging (CT or MR imaging-based). Patients were eligible if they had an infarct volume of less than 70 cc, a penumbra to infarct core ratio of 1.8 or greater, and an absolute penumbra volume of 15 cc or greater. DEFUSE 3 also demonstrated a dramatic treatment effect, with a favorable shift in 90-day mRS compared with medical management.[8]

SYSTEMS OF CARE

The regional system of stroke care is a critical component in diagnosis and timely treatment, as emphasized in the 2019 updated American Heart Association (AHA) guidelines.[11] Important considerations are regional differences in geography, infrastructure, and resources. Generally, there are 3 system models for acute stroke care, which have relevance for patients with LVO: "drip-and-ship," "mothership," and "trip-and-treat."[45] For many regions, it is not feasible to offer EVT at all hospitals. Therefore, hospitals are categorized as "spoke" primary stroke hospitals if they offer IVT without EVT and "hub" comprehensive stroke hospitals if they offer both. Often through Telestroke assessment, patients first presenting to spokes can be evaluated virtually.[38] They can also undergo simple and cost-effective imaging with CT and CTA to allow the rapid exclusion of hemorrhage, identification of LVO, and assessment of collaterals, thereby increasing the efficiency of patients transferred.[39,46,47] Many patients treated with IVT will also benefit from EVT, as in the drip-and-ship

model.[46] Available evidence suggests there are significant benefits to administering IVT a transfer for EVT.[42,43,46] In certain circumstances, the hub ED can be bypassed and patients can present directly to the angio-suite[19] (**Fig. 4**). In contrast, the "mothership" system model offers other advantages, especially in densely populated urban regions.[45] For patients likely to have LVO, they may benefit from direct presentation to a hub comprehensive center, even if it means bypassing a closer spoke hospital that does not offer EVT. Many regions use abbreviated neurologic clinical examinations that first responders can implement in field, such as the Los Angeles Motor Scale.[48] Ongoing research is evaluating the use of in-field portable devices to aid in LVO diagnosis.[49] Another example, while costly for some regions, is a mobile stroke unit, which contains a smaller CT within the ambulance.[50] Finally, the trip-and-treat model is typically limited to only geographies with the densest populations, such as New York City. Under this model, the hub's neurointerventional team is "transferred" to the patient rather than the traditional patient transfer approach.

FUTURE DIRECTIONS

Alteplase has been the standard of care for AIS regardless of the occlusion site for patients who present with a disabling deficit. Recently, there are increasing data supporting the use of tenecteplase as discussed above. An active area of ongoing research is the use of tenecteplase in the extended window beyond 4.5 hours.[51] As

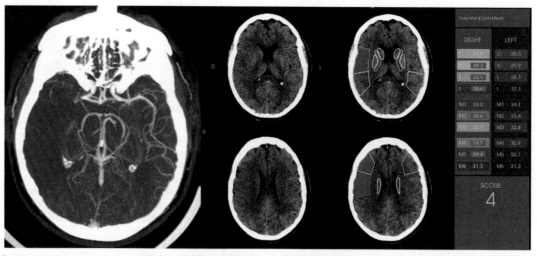

Fig. 5. Large core: A 61-year-old man with hypertension and hyperlipidemia who presented with left-sided weakness and NIHSS 19. He was LKW 2 hours and 10 minutes prior. CT head showed an ASPECTS of 4, suggesting he was a "fast progressor." Given his young age and presentation in the early window, a decision was made to proceed with thrombectomy. A TICI 3 result was achieved. His NIHSS score improved to 5 at discharge.

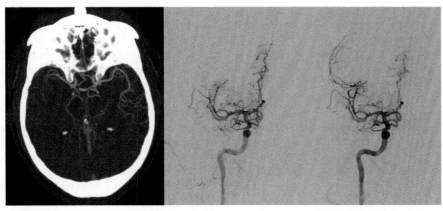

Fig. 6. Distal occlusion: A 50-year-old man without relevant medical history who presented with left-sided weakness and NIHSS 15. He was LKW 5 hours and 50 minutes prior. CT head showed an ASPECTS of 10 and CTA head revealed a right distal M2 occlusion. A decision was made to proceed with thrombectomy given his high NIHSS score, despite the distal location. TICI 2c was achieved, and his NIHSS improved to 1 at discharge.

EVT evolves, certain patients with less severe stroke symptoms (NIHSS <6) and large infarcts (>100 mL or ASPECTS <6) may also be shown to benefit from treatment (**Fig. 5**). For the low NIHSS population, there are mixed data with some studies questioning efficacy[52] while others suggest a treatment effect.[53] Ongoing randomized data are forthcoming with the ENDOLOW and MOSTE trials.[54] In addition to the already published RESCUE-Japan LIMIT study[29], there are several ongoing randomized trials for EVT with large infarcts, including TENSION, LASTE, TESLA, SELECT 2, and ANGEL-ASPECT.[55] Furthermore, more distal occlusions beyond the ICA and M1 are being treated[56] (**Fig. 6**). Finally, the AHA guidelines currently apply only to the anterior circulation. Recent trials comparing basilar artery thrombectomy with medical management alone have been mixed, with the BEST, BASICS, and BAOCHE trials demonstrating mixed results.[57–62]

SUMMARY

AIS diagnosis and treatment is rapidly evolving. NCCT and CTA remain the mainstays of AIS imaging and critical to a hub and spoke system, allowing for rapid diagnosis and accurate disposition, which can decrease treatment times and improve patient outcomes. MR imaging times can be comparable to CT and MR imaging provides accurate infarct core volume assessment, which may improve patient selection criteria for EVT and expand the thrombolysis treatment time for patients with unknown LKW. Collateral imaging can help distinguish between fast and slow progressors as an alternative to perfusion imaging, which may improve patient outcomes.

CLINICS CARE POINTS

- The diagnosis and treatment of acute ischemic stroke is complex, partly due to local differences in care and resources, leading to different regional strategies.

- Neuroimaging is a critical step in the diagnosis and treatment of acute ischemic stroke, although the optimal imaging strategy varies by region and system of care.

- Intravenous and endovascular thrombolysis are effective treatment strategies and current trials aim to expand treatment selection criteria.

DISCLOSURES

R.W. Regenhardt: Rapid Medical–DSMB; Microvention–Site PI; Penumbra–Site PI; NINDS–Grant; SVIN–Grant; Heitman Foundation–Grant C.A. Potter: None; S.S. Huang: None; M.H. Lev: Consultant GE Healthcare, Consultant Takeda/Roche-Genentech/Seagen Pharm.

REFERENCES

1. Tsao CW, Aday AW, Almarzooq ZI, et al. Heart disease and stroke statistics-2022 update: a report from the american heart association. Circulation 2022;145(8):e153–639.
2. Leslie-Mazwi TM, Lev MH, Schaefer PW, et al. MR imaging selection of acute stroke patients with emergent large vessel occlusions for thrombectomy. Neuroimaging Clin 2018;28(4):573–84.

3. Kamalian S, Lev MH. The adult patient with acute neurologic deficit: an update on imaging trends. Neuroimaging Clin 2018;28(3):319–34.

4. Thomalla G, Simonsen CZ, Boutitie F, et al. MRI-guided thrombolysis for stroke with unknown time of onset. N Engl J Med 2018;397(7):611–22.

5. Schwamm LH, Wu O, Song SS, et al. Intravenous thrombolysis in unwitnessed stroke onset: MR WITNESS trial results. Ann Neurol 2018;83(5):980–93.

6. Ma H, Campbell BCV, Parsons MW, et al. Thrombolysis Guided by Perfusion Imaging up to 9 hours after onset of stroke. N Engl J Med 2019;380(19): 1795–803.

7. Nogueira RG, Jadhav AP, Haussen DC, et al. Thrombectomy 6 to 24 hours after stroke with a mismatch between deficit and infarct. N Engl J Med 2018; 378(1):11–99.

8. Albers GW, Marks MP, Kemp S, et al. Thrombectomy for stroke at 6 to 16 hours with selection by perfusion imaging. N Engl J Med 2018;378(8):708–18.

9. Nogueira RG, Haussen DC, Liebeskind D, et al. Stroke imaging selection modality and endovascular therapy outcomes in the early and extended time windows. Stroke 2021;52(2):491–7, 00392499.

10. Potter CA, Vagal AS, Goyal M, et al. CT for treatment selection in acute ischemic stroke: a code stroke primer. Radiographics 2019;39(6):1717–38.

11. Powers WJ, Rabinstein AA, Ackerson T, et al. Guidelines for the early management of patients with acute ischemic stroke: 2019 update to the 2018 guidelines for the early management of acute ischemic stroke: a guideline for healthcare professionals from the american heart association/american stroke association. Stroke 2019;50(12):e344–418. published correction appears in Stroke. 2019 Dec;50(12): e440-e441.

12. Dittrich R, Akdeniz S, Kloska SP, et al. Low rate of contrast-induced Nephropathy after CT perfusion and CT angiography in acute stroke patients. J Neurol 2007;254(11):1491–7.

13. Schaefer PW, Souza L, Kamalian S, et al. Limited reliability of computed tomographic perfusion acute infarct volume measurements compared with diffusion-weighted imaging in anterior circulation stroke. Stroke 2015;46(2):419–24, 00392499.

14. Kudo K, Sasaki M, Yamada K, et al. Differences in CT perfusion maps generated by different commercial software: quantitative analysis by using identical source data of acute stroke patients. Radiology 2010;254(1):200–9.

15. Souza LC, Yoo AJ, Chaudhry ZA, et al. Malignant CTA collateral profile is highly specific for large admission DWI infarct core and poor outcome in acute stroke. AJNR Am J Neuroradiol 2012;33(7): 1331–6.

16. Tong E, Patrie J, Tong S, et al. Time-resolved CT assessment of collaterals as imaging biomarkers to predict clinical outcomes in acute ischemic stroke. Neuroradiology 2017;59(11):1101–9.

17. Schaefer PW, Hassankhani A, Putman C, et al. Characterization and evolution of diffusion MR imaging abnormalities in stroke patients undergoing intra-arterial thrombolysis. AJNR Am J Neuroradiol 2004;25(6):951–7.

18. Campbell BCV, Majoie CBLM, Albers GW, et al. Penumbral imaging and functional outcome in patients with anterior circulation ischaemic stroke treated with endovascular thrombectomy versus medical therapy: a meta-analysis of individual patient-level data. Lancet Neurol 2019;18(1):46–55.

19. Regenhardt RW, Rosenthal JA, Dmytriw AA, et al. Direct to angio-suite large vessel occlusion stroke transfers achieve faster arrival-to-puncture times and improved outcomes. Stroke: Vascular and Interventional Neurology 2022;0:e000327.

20. National Institute of Neurological Disorders and Stroke rt-PA Stroke Study Group. Tissue plasminogen activator for acute ischemic stroke. N Engl J Med 1995;333(24):1581–7.

21. Hacke W, Kaste M, Bluhmki E, et al. Thrombolysis with alteplase 3 to 4.5 hours after acute ischemic stroke. N Engl J Med 2008 Sep 25;359(13):1317–29.

22. Marshall RS. Image-Guided intravenous alteplase for stroke - shattering a time window. N Engl J Med 2019;380(19):1865–6.

23. Regenhardt RW, Bretzner M, Zanon Zotin MC, et al. Radiomic signature of DWI-FLAIR mismatch in large vessel occlusion stroke. J Neuroimaging 2022;32(1): 63–7.

24. Parsons M, Spratt N, Bivard A, et al. A randomized trial of tenecteplase versus alteplase for acute ischemic stroke. N Engl J Med 2012;366(12): 1099–107.

25. Kvistad CE, Næss H, Helleberg BH, et al. Tenecteplase versus alteplase for the management of acute ischaemic stroke in Norway (NOR-TEST 2, part A): a phase 3, randomised, open-label, blinded endpoint, non-inferiority trial. Lancet Neurol 2022;21(6):511–9.

26. Bivard A, Zhao H, Churilov L, et al. Comparison of tenecteplase with alteplase for the early treatment of ischaemic stroke in the Melbourne Mobile Stroke Unit (TASTE-A): a phase 2, randomised, open-label trial. Lancet Neurol 2022;21(6):520–7.

27. Goyal M, Menon BK, van Zwam WH, et al. Endovascular thrombectomy after large-vessel ischaemic stroke: a meta-analysis of individual patient data from five randomised trials. Lancet 2016;387(10029):1723–31.

28. Turk AS 3rd, Siddiqui A, Fifi JT, et al. Aspiration thrombectomy versus stent retriever thrombectomy as first-line approach for large vessel occlusion (COMPASS): a multicentre, randomised, open label, blinded outcome, non-inferiority trial. Lancet 2019; 393(10175):998–1008.

29. Yoshimura S, Sakai N, Yamagami H, et al. Endovascular Therapy for Acute Stroke with a Large Ischemic Region. N Engl J Med 2022;386(14):1303–13.

30. Jahan R, Saver JL, Schwamm LH, et al. Association between time to treatment with endovascular reperfusion therapy and outcomes in patients with acute ischemic stroke treated in clinical practice. JAMA 2019;322(3):252–63.

31. Leslie-Mazwi TM, Hirsch JA, Falcone GJ, et al. Endovascular stroke treatment outcomes after patient selection based on magnetic resonance imaging and clinical criteria. JAMA Neurol 2016;73(1):43–9.

32. Regenhardt RW, González RG, He J, et al. Symmetric CTA collaterals identify patients with slow-progressing stroke likely to benefit from late thrombectomy. Radiology 2022;302(2):400–7.

33. Regenhardt RW, Bonkhoff AK, Bretzner M, et al. Association of infarct topography and outcome after endovascular thrombectomy in patients with acute ischemic stroke. Neurology 2022;98(11):e1094–103.

34. Regenhardt RW, Etherton MR, Das AS, et al. White matter acute infarct volume after thrombectomy for anterior circulation large vessel occlusion stroke is associated with long term outcomes. J Stroke Cerebrovasc Dis 2021;30(3):e153–639.

35. Nguyen TN, Abdalkader M, Nagel S, et al. Noncontrast computed tomography vs computed tomography perfusion or magnetic resonance imaging selection in late presentation of stroke with large-vessel occlusion. JAMA Neurol 2022;79(1):22–31.

36. Román LS, Menon BK, Blasco J, et al. Imaging features and safety and efficacy of endovascular stroke treatment: a meta-analysis of individual patient-level data. Lancet Neurol 2018;17(10):895–904.

37. Regenhardt RW, Young MJ, Etherton MR, et al. Toward a more inclusive paradigm: thrombectomy for stroke patients with pre-existing disabilities. J Neurointerventional Surg 2021;13(10):865–8.

38. Akbik F, Hirsch JA, Chandra RV, et al. Telestroke-the promise and the challenge. Part one: growth and current practice. J Neurointerv Surg 2017;9(4):357–60.

39. Yu AT, Regenhardt RW, Whitney C, et al. CTA protocols in a telestroke network improve efficiency for both spoke and hub hospitals. AJNR American journal of neuroradiology 2021;42(3):435–40.

40. Yang P, Zhang Y, Zhang L, et al. Endovascular Thrombectomy with or without Intravenous Alteplase in Acute Stroke. N Engl J Med 2020;382(21):1981–93.

41. Masoud HE, Havenon A, Castonguay AC, et al. 2022 brief practice update on intravenous thrombolysis before thrombectomy in patients with large vessel occlusion acute ischemic stroke: a statement from society of vascular and interventional neurology guidelines and practice standards (gaps)

42. Kraft AW, Awad A, Rosenthal JA, et al. In a hub-and-spoke network, spoke-administered thrombolysis reduces mechanical thrombectomy procedure time and number of passes. Intervent Neuroradiol 2022 [Epub ahead of print]. 15910199221087498.

43. Regenhardt RW, Rosenthal JA, Awad A, et al. Drip-and-ship' intravenous thrombolysis and outcomes for large vessel occlusion thrombectomy candidates in a hub-and-spoke telestroke model. J Neurointerv Surg 2022;14(7):650–3.

44. Regenhardt RW, Das AS, Stapleton CJ, et al. Blood pressure and penumbral sustenance in stroke from large vessel occlusion. Front Neurol 2017;8:317.

45. Romoli M, Paciaroni M, Tsivgoulis G, et al. Mothership versus drip-and-ship model for mechanical thrombectomy in acute stroke: a systematic review and meta-analysis for clinical and radiological outcomes. J Stroke 2020;22(3):317–23.

46. Regenhardt RW, Awad A, Kraft AW, et al. Characterizing Reasons for Stroke Thrombectomy Ineligibility Among Potential Candidates Transferred in a Hub-and-Spoke Network. Stroke: Vascular and Interventional Radiology 2022;e000282.

47. Mitchell PJ, Yan B, Churilov L, et al. Endovascular thrombectomy versus standard bridging thrombolytic with endovascular thrombectomy within 4·5 h of stroke onset: an open-label, blinded-endpoint, randomised non-inferiority trial. Lancet 2022;400(10346):116–25.

48. Behnke S, Schlechtriemen T, Binder A, et al. Effects of state-wide implementation of the Los Angeles Motor Scale for triage of stroke patients in clinical practice. Neurological Research and Practice 2021;3(1):1–8.

49. Chennareddy S, Kalagara R, Smith C, et al. Portable stroke detection devices: a systematic scoping review of prehospital applications. BMC Emerg Med 2022;22(1):111.

50. Grotta JC, Yamal JM, Parker SA, et al. Prospective, Multicenter, Controlled Trial of Mobile Stroke Units. N Engl J Med 2021;385(11):971–81.

51. Campbell B. and Parsons M. Extending the time window for tenecteplase by effective reperfusion in patients with large vessel occlusion (ETERNAL-LVO). ClinicalTrials.gov [Internet], Available at: https://clinicaltrials.gov/ct2/show/NCT04454788. Accessed Auguest 30, 2022.

52. Volny O, Zerna C, Tomek A, et al. Thrombectomy vs medical management in low NIHSS acute anterior circulation stroke. Neurology 2020;95:e3364–72.

53. Nagel S, Bouslama M, Krause LU, et al. Mechanical thrombectomy in patients with milder strokes and large vessel occlusions. Stroke 2018;49:2391–7.

54. McCarthy DJ, Tonetti DA. Stone J et al. More expansive horizons: a review of endovascular therapy for

committee. Stroke: Vascular and Interventional Neurology 2022;2:e000276.

patients with low NIHSS scores. J Neurointerv Surg 2021;13:146–51.

55. Jadhav AP, Hacke W, Dippel DWJ, et al. Select wisely: the ethical challenge of defining large core with perfusion in the early time window. J Neurointerv Surg 2021;13:497–9.

56. Renieri L, Valente I, Dmytriw AA, et al. Mechanical thrombectomy beyond the circle of Willis: efficacy and safety of different techniques for M2 occlusions. J Neurointerv Surg 2022;14(6):546–50.

57. Ahmed RA, Dmytriw AA, Patel AB, et al. Basilar artery occlusion: a review of clinicoradiologic features, treatment selection, and endovascular techniques. Intervent Neuroradiol 2022 [Epub ahead of print]. 15910199221106048.

58. Leslie-Mazwi TM. Invited commentary on "imaging-based selection for endovascular treatment in stroke. Radiographics 2019;39(6):1714–6.

59. Wu X, Hughes DR, Gandhi D, et al. CT angiography for triage of patients with acute minor stroke: a cost-effectiveness analysis. Radiology 2020;294(3):580–8.

60. Alawieh A, Starke RM, Rano Chatterjee A, et al. Outcomes of endovascular thrombectomy in the elderly: a "real-world" multicenter study. J Neurointerventional Surg 2019;11(6):545–53.

61. Regenhardt RW, Nolan NM, Rosenthal JA, et al. Understanding delays in MRI-based selection of large vessel occlusion stroke patients for endovascular thrombectomy, Clin Neuroradiol, 2022. [Epub ahead of print].

62. Nolan NM, Regenhardt RW, Koch MJ, et al. Treatment Approaches and Outcomes for Acute Anterior Circulation Stroke Patients with Tandem Lesions. J Stroke Cerebrovasc Dis 2021;30(2):e153–639.

Modern Imaging of Aneurysmal Subarachnoid Hemorrhage

Simon Levinson, MD[a], Arjun V. Pendharkar, MD[a],
Andrew J. Gauden, MD, PhD[a], Jeremy J. Heit, MD, PhD[b,c],*

KEYWORDS

• Aneurysm • Hemorrhage • Imaging • Brain • CT • AI

KEY POINTS

- Non-contrast head computed tomography (CT) should be ordered in any patient who presents to the emergency department with sudden onset of "thunderclap headache" and/or headache with new neurologic deficits as it is an excellent screening tool for subarachnoid hemorrhage (SAH).
- Computed tomography angiography (CTA) has excellent sensitivity for detecting aneurysms>3 mm in size. For smaller aneurysms or CTA-negative SAH, diagnostic cerebral angiography is often necessary.
- Vasospasm and delayed cerebral ischemia are distinct pathologies; delayed cerebral ischemia contributes approximately 50% of the morbidity of SAH.
- Transcranial Doppler and CT perfusion can detect vasospasm and cerebral ischemia; vasospasm can be intervened on in the neuroendovascular suite with balloon angioplasty or transarterial vasodilator infusion.
- Advancements in the field including artificial intelligence for aneurysm detection and using MR imaging and PET to predict outcomes in SAH will likely improve patient outcomes by increasing diagnostic accuracy and optimizing critical care.

INTRODUCTION

Subarachnoid hemorrhage (SAH) is a life-threatening condition that requires prompt diagnosis and treatment. SAH is most often caused by intracranial aneurysm rupture, which subsequently leads to blood, under high pressure, entering the subarachnoid space. This hemorrhage results in a series of events that can lead to serious neurologic injury including hydrocephalus, vasospasm, and delayed cerebral ischemia (DCI). Aneurysmal SAH has an approximately 35% 30-day mortality rate, and many of those who do survive have permanent neurologic deficits. Although the incidence of SAH in the United States has not changed in the past 30 years (9/100,000 per year), patient outcomes have significantly improved, which likely reflects advances in prompt diagnosis and medical treatment.

Neuroimaging plays a central role in the diagnosis and subsequent management of SAH. In this review, we examine the recent advances in how SAH and its neurologic sequelae are diagnosed and managed using a combination of

Cerebrovascular Disease issue of Radiologic Clinics 2022.
[a] Department of Neurosurgery, Stanford University School of Medicine, Stanford, CA, USA; [b] Department of Radiology, Stanford University School of Medicine, Stanford, CA, USA; [c] Stanford School of Medicine, 453 Quarry Road, Palo Alto, CA 94304, USA
* Corresponding author. Department of Radiology, Stanford School of Medicine, 453 Quarry Road, Palo Alto, CA 94304.
E-mail address: jheit@stanford.edu
Twitter: @JeremyHeitMDPHD (J.J.H.)

radiologic.theclinics.com

imaging modalities. We focus on computed tomography (CT), MR, and diagnostic cerebral angiography (DSA) in our review.

INITIAL PRESENTATION AND DIAGNOSIS OF SUBARACHNOID HEMORRHAGE

The initial diagnostic study of choice is a non-contrast CT (NCCT) of the head. NCCT is widely available in emergency departments and can be performed rapidly. In addition, it has excellent sensitivity and specificity for SAH (Fig. 1A, B). In a multicenter prospective cohort study of more than 3000 patients who reported the worst headache of their lives, NCCT scan was 93% sensitive for SAH. For the 953 patients who were scanned within 6 h of headache onset, NCCT was successful in identifying all 121 patients with SAH, with a sensitivity and specificity of 100%.[1] Several other studies have confirmed this excellent sensitivity.[2,3]

It can be challenging to rule out SAH, especially in patients who have a delayed presentation or small-volume hemorrhage. In general, three approaches have been validated to rule out SAH (Fig. 2). The classic, though most invasive, is NCCT plus lumbar puncture (LP) to evaluate for xanthochromia.[4] This approach is appropriate in patients with a high pretest probability of SAH but negative or ambiguous NCCT.[4,5] However, with continued advances in CT detectors, many centers consider the LP unnecessary. In a single-center retrospective study of 85 consecutive patients with headache and no neurologic deficit who underwent NCCT and then subsequently underwent LP, there were no instances of LP-positive patients subsequently found to have true aneurysmal SAH.[5]

An alternative approach to LP is the combination of NCCT followed by CTA head to assess for cerebral aneurysm. CTA is approximately 93% sensitive for the detection of an aneurysm>3 mm.[6,7] However, small but symptomatic aneurysms may be under-detected, CTA requires iodinated contrast administration that has the potential for allergic reactions and nephrotoxicity, and it requires additional radiation.

A third approach uses MR imaging and Magnetic Resonance Angiography (MRA). This approach is particularly effective for patients with subacute presentations.[8] In particular, the combination of susceptibility-weighted imaging (SWI) and fluid-attenuated inversion recovery (FLAIR) is superior to NCCT in detecting SAH.[9] MR imaging is also useful in ambiguous cases or where the treating physician suspects another concurrent or underlying pathology as it can rule out SAH and is excellent in detecting other intracranial pathologies.

The downside to MR imaging is longer scan time, higher cost, and limited availability.

In summary, several methods are available to physicians to assess for SAH and for most patients NCCT is an excellent screening test, particularly for those presenting within 6 h of headache onset.

ANEURYSM DETECTION

In patients with SAH on NCCT, the next diagnostic test should be CTA head to determine the underlying cause (Fig. 1C, D). As previously discussed, for aneurysms>3 mm in diameter, CTA has a sensitivity of at least 93%, and in some studies more than 97%.[7,10] Even for aneurysms smaller than 3 mm, CTA, when combined with 3D post-processing tools can have aneurysm detection rates between 85% to 97% depending on the scanner and study methodology.[10–12]

MRA is also an effective tool for the detection of cerebral aneurysms, but it comes with higher cost and longer acquisition time. In a meta-analysis that compared DSA with MRA for cerebral aneurysm detection, time-of-flight (TOF) MRA had 95% sensitivity and 89% specificity for aneurysm detection.[13] Despite the respectable performance of MRA for aneurysm detection, this technique is less frequently performed in the emergency setting.

DSA remains the gold standard for cerebral aneurysm detection. High spatial and temporal resolution of DSA is still unmatched by CTA or MRA. For either very small or complex aneurysms, DSA is essential for treatment decisions.[12,14,15] Even with modern scanners, patients can present with positive NCCT for SAH but negative CTA. The physician then must determine if the hemorrhage is perimesencephalic (caused by rupture of a small vein) or if there is an undetected aneurysm. DSA can detect vascular pathology in CTA-negative, NCCT-positive SAH in 7% to 13%.[14,16] In these cases, DSA should be performed initially and then again in 2 to 4 weeks to exclude an aneurysm as the cause of SAH.

SEQUELAE OF SUBARACHNOID HEMORRHAGE: VASOSPASM AND DELAYED CEREBRAL ISCHEMIA

DCI and angiographic cerebral vasospasm (ACV) are related but distinct post-SAH pathologies that are of great importance because they are thought to be the cause of nearly 30% to 50% of associated morbidity.[17] ACV is a radiographic diagnosis that can be determined by CTA, MRA, transcranial Doppler (TCD), or DSA. It is defined as the narrowing of intracranial intradural arteries

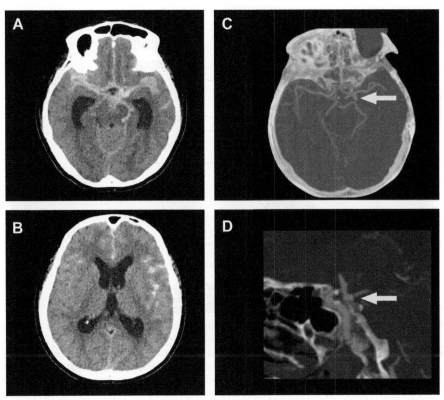

Fig. 1. Aneurysmal SAH. (*A, B*) Axial non-contrast CT showing acute subarachnoid hemorrhage ventricular enlargement consistent with obstructive hydrocephalus. (*C, D*) CTA and 3D reconstruction of a 7-mm left posterior communicating artery origin aneurysm (*yellow arrows*).

and most commonly occurs 5 to 14 days after SAH. DCI is a clinical diagnosis that can be secondary to ACV, but it can also occur in its absence. DCI is defined as a focal neurologic impairment, an increase of two points on the National Institutes of Health Stroke Scale, a decrease of two points on the Glasgow Coma Scale, or new evidence of infarction that is not explained by other causes.[17] It is important to differentiate DCI from ACV because approximately 50% of patients with DCI will not have evidence of ACV.[18] Overall, DCI is the more relevant clinical diagnosis as it has been strongly associated with poor clinical outcomes.[19,20]

DCI is most often diagnosed using a combination of physical examination, CTA, and CT-perfusion (CTP).[19,20,21] MR imaging and DSA can also be used in certain circumstances (**Fig. 3**). In clinical practice, a combination of physical examination and TCDs are used to screen for ACV. Changes on the patient's physical examination are often the impetus to obtain a CTA/CTP to assess for vasospasm as a potentially treatable cause of DCI.

The distribution of infarcts in DCI generally takes on two patterns. Either there is a single cortical

infarction, often near the site of aneurysm rupture or there are multiple widespread cortical and subcortical infarctions. It is therefore hypothesized that there are two distinct mechanisms of DCI. The first type with a single cortical infarct corresponds well to areas of vasospasm, whereas the second appears to have more microvascular perfusion underpinnings related to small vessels at the level of arterioles that likely reflects disrupted cerebral blood flow (CBF) autoregulation.[22]

Transcranial Doppler Ultrasonography

TCDs are a useful noninvasive screening modality and can be used to detect ACV. They are performed at the bedside and do not require radiation. Through the Doppler effect, the blood flow velocity can be calculated for a given vessel and these results can be compared with standardized reference values or trended over several days for an individual patient. As cerebral arteries narrow in caliber due to ACV, the TCD velocities increase. The advantages of TCDs include low cost and relatively wide availability. However, TCDs are highly operator dependent and have a relatively low sensitivity for ACV detection compared with

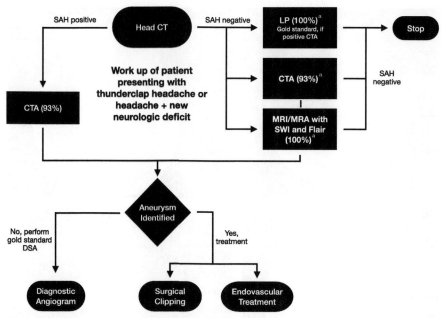

Fig. 2. Workup of a patient presentation concerning aneurysmal SAH. The initial imaging is a non-contrast CT (NCCT) which if positive for SAH is followed by CTA (right side of figure). If an aneurysm is identified a decision regarding treatment is made. If there is no aneurysm but the patient has SAH, the patient should undergo DSA. If the NCCT is negative for SAH, then the patient should either undergo LP or MR imaging/MRA to rule out SAH as these both have a sensitivity of 100%. A patient may also undergo CTA if these other tests are unavailable as CTA has a detection rate for aneurysms greater than 3 mm of at least 93%. [a]Sensitivity for SAH (LP and MR imaging) or aneurysm detection CTA).

DSA or CTA/CTP. TCDs have been well validated to have a high specificity, particularly for MCA vasospasm (99% specificity), but its sensitivity for vasospasm detection is relatively poor and ranges from 42% to 67% depending on the vessel assessed.[23–25]

Conventional values that indicate vasospasm are mean flow velocities in the MCA of >120 cm/s or an increase of greater than 50 cm/s in any one vessel in a 24-h period. Values above 200 cm/s are indicative of severe ACV. An alternative measurement is the Lindegaard ratio, which compares the MCA velocity to the velocity of the extracranial internal carotid artery. Lindegaard ratios control for overall CBF by normalizing the intracranial velocities to that of the internal carotid arteries. Values above 6 are considered severe and below 3 are considered normal.[26]

Computed Tomography Angiography and Perfusion

CTA has a high sensitivity and specificity for proximal artery ACV. Use of CTP allows for improved detection of new infarcts or areas of delayed cerebral perfusion (see **Fig. 3**A).[19] Commonly used CTP parameters include mean-transit-time (MTT), CBF, cerebral blood volume (CBV), and

Time-to-maximum of the residue function (T_{max}), and several of these parameter maps identify the presence of ACV. Evidence suggests that blood-brain-barrier disruption plays a role in DCI, and CTP can compute a permeability surface-area product using MTT and CBF measurements. This measurement has been shown to predict which patients ultimately will develop new ischemic infarcts.[27]

Several meta-analyses have reviewed the literature on CTA/CTP. In the detection of vasospasm, Greenberg and colleagues[28] report 80% sensitivity and 93% specificity for CTA. However, a recent review found interrater reliability to be low for CTA when assessing for ACV, which potentially limits its ability to rule out ACV in the absence of other studies.[29] CTP has a pooled sensitivity of 84% and specificity of 77% for DCI.[30] Additionally, both Tmax and MTT prolongation were found to correlate well with DCI in separate studies.[31,32] The use of both CTA and CTP leads to an increased sensitivity for ACV detection of 93%.[33]

The cost-effectiveness and additional radiation exposure of using CTA/CTP to screen for ACV and DCI in patients with SAH was modeled, and the study authors concluded that CTA/CTP was the preferred imaging modality compared with TCDs given superior prevention of detrimental

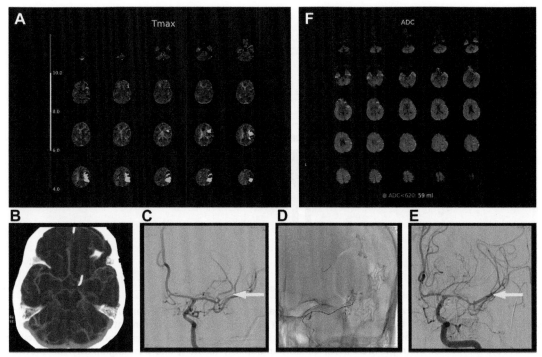

Fig. 3. Vasospasm and delayed cerebral ischemia. (*A*) CT-perfusion showing delayed perfusion in the territory of the left middle cerebral artery (MCA). (*B*) CTA from the same scan showing ACV of the distal left MCA. Angiography of the left internal cerebral artery (*C*) showed severe ACV in a middle branch of the left MCA (*yellow arrow*), which corresponded to the area of delayed perfusion. This was followed by balloon angioplasty (*D*) of the affected artery. Repeat angiography (*E*) shows improved vessel caliber (*yellow arrow*). However, this patient continued to experience vasospasm despite several further treatments and MR imaging (*F*) ultimately showed infarct in the downstream territory.

complications.[34] Whether this model applies in clinical settings remains to be investigated.

MR Imaging

MR imaging is excellent at detecting acute stroke using diffusion-weighted imaging (DWI), which is useful to confirm the diagnosis of DCI (see **Fig. 3**B). Traditionally, MR imaging was viewed as less useful in the management of patients with SAH due to its long scan times and higher cost. However, MR imaging may better predict which patients will develop DCI. Recent advances using intravoxel incoherent motion (IVIM) imaging to extract microvascular perfusion from DWI correlate with subsequent DCI, which suggests that IVIM may be a useful screening tool in high-risk patients.[35]

Diagnostic Cerebral Angiography

Considered the standard for evaluating ACV, DSA is also particularly useful because endovascular ACV treatment can be performed following diagnostic DSA (see **Fig.** 3D–F). A decrease in the diameter of 25% is considered mild, 25% to 50% moderate, and >50% severe ACV. However, ACV development does not correlate well with clinical outcomes, which likely reflects the complex and incompletely understood pathophysiology of DCI. The true benefit of DSA in the assessment of ACV and DCI is the ability to intervene immediately in patients in which these pathologies are identified. The high cost, technical complexity, and radiation exposure of DSA means that it should only be used in patients with a high pretest probability of moderate or severe vasospasm or those at high risk of DCI that are most likely to benefit from treatment.[17,20]

Circulating Biomarkers

Although outside the specific scope of this review, it is important to note that there are nonimaging biomarkers to ACV and DCI. cerebrospinal fluid levels of interleukin-1 (IL-1), IL-18, and tumor necrosis factor α (TNF-α) were shown to have poor prognostic implications in patients with DCI or ACV.[36] Although these and several other substances remain under investigation, their utility in the clinical setting has yet to be determined.

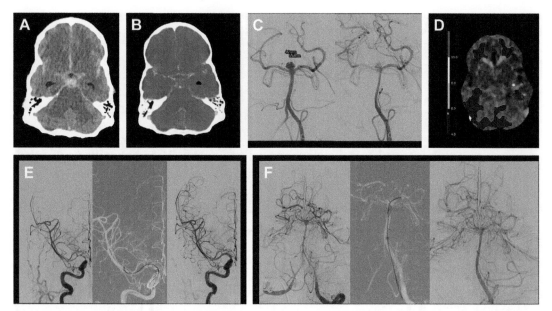

Fig. 4. Clinical vignette illustrative case of a patient with a ruptured 5 mm basilar tip aneurysm. (*A*) NCCT showing SAH. (*B*) CTA showing basilar tip aneurysm. (*C*) Initial DSA (*left*) and WEB device placement (*right*). Five days later, the patient developed increased somnolence. (*D*) CT-perfusion showed moderate perfusion delay in watershed distribution. (*E*) ACV of the right MCA (*left*), balloon angioplasty (*center*), and post-angioplasty run showing improved vessel caliber, the patient also received intra-arterial nicardipine. (*F*) Basilar artery vasospasm (*left*), balloon angioplasty (*center*), and post-angioplasty run showing improved vessel caliber. The patient was discharged 16 days following admission and returned to baseline at a 3-month follow-up.

Treatment of Vasospasm and Delayed Cerebral Ischemia

The mainstay of critical care management of patients with SAH after ruptured aneurysm treatment has been hypertension, hypervolemia, and hemodilution (triple-H therapy). However, there is no strong evidence to support the use of these measures to prevent DCI or improve long-term outcomes.[37] The use of nimodipine may improve long-term clinical outcomes; however, there is still much debate on its effectiveness, and a substantial portion of patients receiving nimodipine will still develop DCI.[38]

There are two commonly used endovascular treatments for ACV and DCI. The first is balloon angioplasty, in which a catheter is passed through a spastic vessel and then inflated to mechanically dilate the vessel. The second is chemical angioplasty, which refers to trans-arterial calcium channel blocker infusion into the ACV vascular bed.[19] Many neurointerventionalists use balloon angioplasty for proximal vessel ACV treatment and chemical angioplasty for both proximal and distal ACV treatment. A recent study found that in comparison with chemical angioplasty, distal balloon angioplasty resulted in lower rates of DCI and had a favorable safety profile.[39] Although several studies have found

no significant difference in the treatment modality used, it should be noted that there is limited evidence for either in reducing the rate of DCI or long-term clinical outcomes.[19] **Fig. 4** highlights a clinical management vignette.

Future Directions

Current neuroimaging research in patients with aneurysmal SAH often focuses on the prediction of DCI development to identify patients at high and low risk of this complication. Advanced MR imaging including DWI, functional MR imaging (fMRI), IVIM, and arterial spin labeling (ASL) have been investigated and show promise in predicting DCI development.[35,40–43] Additionally, cutting-edge artificial intelligence (AI) applications seek to improve radiologist aneurysm detection and to facilitate appropriate treatment planning.

Emerging MR Imaging Techniques

Some authors have shown that DWI changes detected within 24 h of SAH predicted poor outcomes, likely by identifying those patients who had already suffered an irrecoverable brain injury.[42,43] Rowland and colleagues[42] reported that with DWI brain volume measurements 72 h post-SAH (thought to be a proxy for vasogenic edema), good functional recovery at 3 months could be predicted with 84% accuracy.

fMRI is a widely used research imaging modality, but has relatively few acute care indications. It measures changes in CBF in real time, with the assumption that blood flow is a proxy for neuronal activation. Although still in very early stages, several studies using fMRI have found increased blood flow to areas involved in working memory after SAH, which may represent a decreased efficiency in neural processing and disruption of subcortical connections.[41] fMRI may ultimately serve as another useful tool for prognostication in patients with SAH and help better allocate resources toward the patients with the highest chance of functional recovery.

The ability to predict which unruptured aneurysms are at higher rupture risk remains a vexing clinical problem, and it is possible that advanced imaging techniques may better stratify risk. High-resolution vessel wall MR imaging based on its ability to represent aneurysm wall enhancement, a marker for wall inflammation, may help determine aneurysms at the highest rupture risk.[40,44] This technique may be particularly useful when there are multiple aneurysms and the treating physician must determine which aneurysm ruptured or is at the highest risk for rupture.[40]

Lastly, MR imaging morphometry has been investigated as another means of prognostication by using volumetric MR imaging to estimate temporomesial volume.[45] Measurements of both pituitary and hippocampal volume reduction after SAH are associated with decreased cognitive scores at several months post-hemorrhage.[46,47]

Artificial Intelligence

AI holds tremendous promise as a transformative technology in medicine, and the application of AI to imaging is a rapidly evolving area of research. Several studies have applied AI networks to CTA and MRA for the detection of cerebral aneurysms. Many developed AI algorithms have aneurysm detection rates between 92% and 98%.[48–50] Although some pair the algorithm with radiologists to increase overall accuracy, others are able to detect aneurysms independently.[48,50,51] These approaches hold promise to both increase the speed and accuracy of aneurysm detection and may be particularly helpful in lower resource settings where lack of highly trained radiologists may delay patient treatment.

SUMMARY

Neuroimaging is essential in both the diagnosis and management of SAH. An NCCT remains the mainstay of initial diagnosis and patients with thunderclap headache or headache with new neurologic deficits, but negative NCCT should undergo further evaluation with CTA, LP, or MR imaging. Image acquisition and post-processing advancements, including the use of AI are making CTA and MRA aneurysm detection more effective. However, patients with SAH and negative noninvasive imaging still require a DSA for definitive diagnosis. Lastly, once the diagnosis and initial treatments have been completed, patients must be monitored for DCI through a combination of screening with TCDs and the physical examination and prudent use of perfusion imaging. New research focusing on cerebral oxygen delivery and imaging modalities that help predict outcomes in SAH may help clinicians more effectively apply resources to benefit.

CLINICS CARE POINTS

- Subarachnoid hemorrhage detected on CT can be a sign of a medical emergency and the appropriate work up is to investigate the underlying cause with CTA, and/or MRI or DSA if indicated.
- Delayed cerebral ischemia and vasospasm are district clinical and radiographic entities. Both contribute significantly to the morbidity from aneurysmal subarachnoid hemorrhage.
- CT Perfusion imaging should be the initial diagnostic study of choice in most centers to evaluate patients with suspected vasospasm. MRI and DSA are also excellent tests but their availability and timeliness may be more limited.

FUNDING

Funding for this work was provided by a generous donation from Doris and Robert Rivett to Dr JJH.

REFERENCES

1. Perry JJ, Stiell IG, Sivilotti ML, et al. Sensitivity of computed tomography performed within six hours of onset of headache for diagnosis of subarachnoid haemorrhage: prospective cohort study. Bmj 2011; 343:d4277.
2. Byyny RL, Mower WR, Shum N, et al. Sensitivity of noncontrast cranial computed tomography for the emergency department diagnosis of subarachnoid hemorrhage. Ann Emerg Med 2008;51(6):697–703.

3. Long B, Koyfman A, Runyon MS. Subarachnoid Hemorrhage: Updates in Diagnosis and Management. Emerg Med Clin North Am 2017;35(4):803–24.

4. Perry JJ, Spacek A, Forbes M, et al. Is the combination of negative computed tomography result and negative lumbar puncture result sufficient to rule out subarachnoid hemorrhage? Ann Emerg Med 2008;51(6):707–13.

5. Valle Alonso J, Fonseca Del Pozo FJ, Vaquero Álvarez M, et al. Sudden headache, lumbar puncture, and the diagnosis of subarachnoid hemorrhage in patients with a normal computed tomography scans. Emergencias 2018;30(1):50–3.

6. McCormack RF, Hutson A. Can computed tomography angiography of the brain replace lumbar puncture in the evaluation of acute-onset headache after a negative noncontrast cranial computed tomography scan? Acad Emerg Med 2010;17(4):444–51.

7. McKinney AM, Palmer CS, Truwit CL, et al. Detection of aneurysms by 64-section multidetector CT angiography in patients acutely suspected of having an intracranial aneurysm and comparison with digital subtraction and 3D rotational angiography. AJNR Am J Neuroradiol 2008;29(3):594–602.

8. da Rocha AJ, da Silva CJ, Gama HP, et al. Comparison of magnetic resonance imaging sequences with computed tomography to detect low-grade subarachnoid hemorrhage: Role of fluid-attenuated inversion recovery sequence. J Comput Assist Tomogr 2006;30(2):295–303.

9. Verma RK, Kottke R, Andereggen L, et al. Detecting subarachnoid hemorrhage: comparison of combined FLAIR/SWI versus CT. Eur J Radiol 2013; 82(9):1539–45.

10. Wang H, Li W, He H, et al. 320-detector row CT angiography for detection and evaluation of intracranial aneurysms: comparison with conventional digital subtraction angiography. Clin Radiol 2013;68(1):e15–20.

11. Westerlaan HE, van Dijk JM, Jansen-van der Weide MC, et al. Intracranial aneurysms in patients with subarachnoid hemorrhage: CT angiography as a primary examination tool for diagnosis–systematic review and meta-analysis. Radiology 2011;258(1): 134–45.

12. Yang ZL, Ni QQ, Schoepf UJ, et al. Small Intracranial Aneurysms: Diagnostic Accuracy of CT Angiography. Radiology 2017;285(3):941–52.

13. Sailer AM, Wagemans BA, Nelemans PJ, et al. Diagnosing intracranial aneurysms with MR angiography: systematic review and meta-analysis. Stroke 2014; 45(1):119–26.

14. Heit JJ, Pastena GT, Nogueira RG, et al. Cerebral Angiography for Evaluation of Patients with CT Angiogram-Negative Subarachnoid Hemorrhage: An 11-Year Experience. AJNR Am J Neuroradiol 2016;37(2):297–304.

15. Larson AS, Brinjikji W. Subarachnoid Hemorrhage of Unknown Cause: Distribution and Role of Imaging. Neuroimaging Clin N Am 2021;31(2):167–75.

16. Nguyen I, Caton MT, Tonetti D, et al. Angiographically Occult Subarachnoid Hemorrhage: Yield of Repeat Angiography, Influence of Initial CT Bleed Pattern, and Sources of Diagnostic Error in 242 Consecutive Patients. AJNR Am J Neuroradiol 2022;43(5):731–5.

17. Diringer MN, Bleck TP, Claude Hemphill J 3rd, et al. Critical care management of patients following aneurysmal subarachnoid hemorrhage: recommendations from the Neurocritical Care Society's Multidisciplinary Consensus Conference. Neurocrit Care 2011;15(2):211–40.

18. Vergouwen MD, Vermeulen M, Coert BA, et al. Microthrombosis after aneurysmal subarachnoid hemorrhage: an additional explanation for delayed cerebral ischemia. J Cereb Blood Flow Metab 2008;28(11):1761–70.

19. Ivanidze J, Sanelli PC. Vasospasm: Role of Imaging in Detection and Monitoring Treatment. Neuroimaging Clin N Am 2021;31(2):147–55.

20. Connolly ES Jr, Rabinstein AA, Carhuapoma JR, et al. Guidelines for the management of aneurysmal subarachnoid hemorrhage: a guideline for healthcare professionals from the American Heart Association/american Stroke Association. Stroke 2012; 43(6):1711–37.

21. Sanelli PC, Ugorec I, Johnson CE, et al. Using quantitative CT perfusion for evaluation of delayed cerebral ischemia following aneurysmal subarachnoid hemorrhage. Am J Neuroradiol 2011;32(11): 2047–53.

22. Rabinstein AA, Weigand S, Atkinson JL, Wijdicks EF. Patterns of cerebral infarction in aneurysmal subarachnoid hemorrhage. Stroke 2005;36(5):992–7.

23. Lysakowski C, Walder B, Costanza MC, Tramèr MR. Transcranial Doppler versus angiography in patients with vasospasm due to a ruptured cerebral aneurysm: a systematic review. Stroke 2001;32(10): 2292–8.

24. Sharma S, Lubrica RJ, Song M, et al. The role of transcranial Doppler in cerebral vasospasm: a literature review. Subarachnoid Hemorrhage: Neurological Care and Protection 2020;201–5.

25. Wozniak MA, Sloan MA, Rothman MI, et al. Detection of vasospasm by transcranial Doppler sonography. J Neuroimaging 1996;6(2):87–93.

26. Samagh N, Bhagat H, Jangra K. Monitoring cerebral vasospasm: How much can we rely on transcranial Doppler. J Anaesthesiol Clin Pharmacol 2019; 35(1):12–8.

27. Ivanidze J, Kesavabhotla K, Kallas ON, et al. Evaluating blood-brain barrier permeability in delayed cerebral infarction after aneurysmal subarachnoid

hemorrhage. AJNR Am J Neuroradiol 2015;36(5): 850–4.

28. Greenberg ED, Gold R, Reichman M, et al. Diagnostic accuracy of CT angiography and CT perfusion for cerebral vasospasm: a meta-analysis. AJNR Am J Neuroradiol 2010;31(10):1853–60.

29. Letourneau-Guillon L, Farzin B, Darsaut TE, et al. Reliability of CT Angiography in Cerebral Vasospasm: A Systematic Review of the Literature and an Inter- and Intraobserver Study. AJNR Am J Neuroradiol 2020;41(4):612–8.

30. Mir DI, Gupta A, Dunning A, et al. CT perfusion for detection of delayed cerebral ischemia in aneurysmal subarachnoid hemorrhage: a systematic review and meta-analysis. AJNR Am J Neuroradiol 2014;35(5):866–71.

31. Fragata I, Alves M, Papoila AL, et al. Temporal evolution of cerebral computed tomography perfusion after acute subarachnoid hemorrhage: a prospective cohort study. Acta Radiol 2020;61(3):376–85.

32. Murphy A, Lee TY, Marotta TR, et al. Prospective Multicenter Study of Changes in MTT after Aneurysmal SAH and Relationship to Delayed Cerebral Ischemia in Patients with Good- and Poor-Grade Admission Status. AJNR Am J Neuroradiol 2018; 39(11):2027–33.

33. Wintermark M, Ko NU, Smith WS, et al. Vasospasm after subarachnoid hemorrhage: utility of perfusion CT and CT angiography on diagnosis and management. AJNR Am J Neuroradiol 2006;27(1):26–34.

34. Ivanidze J, Charalel RA, Shuryak I, et al. Effects of Radiation Exposure on the Cost-Effectiveness of CT Angiography and Perfusion Imaging in Aneurysmal Subarachnoid Hemorrhage. AJNR Am J Neuroradiol 2017;38(3):462–8.

35. Heit JJ, Wintermark M, Martin BW, et al. Reduced Intravoxel Incoherent Motion Microvascular Perfusion Predicts Delayed Cerebral Ischemia and Vasospasm After Aneurysm Rupture. Stroke 2018;49(3): 741–5.

36. Lv SY, Wu Q, Liu JP, et al. Levels of Interleukin-1β, Interleukin-18, and Tumor Necrosis Factor-α in Cerebrospinal Fluid of Aneurysmal Subarachnoid Hemorrhage Patients May Be Predictors of Early Brain Injury and Clinical Prognosis. World Neurosurg 2018;111:e362–73.

37. Loan JJ, Wiggins AN, Brennan PM. Medically induced hypertension, hypervolaemia and haemodilution for the treatment and prophylaxis of vasospasm following aneurysmal subarachnoid haemorrhage: systematic review. B. J Neurosurg 2018;32(2):157–64.

38. Pickard JD, Murray GD, Illingworth R, et al. Effect of oral nimodipine on cerebral infarction and outcome after subarachnoid haemorrhage: British aneurysm nimodipine trial. Bmj 1989;298(6674):636–42.

39. Labeyrie MA, Gaugain S, Boulouis G, et al. Distal Balloon Angioplasty of Cerebral Vasospasm Decreases the Risk of Delayed Cerebral Infarction. AJNR Am J Neuroradiol 2019;40(8):1342–8.

40. Cornelissen BMW, Leemans EL, Slump CH, et al. Vessel wall enhancement of intracranial aneurysms: fact or artifact? Neurosurg Focus 2019;47(1):E18.

41. Maher M, Churchill NW, de Oliveira Manoel AL, et al. Altered Resting-State Connectivity within Executive Networks after Aneurysmal Subarachnoid Hemorrhage. PLoS One 2015;10(7):e0130483.

42. Rowland MJ, Garry P, Ezra M, et al. Early brain injury and cognitive impairment after aneurysmal subarachnoid haemorrhage. Sci Rep 2021;11(1):23245.

43. Sato K, Shimizu H, Fujimura M, et al. Acute-stage diffusion-weighted magnetic resonance imaging for predicting outcome of poor-grade aneurysmal subarachnoid hemorrhage. J Cereb Blood Flow Metab 2010;30(6):1110–20.

44. Hudson JS, Zanaty M, Nakagawa D, et al. Magnetic Resonance Vessel Wall Imaging in Human Intracranial Aneurysms. Stroke 2019;50(1):e1.

45. de Oliveira Manoel AL, Mansur A, Murphy A, et al. Aneurysmal subarachnoid haemorrhage from a neuroimaging perspective. Crit Care 2014;18(6):557.

46. Bendel P, Koivisto T, Niskanen E, et al. Brain atrophy and neuropsychological outcome after treatment of ruptured anterior cerebral artery aneurysms: a voxel-based morphometric study. Neuroradiology 2009;51(11):711–22.

47. Rass V, Schoenherr E, Ianosi BA, et al. Subarachnoid Hemorrhage is Followed by Pituitary Gland Volume Loss: A Volumetric MRI Observational Study. Neurocrit Care 2020;32(2):492–501.

48. Joo B, Ahn SS, Yoon PH, et al. A deep learning algorithm may automate intracranial aneurysm detection on MR angiography with high diagnostic performance. Eur Radiol 2020;30(11):5785–93.

49. Joo B, Choi HS, Ahn SS, et al. A Deep Learning Model with High Standalone Performance for Diagnosis of Unruptured Intracranial Aneurysm. Yonsei Med J 2021;62(11):1052–61.

50. Shahzad R, Pennig L, Goertz L, et al. Fully automated detection and segmentation of intracranial aneurysms in subarachnoid hemorrhage on CTA using deep learning. Sci Rep 2020;10(1):21799.

51. Heit JJ, Honce JM, Yedavalli VS, et al. RAPID Aneurysm: Artificial intelligence for unruptured cerebral aneurysm detection on CT angiography. J Stroke Cerebrovasc Dis 2022;31(10):106690.

Vascular Injuries in Head and Neck Trauma

Andres Rodriguez, MD, Luis Nunez, MD, Roy Riascos, MD, FACR*

KEYWORDS

• Head and neck • Trauma • Vascular injury • CT angiography • MR angiography

KEY POINTS

- Traumatic vascular injuries of the head and neck represent a life-threatening complication. The Biffl scale is the most commonly used classification for traumatic cerebrovascular injuries.
- Computed tomography angiography is a fast, widely available, and reliable imaging modality that has become the primary modality for evaluating traumatic vascular injuries of the head and neck.
- Low-grade vessel wall injuries may be overlooked and must be assessed under the suspicion of vascular injury.
- Anatomic variants, artifacts, and mimics may simulate vessel-wall injuries.

INTRODUCTION

Blunt and penetrating vascular injuries of the head and neck can represent life-threatening emergencies that require accurate detection and characterization by the radiologist.[1,2] Though vascular injuries can be suspected based on the patient's signs and symptoms, a latent period between the time of injury and the onset of clinical manifestations can delay a prompt diagnosis and therapy. The aim of this review is to highlight, through imaging cases, the different types of vascular injuries that occur in the setting of trauma.[1]

Blunt and penetrating vascular injuries generally occur in the setting of polytrauma and may be overlooked under the scope of more visible lesions during an initial evaluation. Although the prevalence of vascular injuries is difficult to ascertain due to the asymptomatic presentation of minor injuries or during the early stages of the injury, previous studies have described the presence of vascular injuries to be found in 1.6% to 20% of cases.[3,4]

The main proposed mechanism of trauma in blunt cerebrovascular injury (BCVI) is mechanical outstretching of the vessel thus leading to mural vessel damage. Clinical manifestations occur secondary to hemodynamic instability resulting in cerebral or cerebellar infarctions, which can be classified either as embolic when an intraluminal thrombus occurs at the site of the injury, or mechanical when a pseudoaneurysm or mural hematoma compresses the vessel lumen.[4,5]

Carotid artery injuries can occur due to direct blow, hyperextension with rotation, intraoral trauma, or in association with skull base fractures. Arterial dissection locations typically include the bifurcation, petrous, cavernous, and clinoid internal carotid segments. Vertebral artery injuries, generally occlusion and dissection, are commonly due to shearing forces and direct trauma against adjacent bony structures secondary to rotational forces or penetrating injury from fracture fragments. Cervical transverse foramen fractures, cervical facet joint dislocations, and C1–C2 fractures have been associated with vertebral artery injuries.[6] Trivial trauma, including chiropractic manipulation, coughing, yoga, vomiting, and rapid head movement, have also been described as a cause of head and neck vascular injury.[7]

Penetrating injuries are mostly related to motor vehicle accidents, gunshots, and other weapons. Penetrating lesions derived from projectiles can generate a vascular lesion from the shockwave or direct injury. These lesions are generally associated

Department of Diagnostic and Interventional Imaging, Neuroradiology Section, The University of Texas Health Science Center at Houston, Houston, TX, USA
* Corresponding author.
E-mail address: roy.f.riascos@uth.tmc.edu

Radiol Clin N Am 61 (2023) 467–477
https://doi.org/10.1016/j.rcl.2023.01.012

with multiple injuries in the trajectory of the wound. In penetrating neck lesions, approximately 15% to 25% result in arterial compromise, whereas 16% to 18% result in venous injury.[8]

Rationale for Imaging

There is no general rule on screening trauma patients for BCVI, as approximately 80% of patients with BCVI present with a latent, asymptomatic period. The Eastern Association for the Surgery of Trauma (EAST) established imaging recommendations in 2010, based on a systematic review from 1965 to 2005 (Box 1). In recent years, additional risk factors such as complex skull fractures, mandible fractures, scalp degloving, and thoracic vascular injuries, have been added to the screening criteria.[9,10]

Among penetrating injuries, blood vessels are the most commonly affected structure in the neck, followed by the aerodigestive tract and the spinal cord. As the surgical exploration of penetrating wounds of the neck usually depends on the patient's clinical status, a physical examination has been shown to be a good predictor of vascular injury.[11,12]

Box 1
Expanded Denver criteria

Signs/Symptoms

    Arterial hemorrhage from neck, mouth, or nose

    Cervical bruit in patients <50 years

    Expanding cervical hematoma

    Focal neurologic deficit

    Neurologic status not associated with head CT findings

    Stroke on imaging

Risk Factors (High-Energy Trauma)

    Le Fort fracture II or III

    Mandible fracture

    Base of skull fracture

    TBI with GCS < 6

    Cervical spine fracture, subluxation, or ligamentous lesion at any level

    Anoxia secondary to near hanging

    Thoracic vascular injury

    TBI with thoracic injury

    Seat belt abrasion with swelling, pain, or altered mental status

Imaging indicated if one or more criteria are present.

To standardize penetrating lesions of the neck and improve outcomes, the neck has been divided into three zones: zone 1, extending from the clavicles and sternal notch to the cricoid cartilage; zone 2, extending from the cricoid cartilage to the mandibular angle; and zone 3, extending from the mandibular angle up to the skull base. With the use of images and an overall reduction in exploratory cervicotomy in penetrating trauma due to a high percentage of negative explorations and significant morbidity, this classification is mainly used as a descriptive and anatomic classification rather than a management-related classification.[13,14]

IMAGING TECHNIQUES
Digital Subtraction Angiography

Digital subtraction angiography (DSA) has historically been the gold standard for detecting vascular head and neck trauma, given its high sensitivity, cost-effectiveness, and ability to perform a vascular therapeutic intervention in a selected group of patients.[7,10,15] However, its invasiveness carries a higher rate of complications, including stroke, compared with other imaging techniques. Additionally, DSA relies on intraluminal blood vessel opacification, limiting vessel wall and extraluminal assessment.[7]

Computed Tomography Angiography

Although DSA is considered the gold standard, multidetector computed tomography angiography has become the initial modality of choice due to its availability, readiness, noninvasiveness, and ability to detect extravascular abnormalities.[11,14]

High-resolution computed tomography angiography (CTA) performed with isovolumetric acquisition ideally of 1 mm or less can accurately diagnose head and neck traumatic vascular injuries with a specificity of 92% to 100% but limited sensitivity of 66% to 98%. However, most of the lesions missed on CTA constitute low-grade injuries. In external carotid artery lesions where sensitivity is lower, injuries usually are visualized as occlusions, which require no further management.[3,7,16–18]

Although CTA advantages outweigh disadvantages, special attention should be taken in patients who may ultimately need DSA, due to the contrast material overload, particularly in those patients at risk for contrast material-induced nephropathy.[8]

CTA limitations and pitfalls include artifacts and imaging techniques. Bolus timing errors lead to suboptimal vessel opacification and misdiagnosis; beam hardening due to amalgams, spinal hardware, metal or projectile fragments may obscure adjacent vessels, and additional imaging techniques or indirect signs must be considered to make a diagnosis; motion artifact in non-collaborative patients can obscure or mimic injuries; and body habitus can affect image quality, especially in the lower neck segment.[8]

MR Imaging

Though MR imaging is the most sensitive imaging modality in evaluating brain injury, it is not the first-line screening study in acute head and neck vascular injury. Magnetic resonance angiography (MRA) can be an alternative in head and neck vascular traumatic lesions in some circumstances, using time of flight (TOF) or contrasted three-dimensional (3D) MRA. The lack of ionizing radiation and lower incidence of gadolinium allergies compared with iodinated agents is advantageous compared with DSA and CTA. However, in the acute setting, longer acquisition times, lower resolution compared with CT to detect small lesions, and risk of motion artifact, limit MR imaging use.[7,19]

3D and 2D T1-weighted and proton-density-weighted sequences help delineate arterial dissection. Brain MR imaging with DWI is highly sensitive in detecting internal carotid artery dissections and secondary stroke lesions.[20] High-resolution vessel wall imaging (VWI) with blood suppression may help evaluate equivocal CTA cases and could serve as a follow-up imaging examination in subacute settings.[21] For example, VWI performs well as a tool that evaluates the lumen, wall, and periadventitial; detects intimal flaps and wall thickening; and serves as an initial evaluation tool or adjunct in inconclusive cases.[22,23]

In penetrating trauma, metallic foreign bodies can constitute a contraindication to performing an MR imaging and should be considered.[8]

IMAGING FINDINGS

Head and neck traumatic vascular injuries range from minor lesions requiring no treatment to more severe ones requiring immediate surgical or endovascular management. Different scales for head and neck vascular injuries are available, with the Biffl scale being the most commonly used. The higher the grade on the Biffl scale, the higher the risk of complications and worse prognosis (Fig. 1, Table 1).[1,24]

Vessel Wall Irregularity

Vessel wall irregularity corresponds to grade I lesion. Subtle findings are better visualized in 3D reformatted images. On DSA and CTA, acquisitions seem as undulation, slight irregularity of the vessel wall, or minimal focal thickening of the wall; that do not typically cause luminal stenosis, which can be challenging to differentiate from posttraumatic vasospasm or artifact (Fig. 2).[7,9,15]

MRA shows similar findings as DSA and CTA, being less sensitive in detecting grade I lesions. VWI has shown good performance and might be helpful in equivocal cases, isolating the vessel wall and lumen, and useful differentiating between an intramural hematoma and an intraluminal thrombus.[7,22]

In general, vessel wall irregularities and grade I lesions require no direct intervention and will heal over time.[24]

Intramural Hematomas

Depending on the luminal stenosis caused by intramural hematomas, they are classified as grade I, II, or IV. Luminal stenosis <25% is classified as grade I, stenosis ≥25% is considered grade II, and if there is complete occlusion of the vessel lumen, it is categorized as a grade IV traumatic injury.[7]

Mural hematomas are seen as focal or circumferential wall thickening. In theory, these lesions would not compromise the intima; however, this differentiation can be challenging in cross-sectional imaging. VWI will show a crescentic or oval-shaped intramural lesion that displays signal intensity related to the paramagnetic effect of hemoglobin aging and degradation. Usually, acute and chronic lesions will be shown as T1 isointense and subacute lesions with T1 hyperintensity. Consequently, acute and chronic lesions are more likely to be missed due to the isointensity of the surrounding soft tissues (Fig. 3).[25–27]

Dissection

Arterial dissections represent grade II lesions, usually treated with heparin or endovascular therapy due to platelet aggregation after the endothelial damage occurs, leading to thrombus formation and embolization. These lesions occur secondary to a tear in the intima that leads to the entry of blood flow into deeper layers creating a false lumen with a progressive intimal dissection resulting in vessel lumen stenoses. Progression of dissections into the media and thinner adventitia could lead to pseudoaneurysm formation (grade III) and extravasation (grade V).[9,28]

The intimal flap can be visualized as a linear intraluminal defect with a double lumen, the false lumen filled entirely or partially with contrast media. The intimal flap might not be seen in smaller caliber vessels, and tapering of these vessels

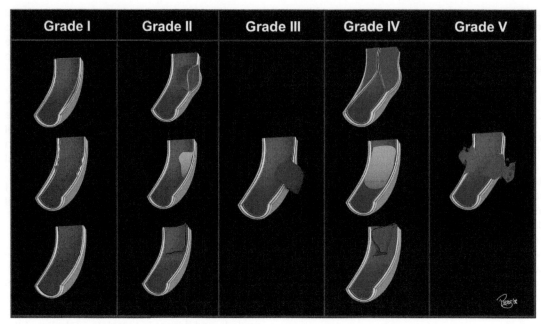

Fig. 1. Visual representation of the Biffl grading scale. (*Courtesy of* R Riascos, MD, Houston, TX.)

can represent a dissection.[7,28] An eccentric crescent focus of hyperdensity paired with a thin layer of peripheral enhancement is a very specific sign of dissection (**Fig. 4**).[29]

MR T1-weighted and proton-density fat-saturated sequences show a T1 hyperintensity in the false lumen due to slow flow and/or subacute thrombus formation. DWI in routine brain protocol show acute blood thrombus as a hyperintense eccentric ring encompassing the false lumen. VWI may provide more accurate detection of intimal flaps compared with CTA, with direct visualization of the intimal lesion and adjacent hemorrhage.[7,20,22]

Intraluminal Thrombus

The presence of an intraluminal thrombus corresponds to a grade II lesion. Endothelial damage at the injury site activates the coagulation cascade resulting in thrombus formation. Potential distal embolization with resultant stroke constitutes the most significant risk of such lesions. Images show a focal intraluminal opacification defect at the injury site, corresponding to the thrombus (**Fig. 5**).

Pseudoaneurysm

When blood flows through the intimal defect resulting from the initial trauma, it is contained between any of the outer vessel layers or adjacent soft tissue, creating a focal eccentric outpouching or pseudoaneurysm. These lesions, classified as grade III injuries, lack a true wall and are held by fragile connective tissue. Intracranial pseudoaneurysms are particularly more prone to bleeding due to a thinner media and adventitia, and the absence of an external elastic lamina. Pseudoaneurysm may be asymptomatic or become symptomatic after rupture, due to acute hemorrhage, including epistaxis, a common sign of acute internal carotid artery (ICA) pseudoaneurysm bleeding. Acute and chronic lesions may manifest with nerve compression from mass effect and vascular proximity to multiple cranial nerves. Endovascular management of pseudoaneurysm is usually performed due to the anatomic limitation of surgery, as most of these lesions are located at the base

Table 1 Biffl grading scale	
Classification	**Description**
Grade I	Vessel wall irregularity or dissection/intramural hematoma with <25% of lumen stenoses
Grade II	Dissection or intramural hematoma with > 25% of lumen stenoses Any raised intimal flap or intraluminal thrombus
Grade III	Pseudoaneurysm
Grade IV	Vessel occlusion
Grade V	Vessel transection or AVF

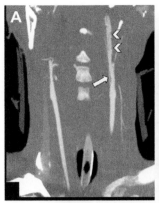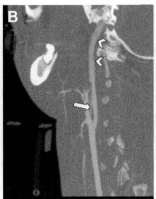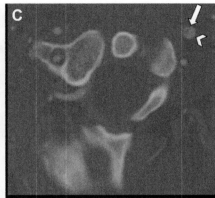

Fig. 2. ICA vessel wall irregularity with associated intimal flap. A 21-year-old patient presented to the ER after a motor vehicle accident. (A) Reformatted coronal. (B) Sagittal MIP CTA. (C) Axial CTA shows left ICA vessel wall irregularity (*arrowheads*) with an associated intimal flap (*arrows*).

of the skull or carotid canal. Conservative management must be cautiously monitored due to thromboembolic risk and the potential of cerebral ischemic events. Anticoagulation is usually indicated until verification of complete recovery is documented.[30,31]

DSA remains the gold standard not only due to its high spatial and temporal resolution but also for its concomitant therapy potential. CTA shows a rounded or fusiform lesion arising from the donor artery that opacifies with contrast media with some areas of nonenhancement secondary to the thrombus (Fig. 6). MR imaging/MRA is helpful in patients with impaired renal function or iodinated contrast media allergy, additionally assessing mural hematomas. High attenuation around the sac may represent a rupture contained by surrounding tissues. Ultrasound performed in cervical arteries demonstrates an anechoic sac arising from the supplying artery, showing lobulations, septa, and/or thrombus. Doppler evaluation shows swirling motion creating the "Yin-yang" sign and a "to-and-fro" spectral waveform.[7,32]

Arterial Occlusion

Arterial occlusions are classified as grade IV injuries; these are challenging to treat as the vessel is thrombosed and cannot be recanalized.[24] Occlusion of cervical segments of the ICA will often show tapering of the vessel before its point of total occlusion. With vertebral arteries, the occlusion will more commonly seem as an abrupt cutoff (Fig. 7). The extent of the occlusion, especially in the vertebral arteries, will be variable secondary to distal recanalization from collateral flow. The normal vessel flow void will disappear on MR imaging, and a T1 intraluminal hyperintensity is seen as a result of an acute thrombus. Owing to flow interruption, TOF MR angiography will note an abrupt cutoff or tapered vessel. However, it has lower sensitivity and can be altered due to slow flow-related artifacts. VWI has shown high sensitivity and specificity, near equivalent to DSA and CTA in recognizing occlusions despite the age of the thrombus, and can be used as an adjunct in inconclusive or non-specific TOF-MRA findings.[7,33]

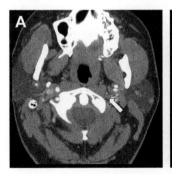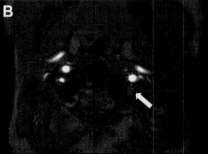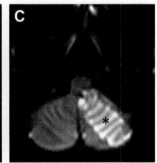

Fig. 3. Intramural hematoma narrowing the left vertebral artery lumen. A 30-year-old patient with vertigo after a soccer match. (A) Axial CTA. (B) Axial MR TOF. (C) Diffusion-weighted MR. There is an intramural thrombus with a narrowing greater than 50% of the left vertebral artery lumen (*arrow*). MR diffusion-weighted images show an acute infarct in the left PICA territory (*asterisk*).

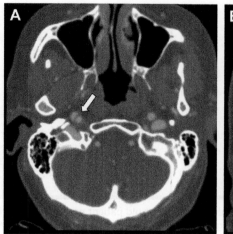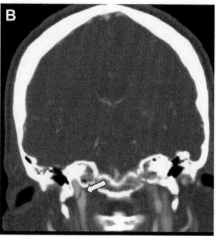

Fig. 4. Right ICA dissection with an intimal flap in a 43-year-old patient who presented with dysarthria after a rapid deceleration trauma. (*A, B*) Axial and coronal CTA images. Images show a raised intimal flap within the lacerum segment of the right ICA (*arrows*).

Arterial Transection and Arterio-Venous Fistula

Arterial transection and arterio-venous fistula (AVF) correspond to the most severe category grade: grade V. Transection is usually secondary to penetrating injuries or high-impact trauma like motor vehicle accidents. Transections show irregular extravasation of the contrast media contiguous to the parent vessel into the surrounding tissues, with an increase in the size of this collection on delayed acquisitions. Immediate surgical or endovascular management is needed, given the high mortality in this type of lesion (**Fig. 8**).[3,34]

AVF is difficult to diagnose on CTA and MR imaging considering the subtle findings. Usually, the primary finding on single-phase CTA might be an engorged vein with early filling during the arterial phase near the injured artery. The fistulous communication is rarely seen on CTA. Time-resolved MRA can help identify AVFs showing early venous opacification. Increased venous outflow in carotid-cavernous fistulas can cause indirect imaging signs that help with diagnosis, including dilatation of the ophthalmic vein and orbital edema with asymmetric engorgement of the cavernous sinus (see **Fig. 7**). A definitive diagnosis is made with DSA, which shows early venous opacification and aberrant communication between the injured artery and vein.

Endovascular intervention is the preferred therapeutic approach because it is a safe, effective, and readily method for shunt interruption in anatomically inaccessible AVFs.[7,15,19] Repair of carotid-

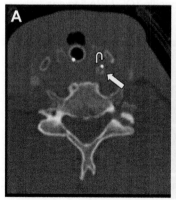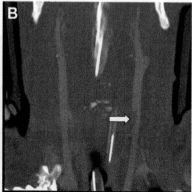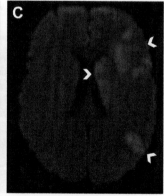

Fig. 5. Left common artery thrombus in a 58-year-old patient with a BB gunshot. (*A*) Axial. (*B*) Reformatted coronal MIP MPR. (*C*) Diffusion-weighted MR. There is a pellet fragment contacting the outer layers of the left common carotid artery (*curved arrow*), with an intraluminal thrombus (*arrows*) and multiple distal infarcts in the territory of the left MCA (*arrowheads*).

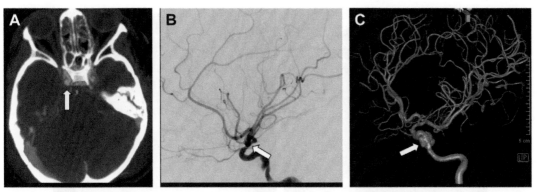

Fig. 6. Pseudoaneurysm of the right ICA. A 40-year-old patient after a motor vehicle accident. (*A*) Axial CTA. (*B*) Lateral DSA after injection in the right ICA. (*C*) Lateral DSA reformatted images after injection in the right ICA. There is a focal lobular saccular dilation of the cavernous segment of the right ICA, representing a pseudoaneurysm (*arrows*).

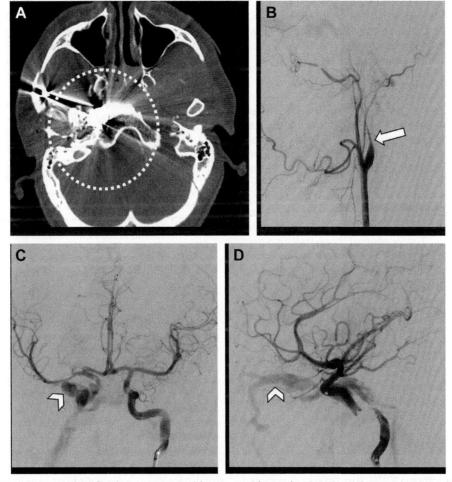

Fig. 7. ICA occlusion and CC-fistula in a 35-year-old patient with gunshot injuries. (*A*) CT axial images. (*B*) Oblique DSA image after right CCA injection. (*C, D*) Left ICA injection DSA images. Multiple bullet fragments located at the base of the skull and right carotid canal generates streak artifact and obscures the carotid canal (*dotted circle*). There is tapering of the ICA with distal occlusion (*arrow*). Opacification through contralateral ICA shows a CC-Fistula with dilation of the ophthalmic vein (*arrowheads*).

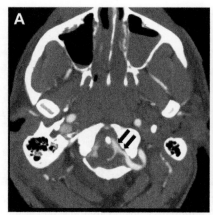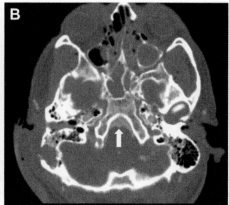

Fig. 8. Left vertebral artery transection. A 35-year-old patient after a high-energy motor-vehicle accident. (*A*) Axial CTA reformatted MIP images. (*B*) Axial CTA. There is a transection of the left vertebral artery in the V3–V4 segment (*black arrows*) with active extravasation into the subarachnoid space (*white arrow*).

cavernous fistulas can be managed by embolization and direct cannulation of the cavernous sinus or using flow-diverting stents.[35,36] If there is active bleeding and a good circle of Willis collateral circulation, the parent vessel can be sacrificed.

Intracranial Aneurysms

Traumatic intracranial aneurysms (TICAs) are rare but may be seen in children. These occur in an acute or delayed manner after a blunt or, more commonly, a penetrating injury. Histologically TICA can be classified as true or false aneurysms; the latter is known as pseudoaneurysms, which have a higher incidence. However, this classification does not affect treatment and thus is not practical to discriminate from a clinical management point of view. The location of these lesions differs on the type of trauma, as ICA and paraclinoid aneurysms are more frequently seen in blunt trauma due to skull base fractures and shearing forces between the vessel and the adjacent bone, distal aneurysms are usually seen secondary to penetrating injuries. Owing to the high risk of rupture and subsequent mortality of up to 50%, imaging and treatment must not be delayed. Skull base fractures, penetrating lesions that cross the midline with fragments near vessels, or delayed neurologic deterioration and unexplained bleeding must prompt a TICA diagnosis.[37–39]

Cerebral Venous Thrombosis

Trauma is a significant risk factor for cerebral venous thrombosis (CVT). It is usually associated with skull fractures that extend into the jugular or dural venous sinuses with associated epidural hematomas near the venous sinus (**Fig. 9**). Additionally, bridge vein thrombosis can be associated with secondary traumatic brain lesions such as the growth of subdural hematomas. This entity should also be considered in the setting of blunt head trauma and venous infarction, increased intracranial pressure, persistent headache, and seizure. MR imaging blood-sensitive sequences can show the bridge vein thrombosis as a tubular structure that blooms and has been described as a "tad-pole, lollipop, or tubular shape" structure. MR venography, TOF, and phase-contrast sequences may show the opacifying defect inside the venous sinus, representing thrombosis. CTA can be used concomitantly to evaluate arterial and venous injuries, depending on imaging timing. Treatment of these lesions must be carefully balanced due to the risk of enlargement of a traumatic hematoma versus thrombus expansion.[40–42]

MIMICS AND PITFALLS
Artifacts

CT beam hardening artifact is a streak-like artifact related to high-density material such as dental amalgams, bullet or metal fragments, spinal hardware, or high-density contrast in the venous system, which results in hypodense linear bands projected from the dense object resulting from photon starvation. Unfortunately, these artifacts are frequent and, in the case of dental amalgams, may obscure sites commonly affected by trauma, such as the skull base (see **Fig. 7**; **Fig. 10**).[7,15,42]

The motion of the carotid artery during the CT acquisition results in superimposition of the carotid density on adjacent structures, leading to a Venn diagram type of overlap appearance, known as a pulsation artifact. It can be visualized as irregularities in the contour of the vessel lumen or the appearance of linear flaplike filling defects on

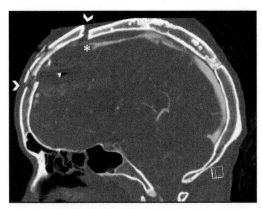

Fig. 9. Multiple skull fractures after a motor vehicle accident with venous thrombosis. Sagittal CTA venous phase image. There are numerous displaced skull fractures involving the frontal and parietal bones (*arrowheads*), with an opacifying defect representing a thrombus in the anterior portion of the superior sagittal sinus (*asterisk*).

reconstructed images, and mainly occur at the thoracic junction, where the carotid artery pulsatility is more marked, and in the common and internal carotid artery, where it lies immediately adjacent to the internal jugular vein.[8,15,42]

Suboptimal timing in the acquisition of images creates poor arterial enhancement obscuring vascular findings or delayed acquisitions creating venous contamination, particularly in the foraminal segments of the vertebral arteries. Patient motion-related artifacts can simulate a double lumen or obscure the vessels. DSA, iterative reconstructions, or open-mouth techniques might help visualize the vessels obscured by these artifacts.

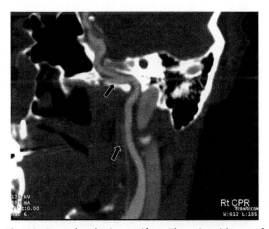

Fig. 10. Beam hardening artifact. There is evidence of streak like artifact (*black arrows*) in the cervical segment of the ICA secondary to dental amalgams, and at the lacerum segment of the ICA due to the skull base bone high density.

Dual-energy CT allows accurate subtraction segmentation, subtracting the non-enhanced images from the enhanced ones in a single acquisition allowing better pathology detection.[7,8,15,43]

Variants

Anatomic variants could simulate or mask an injury. Coiled or looped ICA segments could mimic focal outpouchings or low-grade BCVI lesions; multiplanar reconstructions are essential in differentiating these variants from an injury. Vertebral artery hypoplasia is a relatively common finding that may mimic a dissection or occlusion. Secondary findings aid in diagnosing this variant, such as a small transverse foramen, a diffusely small vertebral artery, or termination of the vertebral artery in posterior inferior cerebellar artery (PICA). ICA hypoplasia is uncommon, with an incidence rate of 0.13%; the presence of an asymmetric or absent carotid canal suggests this variant. Duplication or fenestration can emulate a double-lumen.[7,34]

Mimics

Atherosclerosis is a common condition that can be confused with a traumatic lesion, though consideration of several factors can help differentiate. First, the patient's age, as atherosclerosis mainly occurs in older patients, and second, the location, as atherosclerosis typically involves the carotid or vertebral origins, the outer wall of the carotid bulb, and the cavernous segment of the ICA. VWI and fat-suppressed T1-weighted imaging aid in differentiating between BCVI and atherosclerosis, as an intramural hematoma shows diffuse intrinsic T1 hyperintensity due to subacute hemorrhage compared with atherosclerotic plaques which show focal T1 hyperintensity from intraplaque hemorrhage.[3]

Fibromuscular dysplasia is a non-atherosclerotic, non-inflammatory condition that usually presents in young women and can be confused with dissection. There are alternating focal segments of stenosis and dilation in the internal carotid artery, giving an appearance of a "string of beads". Involvement of the renal arteries should suggest this pathology. Vasospasm is a frequent finding after severe trauma and can be challenging to differentiate from low-grade BCVI injuries; in cases where there is suspicion of vasospasm, follow-up luminal imaging may clarify, as vasospasm often resolves over hours.[7]

FOLLOW-UP

Imaging is considered necessary to determine treatment decision-making. CTA is regarded as the imaging modality of choice for follow-up of vascular injury as it has the highest yield in detecting injury change from the initial assessment. Recent studies have shown that follow-up CTA has the highest yield in treatment change if performed between the first 30 to 90 days after trauma and with no utility in management change if performed beyond 90 days. Imaging follow-up may be unnecessary in low and high-grade lesions because generally, there is no improvement or worsening of these lesions after that period of time.[44,45] VWI could be helpful in the follow-up of intramural hematomas and dissection and patients with equivocal findings on other cross-sectional imaging examinations.[46]

SUMMARY

Vascular injuries in head and neck trauma can present life-threatening emergencies that require a prompt and accurate diagnosis to prevent devastating sequelae. Clinical suspicion and early imaging evaluation are crucial, as timely management reduces the incidence of stroke and death. Although CTA remains the leading imaging technique and DSA remains the gold standard, newer techniques can help discern indeterminate findings, add value in follow-up, and direct treatment decisions.

CLINICS CARE POINTS

- Vascular injuries may be overlooked in the initial evaluation as they may present asymptomatically or due to the presence of more visible injuries in polytrauma.

- This can lead to a delay in prompt diagnosis and treatment.

- CTA and DSA are commonly used techniques, but newer techniques can also provide valuable information for follow-up and treatment decisions.

- Artifacts, variants and mimics of vascular injuries in the head and neck can lead to incorrect diagnosis, and must also be considered to avoid misinterpretation.

- Consideration of multimodality imaging techniques and follow-up scans are important to ensure accurate diagnosis.

DISCLOSURE

The authors have nothing to disclose.

REFERENCES

1. George E, Khandelwal A, Potter C, et al. Blunt traumatic vascular injuries of the head and neck in the ED. Emerg Radiol 2019;26(1):75–85.
2. Schneidereit NP, Simons R, Nicolaou S, et al. Utility of Screening for Blunt Vascular Neck Injuries with Computed Tomographic Angiography. J Trauma Inj Infect Crit Care 2006;60(1):209–16.
3. Sliker CW. Blunt Cerebrovascular Injuries: Imaging with Multidetector CT Angiography. Radiographics 2008;28(6):1689–708.
4. Esnault P, Cardinale M, Boret H, et al. Blunt cerebrovascular injuries in severe traumatic brain injury: incidence, risk factors, and evolution. J Neurosurg 2017;127(1):16–22.
5. Debette S, Leys D. Cervical-artery dissections: predisposing factors, diagnosis, and outcome. Lancet Neurol 2009;8(7):668–78.
6. Kohler R, Vargas MI, Masterson K, et al. CT and MR Angiography Features of Traumatic Vascular Injuries of the Neck. Am J Roentgenol 2011;196(6):W800–9.
7. Rutman AM, Vranic JE, Mossa-Basha M. Imaging and Management of Blunt Cerebrovascular Injury. Radiographics 2018;38(2):542–63.
8. Steenburg SD, Sliker CW, Shanmuganathan K, et al. Imaging Evaluation of Penetrating Neck Injuries. Radiographics 2010;30(4):869–86.
9. So TY, Sawhney A, Wang L, et al. Current Concepts in Imaging Diagnosis and Screening of Blunt Cerebrovascular Injuries. Tomography 2022;8(1):402–13.
10. Bromberg WJ, Collier BC, Diebel LN, et al. Blunt Cerebrovascular Injury Practice Management Guidelines: The Eastern Association for the Surgery of Trauma. J Trauma Inj Infect Crit Care 2010;68(2):471–7.
11. Osborn TM, Bell RB, Qaisi W, et al. Computed Tomographic Angiography as an Aid to Clinical Decision Making in the Selective Management of Penetrating Injuries to the Neck: A Reduction in the Need for Operative Exploration. J Trauma Inj Infect Crit Care 2008;64(6):1466–71.
12. Borsetto D, Fussey J, Mavuti J, et al. Penetrating neck trauma: radiological predictors of vascular injury. Eur Arch Oto-Rhino-Laryngol 2019;276(9):2541–7.
13. Munera F, Soto JA, Nunez D. Penetrating injuries of the neck and the increasing role of CTA. Emerg Radiol 2003;1(1):1.
14. Offiah C, Hall E. Imaging assessment of penetrating injury of the neck and face. Insights Imaging 2012;3(5):419–31.
15. Abu Mughli R, Wu T, Li J, et al. An Update in Imaging of Blunt Vascular Neck Injury. Can Assoc Radiol J 2020;71(3):281–92.
16. Roberts DJ, Chaubey VP, Zygun DA, et al. Diagnostic Accuracy of Computed Tomographic Angiography

for Blunt Cerebrovascular Injury Detection in Trauma Patients: A Systematic Review and Meta-Analysis. Ann Surg 2013;257(4):621–32.

17. Bodanapally UK, Dreizin D, Sliker CW, et al. Vascular Injuries to the Neck After Penetrating Trauma: Diagnostic Performance of 40- and 64-MDCT Angiography. Am J Roentgenol 2015;205(4):866–72.

18. Liang T, Tso DK, Chiu RYW, et al. Imaging of Blunt Vascular Neck Injuries: A Review of Screening and Imaging Modalities. Am J Roentgenol 2013;201(4):884–92.

19. Stallmeyer MJB, Morales RE, Flanders AE. Imaging of Traumatic Neurovascular Injury. Radiol Clin North Am 2006;44(1):13–39.

20. Adam G, Darcourt J, Roques M, et al. Standard Diffusion-Weighted Imaging in the Brain Can Detect Cervical Internal Carotid Artery Dissections. Am J Neuroradiol 2020;41(2):318–22.

21. Vranic JE, Huynh TJ, Fata P, et al. The ability of magnetic resonance black blood vessel wall imaging to evaluate blunt cerebrovascular injury following acute trauma. J Neuroradiol J Neuroradiol 2020;47(3):210–5.

22. Hunter MA, Santosh C, Teasdale E, et al. High-Resolution Double Inversion Recovery Black-Blood Imaging of Cervical Artery Dissection Using 3T MR Imaging. Am J Neuroradiol 2012;33(11):E133–7.

23. Edjlali M, Roca P, Rabrait C, et al. 3D Fast Spin-Echo T1 Black-Blood Imaging for the Diagnosis of Cervical Artery Dissection. Am J Neuroradiol 2013;34(9):E103–6.

24. Go JL, Acharya J, Branchcomb JC, et al. Traumatic Neck and Skull Base Injuries. Radiographics 2019;39(6):1796–807.

25. Yun SY, Heo YJ, Jeong HW, et al. Spontaneous intracranial vertebral artery dissection with acute ischemic stroke: High-resolution magnetic resonance imaging findings. NeuroRadiol J 2018;31(3):262–9.

26. Heldner MR, Nedelcheva M, Yan X, et al. Dynamic Changes of Intramural Hematoma in Patients with Acute Spontaneous Internal Carotid Artery Dissection. Int J Stroke 2015;10(6):887–92.

27. Habs M, Pfefferkorn T, Cyran CC, et al. Age determination of vessel wall hematoma in spontaneous cervical artery dissection: A multi-sequence 3T Cardiovascular Magnetic resonance study. J Cardiovasc Magn Reson 2011;13(1):76.

28. Uyeda JW, Anderson SW, Sakai O, et al. CT Angiography in Trauma. Radiol Clin North Am 2010;48(2):423–38.

29. Madhuripan N, Atar OD, Zheng R, et al. Computed Tomography Angiography in Head and Neck Emergencies. Semin Ultrasound CT MRI 2017;38(4):345–56.

30. Zheng Y, Lu Z, Shen J, et al. Intracranial Pseudoaneurysms: Evaluation and Management. Front Neurol 2020;11:582.

31. Berne JD, Reuland KR, Villarreal DH, et al. Internal Carotid Artery Stenting for Blunt Carotid Artery Injuries With an Associated Pseudoaneurysm. J Trauma Inj Infect Crit Care 2008;64(2):398–405.

32. Saad NEA, Saad WEA, Davies MG, et al. Pseudoaneurysms and the Role of Minimally Invasive Techniques in Their Management. Radiographics 2005;25(suppl_1):S173–89.

33. Al-Smadi AS, Abdalla RN, Elmokadem AH, et al. Diagnostic Accuracy of High-Resolution Black-Blood MRI in the Evaluation of Intracranial Large-Vessel Arterial Occlusions. Am J Neuroradiol 2019;40(6):954–9.

34. Liang T, Tso DK, Chiu RYW, et al. Imaging of Blunt Vascular Neck Injuries: A Clinical Perspective. Am J Roentgenol 2013;201(4):893–901.

35. Bernath MM, Mathew S, Kovoor J. Craniofacial Trauma and Vascular Injury. Semin Interv Radiol 2021;38(01):045–52.

36. Loggini A, Kass-Hout T, Awad IA, et al. Case Report: Management of Traumatic Carotid-Cavernous Fistulas in the Acute Setting of Penetrating Brain Injury. Front Neurol 2022;12:715955.

37. Larson PS, Abdulhadi B. Traumatic intracranial aneurysms. Neurosurg Focus 2000;8:6.

38. Niu Y, Zhou S, Tang J, et al. Treatment of traumatic intracranial aneurysm: Experiences at a single center. Clin Neurol Neurosurg 2020;189:105619.

39. Dubey A, Sung WS, Chen YY, et al. Traumatic intracranial aneurysm: A brief review. J Clin Neurosci 2008;15(6):609–12.

40. Delgado Almandoz JE, Kelly HR, Schaefer PW, et al. Prevalence of Traumatic Dural Venous Sinus Thrombosis in High-Risk Acute Blunt Head Trauma Patients Evaluated with Multidetector CT Venography. Radiology 2010;255(2):570–7.

41. Netteland DF, Mejlænder-Evjensvold M, Skaga NO, et al. Cerebral venous thrombosis in traumatic brain injury: a cause of secondary insults and added mortality. J Neurosurg 2021;134(6):1912–20.

42. Vilanilam GK, Jayappa S, Desai S, et al. Venous injury in pediatric abusive head trauma: a pictorial review. Pediatr Radiol 2021;51(6):918–26.

43. Postma AA, Das M, Stadler AAR, et al. Dual-Energy CT: What the Neuroradiologist Should Know. Curr Radiol Rep 2015;3(5):16.

44. Wu L, Christensen D, Call L, et al. Natural History of Blunt Cerebrovascular Injury: Experience Over a 10-year Period at a Level I Trauma Center. Radiology 2020;297(2):428–35.

45. Brommeland T, Helseth E, Aarhus M, et al. Best practice guidelines for blunt cerebrovascular injury (BCVI). Scand J Trauma Resusc Emerg Med 2018;26(1):90.

46. Bachmann R, Nassenstein I, Kooijman H, et al. High-Resolution Magnetic Resonance Imaging (MRI) at 3.0 Tesla in the Short-Term Follow-up of Patients With Proven Cervical Artery Dissection. Invest Radiol 2007;42(6):460–6.

Current Evaluation of Intracerebral Hemorrhage

Javier M. Romero, MD[a],*, Luisa F. Rojas-Serrano, MD[b]

KEYWORDS

- Intracerebral hemorrhage • Computed tomography • MRI • Digital subtraction angiography
- Multidetector computed tomography angiography • Stroke

KEY POINTS

- The prevalence of ICH in the US has increased by 11% in the last 15 years, largely due to increased usage of anticoagulant and antiplatelet medication.
- ICH is associated with the highest morbidity and mortality among patients with stroke.
- The rapid and accurate assessment of patients is clinically crucial, as re-bleeding and hematoma expansion can occur in up to 38% of ICH patients and increase the risk of a poorer prognosis.
- Multidetector CT angiography is highly sensitive in the detection of ICH vascular etiologies, as well as identifying the spot sign a biomarker of patient outcome.
- Determining early expansion has been the cornerstone of significant research in ICH; advanced imaging is able to predict with certain precision which hematomas will expand in the first 24 hours.

INTRODUCTION

Intracerebral hemorrhage (ICH) is associated with high morbidity and mortality worldwide.[1] This subtype of stroke accounts for 10% of all strokes each year in the United States.[2] ICH is a devastating disease that involves blood vessel rupture and subsequent bleeding within the brain parenchyma.[3] ICH is classified as either traumatic or spontaneous, the latter having an incidence of 10 to 30 per 100,000 population.[4] The prevalence of ICH in the United States has increased by 11% in the last 15 years, largely due to increased usage of anticoagulant and antiplatelet medication; therefore, imaging is crucial to screen high-risk patients promptly and accurately.[5]

Neuroradiological imaging is pivotal in determining the diagnosis of ICH through the exclusion of differential diagnoses and establishing the cause of the hematoma.[6] The cause of ICH can be classified into primary and secondary, where primary ICH accounts for 85% of all cases.[3] A primary bleed is typically due to small vessel disease, most commonly chronic hypertension (HTN), or cerebral amyloid angiopathy (CAA). Conversely, secondary ICH indicates underlying structural pathologic condition, such as a vascular malformation, neoplasm, or bleeding diathesis.[6] Imaging is critical for detecting this underlying pathologic condition because there are distinct therapeutic interventions contingent on the cause of the hematoma. The most effective imaging modalities for screening patients who present with ICH include computed tomography (CT), MR imaging, and digital subtraction angiography.[6] The rapid and accurate assessment of patients is clinically crucial because rebleeding and hematoma expansion can occur in up to 38% of patients with ICH and increase the risk of a poorer prognosis.[3]

Although highly effective treatments for ICH have not yet been developed, the detection of expansion has provided clinicians with valuable information regarding prognosis, hemostatic therapy, and palliative care measures.[7] Advanced imaging techniques such as assessing specific biomarkers on multidetector computed tomography angiography (MDCTA) and noncontrast computed tomography (NCCT) scans have

a Radiology Department, Massachusetts General Hospital, Harvard Medical School, 55 Fruit Street, Gray Building, 241G, MA 02114, USA; b Universidad del Rosario, Calle 12C No 6-25 - Bogotá, D.C. Colombia
* Corresponding author.
E-mail address: jmromero@mgh.harvard.edu

Radiol Clin N Am 61 (2023) 479–490
https://doi.org/10.1016/j.rcl.2023.01.005

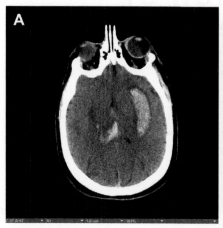
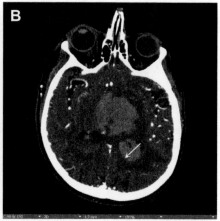

Fig. 1. (*A*) Axial noncontrast CT of the head demonstrates a left basal ganglia intraparenchymal hematoma, associated with a right thalamic hemorrhage. (*B*) Axial CT angiography of the head demonstrates a large intraparenchymal hematoma within the left thalamus with intraventricular extension (*arrow*).

allowed for the prediction of hematoma expansion.[8] Imaging has led to more effective diagnosis of ICH and consequent new trials to explore possible treatment plans.[2]

TYPES OF INTRACEREBRAL HEMORRHAGE

ICH can further be classified into primary and secondary.[9] Primary ICH accounts for 80% to 85% of ICH cases,[3] whereas secondary ICH accounts for 15% to 20% of all ICH.[10] Nilsson and colleagues[11] noted a mortality rate in primary ICH of 36% at 30 days and 47% in the 1-year follow-up. However, only 35% of arteriovenous malformation (AVM) ruptures result in complete recovery for survivors.[12]

PRIMARY

Primary ICH is the most common cause of spontaneous ICH[13] and occurs because of spontaneous rupture of small vessel damage caused by HTN and/or CAA.[14] The most common symptoms at presentation are sudden onset of focal neurological deficit, headache, nausea/vomiting, seizures, and elevation of the diastolic blood pressure.[3] The newest AHA guidelines for the management of patients with spontaneous ICH suggest that the appropriate diagnosis and assessment for this pathologic condition may contain a focused history, physical examination, and neuroimaging to confirm the diagnosis.[15]

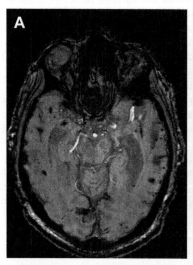
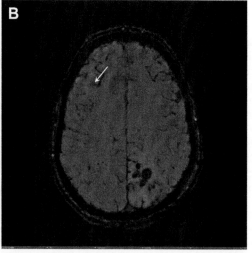

Fig. 2. (*A*) Axial susceptibility images demonstrate increased prevalence of microhemorrhage within the temporal and occipital lobes in CAA. (*B*) Axial susceptibility images demonstrate superficial siderosis within the right frontal lobe (*arrow*) and intraparenchymal hemorrhage within the left upper parietal lobule in a patient with CAA.

Uncontrolled HTN is the most common cause of primary ICH,[16] causing small vessel disease affecting most commonly the penetrating arteries of the basal ganglia (40%–50%; **Fig. 1**A), lobar regions (20%–50%), thalamus (10%–15%; **Fig. 1**B), pons (5%–12%), and cerebellum (5%–10%).[17] The second most frequent cause of primary ICH is CAA. This is a disease characterized by the accumulation of amyloid-beta peptides within the leptomeninges and small-to-medium-sized cortical vessels (**Fig. 2**A).[18] Contrary to the common sites of hemorrhage in primary HTN, CAA is often present in lobar ICH and subarachnoid hemorrhage (SAH)[17] (**Fig. 2**B).

Location of ICH is a predictor of the cause, where a superficial distribution is associated with CAA[19] and characterized by lobar and cortical microbleeds, superficial siderosis (see **Fig. 4**), and microinfarcts.[20] As well, SAH had a high sensitivity for CAA.[21]

Noncontrast Computed Tomography

NCCT, in this context, is most commonly used for the assessment of acute stroke, hemorrhage, and severe headaches.[22] NCCT is the study of choice in emergency settings due to its faster image acquisition, availability, sensitivity, and capability for the measurement of volume, mass effect, and cerebral edema. NCCT also provides differentiation between acute, subacute, or chronic hemorrhage,[9] further making it the gold standard in measuring hematoma volume.[23] ICH score is a clinical scale that allows clear communication of the type of hemorrhage but does not provide a risk stratification of ICH (**Table 1**).[24]

Multidetector Computed Tomography Angiography

MDCTA is highly sensitive in the detection of ICH vascular causes, as well as identifying the spot sign.[25] When compared with CTA, MDCTA allows for technical advantages in speed, volume coverage, and resolution.[26] MDCTA has been shown to accurately identify causes of secondary ICH.[7] In our hospital, it is currently used as the first-line of evaluation for ICH of unknown origin.

MDCTA utility is further illustrated in regards to the identification of the spot sign for the prediction of ICH expansion[27] (**Fig. 3**).

Magnetic Resonance Imaging

MR imaging is a powerful technique in the identification structural lesions causing ICH. High-resolution magnetic resonance image (HR-MRI) helps differentiate hypertensive ICH from CAA ICH by the location and distribution of microhemorrhage[4]

Table 1 ICH score	
Component	**Score**
Age	
>80	1
<80	0
Glasgow score	
3–4	2
5–12	1
13–15	0
ICH volume (cm³)	1
	0
IVH	
Yes	1
No	0
Infratentorial origin of ICH	
Yes	1
No	0
Total score	
0	0%
1	13%
2	26%
3	72%
4	97%
5–6	100%

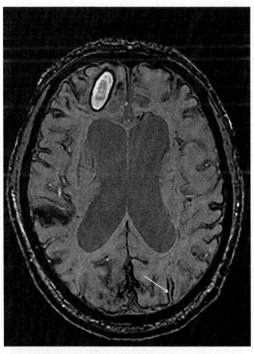

Fig. 3. Axial susceptibility image demonstrates a large intraparenchymal hematoma within the right frontal lobe associated with superficial siderosis (*arrow*).

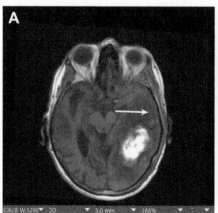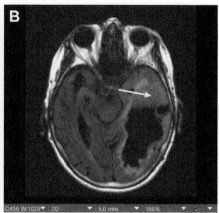

Fig. 4. (*A*) Axial T1-weighted demonstrates hemorrhages with 2 different chronology, a small hyperacute anterior temporal hemorrhage (*arrow*) isointense and a larger posterior subacute lesion with increased T1 signal. (*B*) Axial FLAIR shows the low signal of the most anterior hyperacute lesion (*arrow*) and the low signal of the more subacute lesion posteriorly.

(see **Fig. 2**A). These microhemorrhages on susceptibility-weighted images (SWIs) and gradient echo appear as low signal lesions.[4] Additionally, cortical superficial siderosis as another sign of CAA can be visualized as hypointense on SWI.[4] The presence of many cerebral microhemorrhages in MR imaging is associated with worse outcomes and higher mortality in CAA.[28] MR imaging has the ability to approximate the age of an ICH; for example, hyperacute ICH is visualized as isointense to hyperintense on DWI and T2-weighted image at the central core and as hypointense on DWI and T2 in the periphery (**Fig. 4**).[29]

Decision-making
It should be noted that although there are different options in the approach of a patient with ICH, the appropriate neuroimaging should be selected by considering the cost-effectiveness of each one of them (**Table 2**). However, cost-effectiveness studies are scarce in this field despite being an important area of research.[30]

Chaloui and colleagues[30] concluded that routine use of MR imaging/MRA should not be supported; instead, follow-up MR imaging could be recommended once the hemorrhage has resolved to detect underlying causes.

Secondary intracranial hemorrhage Secondary ICH is a hemorrhagic stroke that is caused by underlying pathologic condition related to structural abnormality, accounting for 15% of all ICH cases.[3] Risk factors for a secondary ICH include but are not limited to family history of vascular pathologic condition, male sex, cigarette smoking, excessive

Table 2
Appropriateness of imaging modality

	Indication
NCCT	First-line assessment[6]
MDCTA	First few hours to identify vascular cause and risk of subsequent ICH[15]
CTV	Cord sign or empty delta sign in NCCT for further evaluation of venous sinus thrombosis[4]
MR imaging	MR imaging is more accurate than CT in patients with acute and chronic ICH[7] without clear cause after an initial assessment with MDCTA[6]

Table 3
Clues in NCCT to identify secondary causes of intracerebral hemorrhage

Sign	Causes
Disproportionate peripheral edema	Metastasis High-grade primary tumor
Calcification/ phleboliths	AVM
Hyperdense tubular structures	AVM
Empty delta sign	Venous sinus thrombosis
Calcification with minimal peripheral edema	Cavernous malformation
Multiple ICH or fluid-fluid levels within the hemorrhage	Coagulopathy or anticoagulation

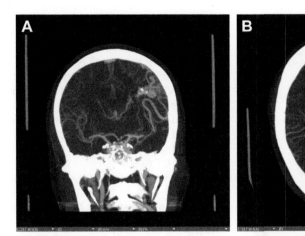

Fig. 5. (*A*) A coronal MPR of a CT angiography showing multiple abnormal tubular structures within the left frontal lobe, likely corresponding to an arteriovenous malformation. (*B*) Axial MPR of a CT angiogram demonstrating multiple tubular abnormalities representing "bag of worms."

alcohol consumption, sympathomimetic drug use, low-density lipoprotein cholesterol, metastatic lesions, recent ischemic infarct, and warfarin/aspirin use.[31] Although imaging findings do not always differ from one cause to the other, we will identify clues in this segment to detect secondary ICH causes (**Table 3**). Imaging is important in this case to determine the risk stratification for underlying vascular lesions and prevent recurrent hemorrhagic stroke.[7]

Vascular Malformations

Vascular malformations within the brain are altered intracranial vessels, which can be acquired or congenital.[32] An AVM causes an abnormal connection between the arterial and venous systems, without capillary exchange.[7,32] Vascular malformations pose a high risk for ICH because these abnormal vessel pathways are more likely to lead to rupture.[33] More specifically, developmental vascular abnormalities, dural arteriovenous fistulas, and cavernous malformations can all lead to secondary ICH, especially in patients aged younger than 45 years.

AVMs are the underlying cause for about 36% to 38% of all secondary ICH cases. The mortality rate for patients with ICH due to a ruptured AVM is about 12.9% as compared with other underlying causes that have a 29% mortality rate.[34]

CT and MR imaging are the most common imaging modalities for initial diagnosis, whereas an angiography remains the gold standard for diagnosis and treatment. On an NCCT, AVMs typically present as tubular hyperdense structures with focal hyperdense calcifications that may represent

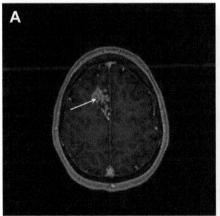
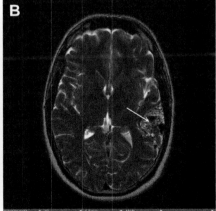

Fig. 6. (*A*) Axial MR imaging, T1 postcontrast shows multiple punctate foci of enhancement within the right frontal lobe (*arrow*), likely representing an arteriovenous malformation. (*B*) Axial MR imaging, T2-weighted images demonstrate multiple focal areas of low signal within the left temporal lobe (*arrow*) likely corresponding to flow voids from an arterial venous malformation.

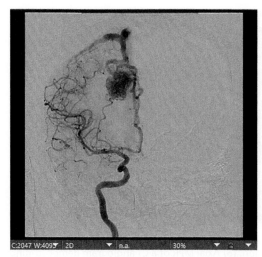

Fig. 7. AP view of the brain, conventional angiogram, demonstrating a nidus of vessels in the right frontal lobe, with feeders from the ACA and MCA and superficial venous drainage through the superior sagittal sinus.

phleboliths. AVMs on postcontrast imaging can easily delineate abnormal feeding arteries and draining veins, often presenting as serpiginous (bag of worms) in appearance (Fig. 5). On MR imaging, this condition will seem as tangled blood vessels with tubular voids, presenting on both T1 and, more prominently, on T2-weighted images (Fig. 6). An angiography allows for an exact recreation of the vessels and specific anatomy of the AVM, making it the gold standard for diagnosis and informing of potential interventions[35] (Fig. 7).

Dural arterial fistulas (DAVF) are vascular malformations that have abnormal vascular connections of the dural arteries with the venous bed, bypassing the brain parenchyma, which creates a fistulous connection. The hallmark finding of DAVF in angiography is the early filling of venous structures at the site of the fistula (Fig. 8). The incidence of DAVF among all AVMs ranges between 10% and 15%.[36] The gold standard for the detection of DAVF is the conventional angiogram due to its high temporal resolution. In a meta-analysis performed by Lin and colleagues,[37] comparison of CT and MR imaging in the detection of DAVF found a high sensitivity for both MR imaging (0.90) and CT (0.80).

A recent small review study evaluated the sensitivity of 4D CTA in the detection of DAVF and detected a sensitivity of 0.77 and a specificity of 1.0.[38]

DAVF are classified depending on the drainage pattern. Cognard classification is the most commonly used (Box 1) and shows a high correlation between rupture risk and clinical outcome.

Cavernous Malformation

Cerebral cavernous malformations (CCMs) are one of the most common vascular pathologic conditions in humans, accounting for 10% to 25% of all vascular abnormalities. CCMs are clusters of low-flow hyalinized capillaries without intervening brain parenchyma.[39] Although sporadic events do occur, 40% to 60% of CCM cases—and up to 50% of cases in Hispanic patients—are familial.[40] The majority of CCM are asymptomatic, with only 25% of cases presenting with ICH.[39] CCMs are often described in macro pathologic condition as "mulberry-like" in appearance, with well-circumscribed, multilobulated vascular lesions with no intervening neural tissue. On NCCT images, CCMs may present with calcification associated with minimal hemorrhage (Fig. 9).

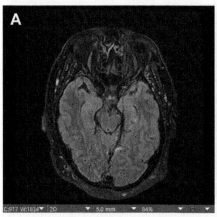
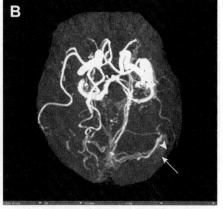

Fig. 8. (A) Axial FLAIR shows multiple enlarged venous structures in the subarachnoid space. (B) Axial 3D-TOF (three dimensional- time of flight) MRA of the brain demonstrates enlarged dural veins (arrow) with early draining into the left sigmoid sinus (arrow head).

CCMs are most easily diagnosed using MR imaging because these lesions have a characteristic hypointense border and hyperintense core on T2-weighted sequences and prominent blooming on graded-echo and SWIs.[41] CCMs have a typical popcorn-like appearance.

Neoplasms

Patients with cancer may present with ICH, typically due to intratumoral bleeding or coagulopathy.[42] Hemorrhage occurs in roughly 3% to 20% of brain metastases and 3% to 7% of primary cerebral gliomas. The most common metastatic hemorrhagic neoplasms are melanoma, renal cell carcinoma, thyroid carcinoma, and pulmonary carcinoma.[43] MR imaging is the most accurate radiological imaging for detecting underlying neoplasms. Research suggests that tumor-related hemorrhages can present with edema measuring more than or equal to the diameter of the hematoma on T2-weighted imaging.[44] Imaging of hemorrhagic neoplasms frequently show different chronological phases of blood product within the same lesion[25] (**Fig. 10**).

Aneurysms

Although most ruptured cerebral aneurysms cause SAHs, research has indicated incidence of up to 18% of patients with secondary ICH.[7] Of all intracranial aneurysms, roughly 20% are located in the middle cerebral artery (MCA; see **Fig. 13**), 50% of which typically lead to ICH if ruptured.[45] Specific radiological clues of ICH secondary to an underlying aneurysm include enlarged vessels or calcifications along the margins of the hematoma on a noncontrast CT image. Additionally, SAH adjacent to the circle of Willis or within the subarachnoid cisterns present a risk for an underlying aneurysm.[46]

Venous Infarction

Although cerebral venous thrombosis (CVT) only accounts for 0.5% of strokes, about one-third of all cases result in ICH. CVT is an occlusion of a cerebral vein or venous sinus due to thrombosis and most typically occurs in younger women, smokers, and those on birth control medications.

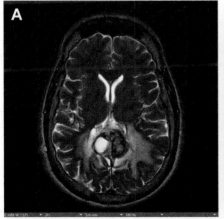 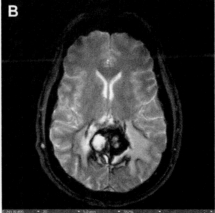

Fig. 9. (*A*) Axial T2-weighted image shows a multilobulated heterogeneous signal lesion in the splenium of the corpus callosum with a hypointense rim, representing a cavernous malformation. (*B*) Axial SWI of the same patient shows extensive peripheral susceptibility blooming of the cavernous malformation and adjacent superficial siderosis.

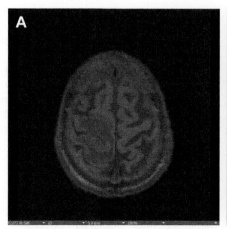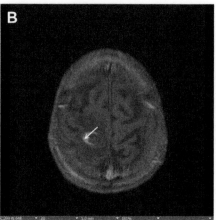

Fig. 10. (*A*) Axial T1-weighted precontrast shows a subacute hemorrhage in the right frontal lobe secondary to a cavernous malformation. (*B*) Axial T1-weighted postcontrast of the same patient demonstrates peripheral enhancement (*arrow*), which is a frequent finding after subacute hemorrhage.

Noncontrast CT imaging of CVT typically displays an "empty delta sign" of triangular enhancement surrounding a hypoattenuated area within either the superior sagittal sinus, straight sinus, or transverse sinus.[47] Additionally, the cord sign, or a hyper attenuation of the thrombosed sinus, is characteristic of CVT and can be appreciated on noncontrast CT imaging (**Fig. 11**). Coronal NCCT reconstructions are particularly helpful in this diagnosis because they provide a direct density comparison of the superior and both transverse sinuses. Research shows that MR imaging and MR venography are effective tools for the diagnosis of CVT because a lack of flow and visualization of the thrombosis can be appreciated[25,48]

(**Fig. 12A and B**). Susceptibility imaging also demonstrates high sensitivity detecting vascular thrombosis with significant low-signal intensity in the venous structure (**Fig. 12C**).[49]

Hemorrhagic Transformation of Ischemic Stroke

Patients might develop ICH through a hemorrhagic conversion of an ischemic stroke, largely spontaneously or due to thrombolytic therapy in order to treat the initial stroke. A hemorrhagic transformation typically occurs in 8% to 15% of ischemic stroke cases and can take the form of either a petechial or parenchymal hemorrhage.[50,51] Stroke patients that are administered anticoagulants are at increased risk of bleeding, typically within 1 to 3 days of the infarct.[25,50] CT imaging is favorable for detecting a hemorrhagic transformation because increased density may be noted at the lentiform nucleus and the insular ribbon when a MCA infarct is present[50] (**Fig. 13**). Larger sized infarcts increase the risk of hemorrhagic transformation.[52]

Coagulopathy

The prevalence of ICH in North America has increased by 11% in the last 15 years, largely due to increased usage of anticoagulant and antiplatelet medication; therefore, imaging is crucial to promptly and accurately screen high-risk patients.[5] Anticoagulant and antiplatelet medication have increased in order to account for the exceedingly high morbidity and mortality of stroke, specifically atrial fibrillation. However, the anticoagulatory nature of these medications puts patients at higher risk for hemorrhage.[53] Although

Fig. 11. NCCT with the cord sign in the right jugular bulb, representing a venous sinus thrombosis.

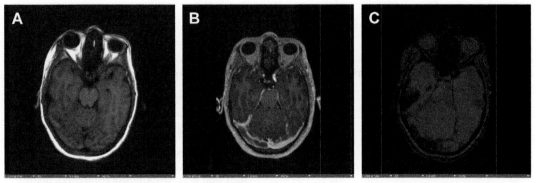

Fig. 12. (A) Axial T1-weighted image shows a hyperintense lesion in the right transverse sinus, likely representing thrombosis. (B) Axial T1 postcontrast image has a filling defect of the right transverse sinus representing thrombosis. (C) Axial SWI of the brain shows significant blooming of the right transverse sinus and cortical veins representing clot formation.

detecting this coagulopathy would be more effective through blood analysis and patient medical history assessment, CT scans of an ICH due to bleeding diathesis are more likely to present with multiple intracranial bleeding sites and fluid-fluid levels.[54]

Advanced imaging in the prediction of intracerebral hemorrhage expansion and clinical outcome

Clinically significant ICH expansion has been determined in various trials as an enlargement of at least 6 mL or 33% of the initial volume. Delgado and colleagues[55] developed and validated the secondary intracerebral hemorrhage (SICH) score, which predicts the risk of a patient with ICH due to underlying vascular cause. It requires NCCT, age,

sex, history of HTN, use of antiplatelet medication, platelet count, INR, and aPTT information.[56]

The first multicenter prospective trial validating the spot sign as a predictor of hematoma expansion was the PREDICT trial that determined the value of this sign in predicting clinically significant expansion.[57] Our laboratory validated these results in a single-center trial that also included a score that increased the specificity of the spot sign.[58,59]

A 90-second delay acquisition demonstrated an increased sensitivity to predict expanders, permitting longer circulation of contrast and improved depiction of the spot sign.[60] Multiple imaging characteristics have been discovered on NCCT and CTA to predict hemorrhage expansion, with high sensitivity and specificity (**Table 4**).

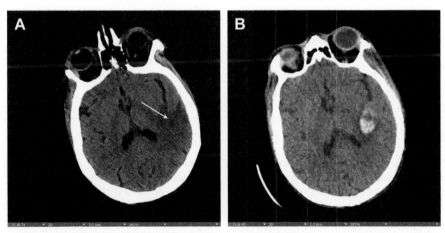

Fig. 13. (A) Axial noncontrast CT of the head demonstrates a wedge-shaped area of low attenuation in the posterior left insular and superior temporal gyrus (arrow), likely representing an acute infarction. (B) Axial noncontrast CT of the head shows a hemorrhagic transformation of the previously noted left MCA stroke.

Table 4
Predictors of intracerebral hemorrhage expansion

	Expansion Measurement	Other Signs
NCCT	Baseline hematoma volume: using ABC/2[6]	• Island signs: specificity of 98.2%[61] • Satellite sign: sensitivity of 54.0% and specificity of 94.0%[61] • Blend sign: specificity (95.5%)[61] • Black hole sign: sensitivity of 30% and specificity of 91%[61] • Hypodensities: sensitivity of 60% and specificity of 78%. With a greater specificity using spot sign and hypodensity combined, being 93%[62]
CTA	Spot sign: with a sensitivity of 62% and specificity 88%[27]	

CLINICS CARE POINTS

- MD-CTA is the first line of evaluation of ICH to detect secondary etiologies of ICH.
- The spot sign score has been proven to be an accurate biomarker for future hematoma expansion and is currently used in multiple trials as a predictor of ICH expansion.
- Early detection of vascular malformations or aneurysms is essential in managing patients with ICH in the intensive care unit.
- MRI and susceptibility weighted imaging have demonstrated high sensitivity in detecting cavernous malformations, vascular malformations, tumors, and stigmata of cerebral amyloid angiopathy.

DECLARATION OF INTERESTS

The authors have nothing to disclose.

ACKNOWLEDGMENTS

Christina Younan, Major in Neuroscience, Boston University, cyounan@bu.edu.

REFERENCES

1. Ziai WC, Carhuapoma, Ricardo J. Intracerebral Hemorrhage. Continuum (Minneap Minn) 2018. https://doi.org/10.1212/CON.0000000000000672.
2. Greenberg SM, Ziai WC, Cordonnier C, et al. 2022 guideline for the management of patients with spontaneous intracerebral hemorrhage: a guideline from the american heart association/american stroke association. Stroke 2022;53(7):e282–361.
3. Rajashekar D, Liang JW. Intracerebral Hemorrhage - StatPearls - NCBI Bookshelf 2022. Available at: https://www.ncbi.nlm.nih.gov/books/NBK553103/. Accessed June 28, 2022.
4. Jain A, Malhotra A, Payabvash S. Imaging of spontaneous intracerebral hemorrhage. Neuroimaging Clin N Am 2021;31(2):193–203.
5. Bako AT, Pan A, Potter T, et al. Contemporary trends in the nationwide incidence of primary intracerebral hemorrhage. Stroke 2022;29(2):E70–4.
6. Sporns PB, Psychogios MN, Boulouis G, et al. Neuroimaging of acute intracerebral hemorrhage. J Clin Med 2021;10(5):1–13.
7. Delgado Almandoz JE, Romero JM. Advanced CT imaging in the evaluation of hemorrhagic stroke. Neuroimaging Clin N Am 2011;21(2):197–213.
8. Morotti A, Boulouis G, Dowlatshahi D, et al. Standards for detecting, interpreting, and reporting noncontrast computed tomographic markers of intracerebral hemorrhage expansion. Ann Neurol 2019;86(4):480–92.
9. Jain A, Malhotra A, Payabvash S. Imaging of Spontaneous Intracerebral Hemorrhage. Neuroimaging Clin N Am 2022;31(2):193–203.
10. Macellari F, Paciaroni M, Agnelli G, et al. Neuroimaging in intracerebral hemorrhage. Stroke 2014;45(3):903–8.
11. Nilsson OG, Lindgren A, Brandt L, et al. Prediction of death in patients with primary intracerebral hemorrhage: a prospective study of a defined population. J Neurosurg 2002;97:531–6.
12. Karlsson B, Jokura H, Yang HC, et al. Clinical outcome following cerebral AVM hemorrhage. Acta Neurochir 2020;162(7):1759–66.
13. Schrag M, Kirshner H. Management of Intracerebral Hemorrhage: JACC Focus Seminar. J Am Coll Cardiol 2020;75(15):1819–31.
14. Kahan J, Ong H, Ch'ang J, et al. Comparing hematoma characteristics in primary intracerebral

hemorrhage versus intracerebral hemorrhage caused by structural vascular lesions. J Clin Neurosci 2022;99:5–9.

15. Greenberg SM, Ziai WC, Cordonnier C, et al. 2022 Guideline for the Management of Patients With Spontaneous Intracerebral Hemorrhage: A Guideline From the American Heart Association/American Stroke Association. Stroke 2022;53(7). https://doi.org/10.1161/STR.0000000000000407.

16. Hong D, Stradling D, Dastur CK, et al. Resistant hypertension after hypertensive intracerebral hemorrhage is associated with more medical interventions and longer hospital stays without affecting outcome. Front Neurol 2017;8(MAY):184.

17. Dastur CK, Yu W. Current management of spontaneous intracerebral haemorrhage. Stroke Vasc Neurol 2017;2(1):21–9.

18. Kuhn J, Sharman T. Cerebral Amyloid Angiopathy - StatPearls - NCBI Bookshelf 2021. Available at: https://www.ncbi.nlm.nih.gov/books/NBK556105/. Accessed June 28, 2022.

19. Pasi M, Pongpitakmetha T, Charidimou A, et al. Cerebellar microbleed distribution patterns and cerebral amyloid angiopathy: a MRI and pathology-based study. Stroke 2019;50(7):1727.

20. Charidimou A, Boulouis G, Gurol ME, et al. Emerging concepts in sporadic cerebral amyloid angiopathy. Brain 2017;140(7):1829–50.

21. Baron JC, Boulouis G, Benzakoun J, et al. Cerebral amyloid angiopathy-related acute lobar intracerebral hemorrhage: diagnostic value of plain CT. J Neurol 2022;269(4):2126–32.

22. Magadán A. Neuroimaging of Hypertension and Related Cerebral Pathology. In: Hypertension and Stroke. Springer International Publishing; 2016. p. 315–42. https://doi.org/10.1007/978-3-319-29152-9_18.

23. Ovesen C, Havsteen I, Rosenbaum S, et al. Prediction and observation of post-admission hematoma expansion in patients with intracerebral hemorrhage. Front Neurol 2014. https://doi.org/10.3389/fneur.2014.00186.

24. Hemphill JC, Bonovich DC, Besmertis L, et al. The ICH Score. Stroke 2001;32(4):891–6.

25. Romero JM, Rosand J. Hemorrhagic cerebrovascular disease. Handb Clin Neurol 2016;135:351–64. https://doi.org/10.1016/B978-0-444-53485-9.00018-0. Elsevier B.V.

26. Yoon DY, Chang SK, Choi CS, et al. Multidetector row CT angiography in spontaneous lobar intracerebral hemorrhage: a prospective comparison with conventional angiography. AJNR Am J Neuroradiol 2009;30(5):962.

27. Xu X, Zhang J, Yang K, et al. Accuracy of spot sign in predicting hematoma expansion and clinical outcome: a meta-analysis. Medicine 2018;97(34). https://doi.org/10.1097/MD.0000000000011945.

28. Martinez-Ramirez S, Greenberg SM, Viswanathan A. Cerebral microbleeds: overview and implications in cognitive impairment. Alzheimer's Res Ther 2014; 6(3). https://doi.org/10.1186/ALZRT263.

29. Iftikhar S, Rossi N, Goyal N, et al. Magnetic resonance imaging characteristics of hyperacute intracerebral hemorrhage. J Vasc Interv Neurol 2016; 9(2):10. Accessed June 29, 2022./pmc/articles/ PMC5094255/.

30. Chalouhi N, Mouchtouris N, Saiegh F al, et al. Analysis of the utility of early MRI/MRA in 400 patients with spontaneous intracerebral hemorrhage. J Neurosurg 2020;132(6):1865–71.

31. Boden-Albala B, Braun LT, Bravata DM, et al. Guidelines for the primary prevention of stroke a statement for healthcare professionals from the american heart association/american stroke association Council on Cardiovascular and Stroke Nursing, Council on Clinical Cardiology, Council on Functional Genomics and Translational Biology, and Council on Hypertension. Stroke 2014. https://doi.org/10.1161/STR.0000000000000046/-/DC1.

32. Whitehead KJ, Smith MCP, Li DY. Arteriovenous malformations and other vascular malformation syndromes. Cold Spring Harb Perspect Med 2013; 3(2). https://doi.org/10.1101/cshperspect.a006635.

33. Zyck S, Gould GC. Cavernous Venous Malformation. 2022 May 9. In: StatPearls [Internet]. Treasure Island (FL): StatPearls Publishing; 2022 Jan -. PMID: 30252265.

34. Murthy SB, Merkler AE, Omran SS, et al. Outcomes after intracerebral hemorrhage from arteriovenous malformations. Neurology 2017 May 16;88(20): 1882–8. https://doi.org/10.1212/WNL.0000000000 0003935. Epub 2017 Apr 19. PMID: 28424275; PMCID: PMC5444313.

35. Bokhari MR, Bokhari SRA. Arteriovenous Malformation Of The Brain. 2022 Sep 6. In: StatPearls [Internet]. Treasure Island (FL): StatPearls Publishing; 2022 Jan. PMID: 28613495.

36. Kwon BJ, Han MH, Kang HS. MR imaging findings of intracranial dural arteriovenous fistulas: relations with venous drainage patterns. AJNR Am J Neuroradiol 2005 Nov-Dec;26(10):2500–7. PMID: 16286391; PMCID: PMC7976221.

37. Lin YH, Wang YF, Liu HM, et al. Diagnostic accuracy of CTA and MRI/MRA in the evaluation of the cortical venous reflux in the intracranial dural arteriovenous fistula DAVF. Neuroradiology 2018;60(1):7–15.

38. Biswas S, Chandran A, Radon M, et al. Accuracy of four-dimensional CT angiography in detection and characterisation of arteriovenous malformations and dural arteriovenous fistulas. NeuroRadiol J 2015;28(4):376–84.

39. Caton MT, Shenoy VS. Cerebral Cavernous Malformations. [Updated 2022 Oct 3]. In: StatPearls [Internet]. Treasure Island (FL): StatPearls

Publishing; 2022. Available from: https://www.ncbi.nlm.nih.gov/books/NBK538144/.

40. Jenson AV, Rodriguez GJ, Alvarado LA, et al. Higher Rate of Intracerebral Hemorrhage in Hispanic Patients with Cerebral Cavernous Malformation. J Vasc Interv Neurol 2015 Oct;8(4):1–4. PMID: 26600922; PMCID: PMC4634773.

41. Wang KY, Idowu OR, Lin DDM. Radiology and imaging for cavernous malformations. Handb Clin Neurol 2017;143:249–66. Elsevier B.V.

42. Velander AJ, DeAngelis LM, Navi BB. Intracranial Hemorrhage in patients with cancer. Curr Atheroscler Rep 2012;14(4):373–81.

43. Ostrowski RP, He Z, Pucko EB, et al. Hemorrhage in brain tumor – An unresolved issue. Brain Hemorrhages 2022;3(2):98–102.

44. Tung GA, Julius BD, Rogg JM. MRI of intracerebral hematoma: value of vasogenic edema ratio for predicting the cause. Neuroradiology. 2003 Jun;45(6):357-62. https://doi.org/10.1007/s00234-003-0994-0. Epub 2003 May 8. PMID: 12736768.

45. Shim YS, Moon CT, Chun Y il, et al. Grading of intracerebral hemorrhage in ruptured middle cerebral artery aneurysms. J Korean Neurosurg Soc 2012;51(5):268–71.

46. Yoon DY, Lim KJ, Choi CS, et al. Detection and characterization of intracranial aneurysms with 16-channel multidetector row CT angiography: a prospective comparison of volume-rendered images and digital subtraction angiography. Am J Neuroradiol 2007;28:60–7. Available at: www.ajnr.org.

47. Canedo-Antelo M, Baleato-González S, Mosqueira AJ, et al. Radiologic clues to cerebral venous thrombosis. Radiographics 2019;39(6):1611–28.

48. Saposnik G, Barinagarrementeria F, Brown RD Jr, Bushnell CD, Cucchiara B, Cushman M, deVeber G, Ferro JM, Tsai FY. American Heart Association Stroke Council and the Council on Epidemiology and Prevention. Diagnosis and management of cerebral venous thrombosis: a statement for healthcare professionals from the American Heart Association/American Stroke Association. Stroke 2011 Apr;42(4):1158–92. https://doi.org/10.1161/STR.0b013e31820a8364. Epub 2011 Feb 3. PMID: 21293023.

49. Haacke EM, Mittal S, Wu Z, et al. Susceptibility-weighted imaging: Technical aspects and clinical applications, part 1. Am J Neuroradiol 2009;30(1):19–30.

50. Zhang J, Yang Y, Sun H, et al. Hemorrhagic transformation after cerebral infarction: Current concepts and challenges. Ann Transl Med 2014;2(8). https://doi.org/10.3978/j.issn.2305-5839.2014.08.08.

51. Unnithan AKA, M Das J, Mehta P. Hemorrhagic Stroke. 2022 Sep 30. In: StatPearls [Internet]. Treasure Island (FL): StatPearls Publishing; 2022 Jan -. PMID: 32644599.

52. Álvarez-Sabín J, Maisterra O, Santamarina E, et al. Factors influencing haemorrhagic transformation in ischaemic stroke. Lancet Neurol 2013;12(7):689–705.

53. Morgan A, Joshy G, Schaffer A, et al. Rapid and substantial increases in anticoagulant use and expenditure in Australia following the introduction of new types of oral anticoagulants. PLoS One 2018;13(12). https://doi.org/10.1371/journal.pone.0208824.

54. Uglietta JP, O'Connor CM, Boyko OB, Aldrich H, Massey EW, Heinz ER. CT patterns of intracranial hemorrhage complicating thrombolytic therapy for acute myocardial infarction. Radiology 1991 Nov;181(2):555–9. https://doi.org/10.1148/radiology.181.2.1924804. PMID: 1924804.

55. Delgado Almandoz JE, Schaefer PW, Goldstein JN, et al. Practical scoring system for the identification of patients with intracerebral hemorrhage at highest risk of harboring an underlying vascular etiology: the secondary intracerebral hemorrhage score. Am J Neuroradiol 2010;31(9):1653–60.

56. Delgado Almandoz JE, Schaefer PW, Goldstein JN, et al. Editor's Choice: Practical Scoring System for the Identification of Patients with Intracerebral Hemorrhage at Highest Risk of Harboring an Underlying Vascular Etiology: The Secondary Intracerebral Hemorrhage Score. AJNR Am J Neuroradiol 2010;31(9):1653.

57. Demchuk AM, Dowlatshahi D, Rodriguez-Luna D, et al. Prediction of haematoma growth and outcome in patients with intracerebral haemorrhage using the CT-angiography spot sign (PREDICT): a prospective observational study. Lancet Neurol 2012;11(4):307–14.

58. Brouwers HB, Chang Y, Falcone GJ, et al. Predicting hematoma expansion after primary intracerebral hemorrhage. JAMA Neurol 2014;71(2):158–64.

59. Delgado Almandoz JE, Yoo AJ, Stone MJ, et al. Systematic characterization of the computed tomography angiography spot sign in primary intracerebral hemorrhage identifies patients at highest risk for hematoma expansion: the spot sign score. Stroke 2009;40(9):2994–3000.

60. Ciura VA, Brouwers HB, Pizzolato R, et al. Spot sign on 90-second delayed computed tomography angiography improves sensitivity for hematoma expansion and mortality: prospective study. Stroke 2014;45(11):3293–7.

61. Lv XN, Deng L, Yang WS, et al. Computed tomography imaging predictors of intracerebral hemorrhage expansion. Curr Neurol Neurosci Rep 2021;21(5):1–8.

62. Morotti A, Boulouis G, Charidimou A, et al. Integration of computed tomographic angiography spot sign and noncontrast computed tomographic hypodensities to predict hematoma expansion. Stroke 2018;49(9):2067.

Vessel Wall Imaging in Cryptogenic Stroke

Bhagya Sannananja, MD[a], Chengcheng Zhu, PhD[b], Mahmud Mossa-Basha, MD[b],*

KEYWORDS

- Stroke • Cryptogenic stroke • Embolic stroke of undetermined source • Vessel wall imaging

KEY POINTS

- Vessel wall imaging has value in the evaluation of various vascular pathologies.
- Vessel wall imaging can detect and differentiate non-stenotic vascular lesions that may elude conventional luminal imaging techniques.
- Vessel wall imaging combined with conventional vascular imaging may elucidate etiologies of cryptogenic stroke and help direct secondary stroke prevention.

INTRODUCTION

Stroke is one of the leading causes of death and long-term disability worldwide.[1] The Trial of Org 10172 in Acute Stroke Treatment (TOAST), first published in 1993, classified ischemic strokes into 5 subtypes based on etiology: large-artery atherosclerosis, cardioembolic disease, small-vessel disease, other determined etiology, and in 10% to 40%, no etiology can be identified after a standard diagnostic evaluation, termed cryptogenic stroke (CS).[2] CS constitutes a significant percentage of total stroke cases and since the etiology remains unknown, no evidence-based targeted therapy can be instituted, which puts them at higher risk of recurrent stroke.

Multiple additional etiologic classification systems for IS have been proposed including embolic stroke of undetermined source (ESUS). ESUS includes non-lacunar infarcts without atherosclerosis causing ≥50% stenosis in arteries supplying the ischemic territory, no cardioembolic source or any other etiology,[3] and accounts for 17% of all IS. Occult atrial fibrillation was thought to represent the primary etiology for ESUS, however, there is evidence to suggest ESUS is a heterogeneous group with multiple potential etiologies beyond atrial fibrillation, including <50%-stenotic atherosclerosis affecting the aortic arch, cervical, and intracranial arteries.

In current practice, luminal imaging such as computed tomography angiography (CTA), MRA or digital subtraction angiography (DSA) are used for stroke etiology, but provide little information of vessel wall abnormalities, whereas vessel wall imaging (VWI) directly visualizes the vessel wall and has shown its value in intra- and extra-cranial vasculopathy assessment.[4,5] In this article, we review the role of VWI in the diagnostic workup of CS.

CONVENTIONAL VASCULAR IMAGING IN ISCHEMIC STROKE

Conventional arterial evaluation of head, neck, and proximal aorta is typically performed with CTA or MRA. Both CTA and MRA, however, have several limitations. Beam hardening artifacts can result from high-density materials including dense calcifications, hardware, dental amalgam, arterial or venous stents, or even highly concentrated iodinated contrast material in the veins that can impede

---

[a] Department of Radiology and Imaging Sciences, Emory University School of Medicine, 1364 Clifton Road Northeast Suite BG20, Atlanta, GA 30322, USA; [b] Department of Radiology, University of Washington School of Medicine, 1959 NE Pacific St, Seattle, WA 98195, USA

* Corresponding author. Department of Radiology, University of Washington School of Medicine, 1959 NE Pacific St, Seattle, WA 98195, USA

E-mail address: mmssab@uw.edu

Twitter: @mossabas (M.M.-B.)

Radiol Clin N Am 61 (2023) 491–500

https://doi.org/10.1016/j.rcl.2023.01.006

the assessment of cervical arteries on CTA. Non-contrast TOF-MRA can overestimate the degree of stenosis with high-grade stenosis secondary to flow dephasing and may be insensitive to slow or in-plane flow.[6,7] Both CTA and MRA are limited for <50%/non-stenotic lesion detection, including intracranial atherosclerotic disease (ICAD) with outward remodeling,[7] that can be the source of ischemia. Another drawback of luminal imaging is the lack of specificity in vasculopathy differentiation,[8] as several vasculopathies present with similar patterns of stenosis and may be impossible to distinguish.[4,5]

VESSEL WALL IMAGING

VWI techniques have increasingly shown utility in the diagnosis and characterization of various vascular pathologies compared with conventional imaging. A survey of the American Society of Neuroradiology (ASNR) membership showed more than half of respondents were performing intracranial VWI, with 71.5% performing it >1 to 2 times per month.[9] ICAD is the most common cause of ischemic stroke worldwide, but due to its proclivity to outwardly remodel, is frequently underestimated, both in terms of disease burden and stroke etiology.[10–17] In addition, other less common stroke etiologies may be non-stenosing, and may be difficult to diagnose or detect with conventional imaging techniques.[18–22] The value of carotid plaque characteristics on VWI, in associating with current stroke and predicting future strokes above luminal imaging has been established in the literature.[23]

VESSEL WALL IMAGING TECHNIQUES

Multiple studies have established VWI as a reliable technique to characterize carotid atherosclerotic plaque morphology and composition.[23–25] The ASNR VWI study group recommends in-plane resolution of at least 0.6 mm and through-plane resolution of 2 mm centered on the carotid bifurcation for plaque imaging.[25] Carotid phased-array coils can be used and will improve SNR but may not be necessary.[26] Three-dimensional (3D) acquisitions enable high-resolution images and multiplanar reconstructions with isotropic acquisitions, whereas 2D acquisitions are susceptible to partial volume averaging and longer scan times. Contrast administration enables improved detection of LRNC and fibrous cap (FC) evaluation and is recommended if there are no contraindications.[25]

Intracranial VWI is technically more challenging given the smaller caliber and tortuous intracranial arteries.[8,27] 3D variable-refocusing flip-angle (VRFA) sequences with intrinsic black blood properties are the most commonly used 3D techniques.[27] VRFA techniques have vendor-specific names: SPACE (Siemens Healthineers, Erlangen, Germany), VISTA (Philips Healthcare, Best, the Netherlands), and CUBE (GE Healthcare, Milwaukee, Wisconsin).[28–30] Recent technical advances have focused on imaging acceleration and preparation pulses for blood and CSF suppression.[31–34] Sannananja and colleagues[32] showed significant improvement in image quality, including blood suppression and artifact extent, with the incorporation of DANTE blood- and CSF-suppression or DANTE and CAIPI T1-SPACE as compared with conventional T1-SPACE.

CAROTID ATHEROSCLEROSIS

Stroke risk assessment based on the degree of stenosis is not sufficient; plaque morphology and composition is beneficial in the management of asymptomatic and symptomatic atherosclerosis (Fig. 1).[35] A meta-analysis (n = 18304 patients) reported prevalence of 51% non-stenotic carotid plaques in patients with acute IS/TIA (95% confidence interval [CI] = 43 to 59) and the prevalence was slightly higher (55%) among patients with ESUS (95% CI = 42 to 68).[35] Non-stenotic carotid plaques were present in 39.1% (54/138) of patients with ESUS in the INTERRSeCT study and were significantly more common ipsilateral to IS compared with contralateral (60.6% vs 29.2%, p = 0.004).[36] Another meta-analysis (n = 323 patients) reported patients with ESUS had a higher prevalence of non-stenotic carotid atherosclerosis with high-risk plaque (HRP) features in the ipsilateral carotid compared with the contralateral side (32.5% vs 4.6%, 95% CI = 0.1 to 13.1).[37]

Increasing evidence supports carotid plaque VWI for assessment of CS/ESUS. The CARE II study (n = 1047) found HRPs were 1.5 times more prevalent than severe (≥50%) luminal stenosis ipsilateral to IS (28% vs 19%).[38] In addition, 56% of HRPs were identified in arteries with <50% stenosis suggesting VWI may be more useful in risk stratification than luminal imaging.[38] Recurrent strokes/TIA were significantly more frequent in CS patients with HRPs identified on baseline VWI than those without (10.92 vs 1.82 per 100 patient-years; p = 0.003),[39] specifically, ruptured FC (hazard ratio [HR] = 4.91; 95% CI = 1.31 to 18.45) or IPH (HR = 4.37; 95% CI = 1.20 to 15.97). The European Society for Vascular Surgery and the European Society of Cardiology incorporated plaque morphology assessment as part of the optimal management of asymptomatic patients.

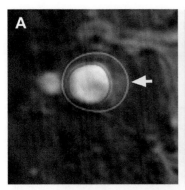 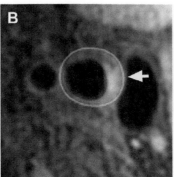 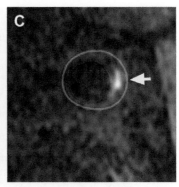

Fig. 1. Stroke with non-stenotic plaque. Axial TOF-MRA (*A*) shows non-stenotic carotid plaque, with outer wall thickening (*short arrow*). Axial T1-weighted VWI pre-contrast (*B*) shows outward remodeling plaque (*short arrow*) with vague internal T1 hyperintensity, whereas on axial T1-MPRAGE (*C*), plaque hyperintensity (*short arrow*) is more defined, more clearly representing intraplaque hemorrhage.

IPH is a key plaque vulnerability feature and is likely due to intraplaque neovessels and/or FC rupture. IPH is the strongest clinical predictor of ischemic stroke. Schindler and colleagues[40] found IPH increased the risk of future ipsilateral stroke in patients with both symptomatic and asymptomatic carotid stenosis, with hazard ratios of 10.2 and 7.9, respectively. Mark and colleagues[41] reported the odds of having IPH ipsilateral to the IS compared with contralateral was 6.92 (95% CI = 3.04 to 15.79) in 354 patients with ESUS. Kopzack and colleagues[39] found ipsilateral IPH had a 4.4-fold increased risk of recurrent IS or TIA compared with those without. MPRAGE is most used for IPH detection with the sensitivity of 80% and specificity of 97% compared with histology and has higher accuracy for IPH than 2D T1-TSE and TOF-MRA (see **Fig. 1**).[42]

LRNC is heterogeneous tissue composed of necrotic debris, apoptotic cells, cholesterol, and cholesteryl esters.[23] Percentage plaque volume of LRNC is significantly larger in plaques ipsilateral to CS (20 ± 23) compared with cardioembolic or small vessel stroke (11 ± 18, $p < 0.05$),[43] with LRNC volume associated with outward remodeling. LRNC appears hypointense on T2-weighted imaging, isointense on proton-density, and does not enhance appreciably.[44]

FC separates thrombogenic plaque components from flowing blood and is composed of fibrous connective tissue, smooth muscles, and macrophages,[23] which when ruptured triggers surface thrombus formation and subsequent thromboembolism. Intact FC is seen as an enhancing juxtaluminal band on post-contrast T1-weighted VWI, with a smooth surface, whereas a thin intact FC shows loss of that enhancing band but with preserved smooth luminal surface. A ruptured FC shows a disrupted or dark band on post-contrast VWI with an irregular luminal surface.[25] Thinning and rupture of the FC (TRFC) increases ischemic stroke risk by sixfold.[25] Multisequence MR imaging has high sensitivity and specificity (0.81 and 0.90, respectively) for FC status compared with histopathology.[45] Unlike luminal imaging, VWI can distinguish between thick and thinned FC, as thinning is also associated with increased future stroke/TIA risk.

EXTRACRANIAL ARTERIAL INJURY

Craniocervical dissection accounts for 20% of stroke in patients under 45 years of age, and can be subadventitial, subintimal, or both in location of wall involvement.[20] 8.5% of blunt cerebrovascular injuries (BCVI) have associated stroke, with higher-grade injuries, carotid injuries and multiple arterial injuries in a patient were associated with higher likelihood of stroke.[22] The classic imaging findings include the presence of luminal stenosis secondary to intramural hemorrhage and/or the presence of a false lumen and dissection flap. On VWI, the dissection flap can be accurately depicted, in addition to visualization to wall hematoma, regardless of the presence or absence of stenosis (**Fig. 2**). Subadventitial dissections without luminal stenosis may not be detectable on luminal imaging (CTA, MRA, or DSA).[21] Vranic and colleagues[21] found that VWI had significantly higher agreement with expert consensus review for the diagnosis of BCVI, compared with CTA with expert consensus review (κ = 0.86 vs 0.36). This difference only increased when considering indeterminate findings on CTA, where VWI can clarify presence or absence of a lesion.

INTRACRANIAL ATHEROSCLEROSIS

ICAD is the leading cause of stroke worldwide.[29] Conventional luminal imaging techniques use

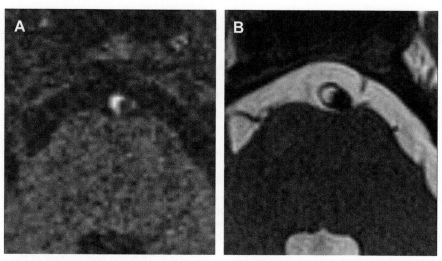

Fig. 2. Non-stenotic dissection. Axial T1-weighted (*A*) and T2-weighted (*B*) VWI show crescentic T1 and T2 hyperintense intramural blood, representing dissection.

stenosis as a surrogate for the identification of ICAD, frequently underestimating its true prevalence.[16] Results of the cadaveric Brain Arterial Remodeling Study showed advanced ICAD changes in greater than 40% of their study population in the absence of significant luminal stenosis.[46] Sun and colleagues[16] found no association between stenosis degree and plaque wall thickness. More than 26% of plaques detected on VWI were not appreciated on DSA, according to Tian and colleagues.[7] This likely results from ICAD initially growing outward with luminal stenosis developing only at advanced disease stages (**Fig. 3**).

In a meta-analysis, the prevalence of ICAD on VWI among patients with acute/subacute ischemic stroke was 50.6% for patients (*n* = 463) without stenosis and 51.2% for patients (*n* = 651) with <50% luminal stenosis.[47] Schaafsma and colleagues[48] found the inclusion of VWI in the stroke diagnostic workup changed the etiologic classification of IS in 55% of patients (112/205), with a decrease in diagnosis of "intracranial arteriopathy not otherwise specified" from 31% to 4% (*p* < 0.001) and increase in the diagnosis of ICAD from 23% to 57% (*p* < 0.001). In 243 patients with ESUS, there was a 63.8% prevalence of ICAD ipsilateral compared with 42.8% contralateral to IS (odds ratio [OR] = 5.25; CI = 2.83 to 9.73), whereas there was no difference in plaque distribution in 160 small vessel infarct patients.[49] Remodeling index, an indicator of outward remodeling, was independently associated with ESUS (OR = 2.33; 95% CI = 1.7 to 3.2).

IS in ICAD could result from plaque rupture and thromboembolism, plaque growth occluding

perforator origins, or progressive stenosis leading to downstream hypoperfusion. As histopathologic validation is difficult to achieve in cases of ICAD, VWI could be an excellent noninvasive diagnostic tool for the identification, characterization, and follow-up of lesions.

Plaque enhancement is one of the most commonly studied ICAD imaging biomarkers and has been shown to be associated with IS irrespective of the degree of luminal stenosis.[13–15,50] Neovascularization, plaque permeability, and inflammation are potential mechanisms for plaque enhancement. The degree of enhancement is frequently graded qualitatively using pituitary stalk enhancement as a reference. Yang and colleagues found symptomatic plaques had a significantly greater degree of enhancement compared with asymptomatic plaques (38.9 ± 18.2 vs 18.2 ± 16.2, *p* < 0.001). Among the symptomatic plaques, the enhancement decreased with increasing time between stroke onset and exam acquisition (*p* = 0.001).[51] Quantitative plaque enhancement has been shown to have an independent association with recurrent stroke as compared with first-time stroke (OR = 2.5, *p* = 0.036).[15] Although the association between plaque enhancement and stroke has been established, approximately 70% of non-culprit plaques may show enhancement as well. A nonenhancing plaque is unlikely to be symptomatic.[52]

ICAD commonly shows outward remodeling, leading to advanced plaque stages before appreciable stenosis. Sun and colleagues[16] recently found that ICA plaques were more likely nonstenotic compared with other segments (80% vs 55%, *p* = 0.03), whereas posterior circulation

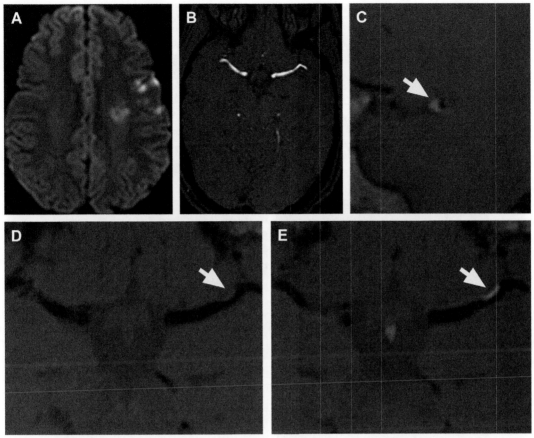

Fig. 3. Stroke with non-stenotic plaque. On axial DWI (*A*), left MCA territory acute ischemic infarcts are present. Axial TOF-MRA of the brain (*B*) shows no evidence of left MCA stenosis. Sagittal (*C*) and axial (*E*) post-contrast and axial (*D*) pre-contrast T1-weighted VWI show an eccentric, non-stenotic, outwardly remodeling, and enhancing atherosclerotic plaque along the anterior wall of the distal left M1 MCA (*short arrow*).

was found to have lower percentages of non-stenotic plaques. A recent meta-analysis ($n = 352$) reported an odds ratio of 5.6 for the presence of outward remodeling in ICAD upstream from stroke (95% CI = 2.2 to 14.0, $P<.001$).[53]

Higher plaque burden has been shown to be associated with recurrent strokes. Sun and colleagues[15] showed that recurrent stroke patients had significantly more intracranial plaques compared with first-time acute or chronic stroke patients ($p < 0.001$). Adequate distinction of plaque components such as LRNC is still challenging in ICAD given the current limitations of spatial resolution. Ex vivo plaque MR imaging-histopathologic studies have validated the presence of LRNCs in intracranial plaques, where LRNC showed shorter T1 relaxation compared with FC and normal wall ($p = 0.01$, $p < 0.0001$, and $p = 0.0026$).[54]

NON-ATHEROSCLEROTIC INTRACRANIAL VASCULOPATHIES

Although rare, non-atherosclerotic intracranial vasculopathies contribute to ESUS, especially considering their diagnostic challenges. Inflammatory vasculopathies frequently present with nonspecific findings on lumbar puncture and CSF analysis.[55] The gold standard for inflammatory vasculopathy diagnosis, brain biopsy, has limited sensitivity, high risk of procedural morbidity, low pretest probability, and attempts to reduce complications through the performance of smaller biopsy samples typically lead to non-diagnostic samples.[56] Diagnostic accuracy of luminal imaging for inflammatory vasculopathies, reversible cerebral vasoconstriction (RCVS), and Moyamoya disease (MMD) are limited, ranging from 31.6 to 36.1%, and typical luminal imaging characteristics, including proximal involvement

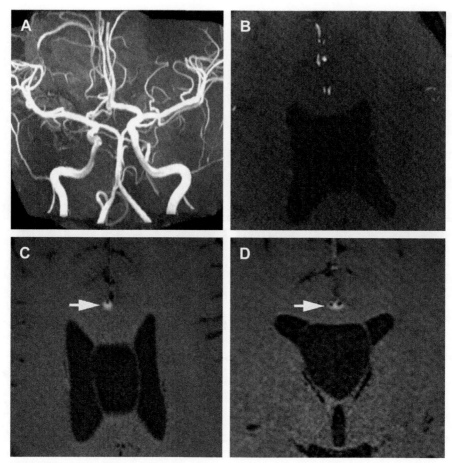

Fig. 4. Non-stenotic vasculitis. 3D-MIP TOF-MRA (*A*) and axial source TOF-MRA (*B*) covering the ACA show no luminal stenosis. Axial T1-weighted post-contrast VWI (*C*) shows eccentric diffusely enhancing lesion involving the pericallosal anterior cerebral artery branch, with blurry margins (*short arrow*). Coronal T1-weighted post-contrast image (*D*) shows circumferential enhancement with blurry margins involving the pericallosal arteries on both sides (*short arrow*). Biopsy revealed primary angiitis of the CNS.

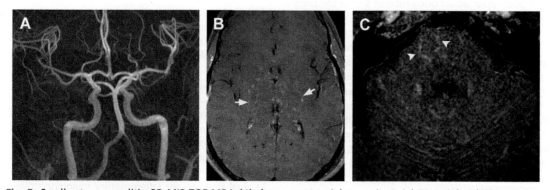

Fig. 5. Small artery vasculitis. 3D-MIP TOF-MRA (*A*) shows no arterial stenosis. Axial T1-weighted post-contrast image (*B*) at the basal ganglia shows multiple punctate foci of enhancement (*short arrows*) along perivascular spaces. Axial post-contrast T1-weighted VWI (*C*) over the pons shows curvilinear enhancement, representing perforator arteries and perivascular soft tissues enhancement (*arrowheads*). Biopsy revealed granulomatous angiitis.

for ICAD and peripheral involvement for inflammatory vasculopathy or RCVS, showed no association with diagnosis.[4,5] These vasculopathies may also present with normal luminal imaging (Fig. 4), especially when considering small artery angiitis (Fig. 5). VWI inclusion significantly improves diagnostic accuracy to 86.8% to 88.8%.[4,5] On VWI ICAD most frequently shows eccentric wall involvement, outward remodeling, variable and heterogeneous lesion enhancement.[19] Inflammatory vasculopathy typically shows intense, homogeneous, circumferential lesion enhancement with blurry margins due to spillover of inflammation into the peri-vascular tissues (see Fig. 4), whereas RCVS shows minimal to no wall thickening or enhancement.[19] Although ICAD may show circumferential involvement, T2-weighted VWI signal characteristics can help differentiate ICAD from other vasculopathies, as ICAD typically shows juxtaluminal T2 hyperintensity with deeper lesion hypointensity. The presence and degree of enhancement and wall thickening can differentiate RCVS from other vasculopathies for concentric lesions. There is heterogeneity in the literature regarding the presence of wall enhancement and wall thickening in MMD.[4,57] This may result from differing pathophysiological processes converging on a luminal phenotype, imaging at different stages of disease evolution, and/or heterogeneity of imaging techniques resulting in flow artifacts mimicking wall enhancement in steno-occlusive pathology. There is consensus, however, that MMD will not show outward remodeling, whereas ICAD will. In addition, T2 signal characteristics can help differentiate the two.[4]

AORTIC DISEASE

Aortic arch atherosclerotic disease (AAAD) is a frequent finding in ischemic stroke patients. A meta-analysis by Macleod and colleagues[58] indicated significant association of IS with AAAD (3.76 [95% CI = 2.58 to 5.48]). An autopsy case-control study (n = 500) found ulcerated aortic arch plaques in 26% of IS patients compared with 5% with other neurologic disease.[59] The NAVIGATE ESUS trial showed AAAD in 29% of patients with ESUS, who underwent transesophageal echocardiography (TEE), and of these 8% had ≥1 complex feature (ulcerated, ≥4 mm in thickness or mobile thrombus).[60] Harloff and colleagues[61] reported significantly higher detection of HRPs using MR imaging compared with TEE in their CS cohort. MR imaging detected an additional aortic high-risk embolic source in 30.8% (8/26) of patients with CS whose prior evaluation also included TEE. In addition, visualization of the ascending aorta and aortic arch by TEE was limited in 11/74 (14.9%) and 45/74 (60.8%) patients, respectively.

Retrograde flow approximating distal aortic arch and proximal thoracic aorta plaques has been shown to flow into the left subclavian artery in 31.7% (20/63) of patients with acute retinal or cerebral ischemia in which the standard diagnostic evaluation was unrevealing.[62] Four of these 20 patients had embolic pattern infarcts within the posterior circulation, the etiology of which could not be explained by other processes.

SUMMARY

In current clinical practice, a significant percentage of patients presenting with ischemic strokes are classified as cryptogenic following standard diagnostic evaluation. VWI techniques with their capability to directly visualize the vessel wall have the potential to identify <50%/non-stenotic vascular lesions responsible for stroke and differentiate vasculopathies. Potential applications of VWI in the stroke workup may include identifying and characterizing high-risk plaques in non-stenotic cervical and intracranial arteries as well as in the aorta. Broader yet judicious application of VWI as an adjunct to conventional imaging may better categorize stroke etiology, and reduce the number of cryptogenic cases.

CLINICS CARE POINTS

- Intracranial and extracranial non-stenotic atherosclerotic plaque is likely a major contributing etiology for cryptogenic stroke.
- Non-stenotic atherosclerotic plaques along the superior wall the of middle cerebral arteries is associated with acute basal ganglia infarcts, as compared to plaque along the inferior wall of the MCA.
- Dissections with intramural hematoma are better depicted on vessel wall MRI as compared to luminal imaging techniques.
- Vulnerable characteristics of non-stenotic extracranial carotid atherosclerosis can be readiy depicted on vessel wall MRI, and are associated with current, future and recurrent symptoms.

ACKNOWLEDGMENTS

Funding support:-NIH R01NS125635, NIH R01NS092207

DISCLOSURE

The authors have nothing to disclose.

REFERENCES

1. Katan M, Luft A. Global burden of stroke. Semin Neurol 2018;38(2):208–11.
2. Adams HP Jr, Bendixen BH, Kappelle LJ, et al. Classification of subtype of acute ischemic stroke. Definitions for use in a multicenter clinical trial. TOAST. Trial of Org 10172 in Acute Stroke Treatment. Stroke 1993;24(1):35–41.
3. Hart RG, Diener HC, Coutts SB, et al. Embolic strokes of undetermined source: the case for a new clinical construct. Lancet Neurol 2014;13(4): 429–38.
4. Mossa-Basha M, de Havenon A, Becker KJ, et al. Added value of vessel wall magnetic resonance imaging in the differentiation of moyamoya vasculopathies in a non-asian cohort. Stroke 2016;47(7): 1782–8.
5. Mossa-Basha M, Shibata DK, Hallam DK, et al. Added value of vessel wall magnetic resonance imaging for differentiation of nonocclusive intracranial vasculopathies. Stroke 2017;48(11):3026–33.
6. Sarikaya B, Colip C, Hwang WD, et al. Comparison of time-of-flight MR angiography and intracranial vessel wall MRI for luminal measurements relative to CT angiography. Br J Radiol 2021;94(1118): 20200743.
7. Tian X, Tian B, Shi Z, et al. Assessment of intracranial atherosclerotic plaques using 3D Black-Blood MRI: comparison with 3D time-of-flight MRA and DSA. J Magn Reson Imaging 2021;53(2):469–78.
8. Mossa-Basha M, Alexander M, Gaddikeri S, et al. Vessel wall imaging for intracranial vascular disease evaluation. J Neurointerventional Surg 2016;8(11): 1154–9.
9. Mossa-Basha M, Zhu C, Yuan C, et al. Survey of the american society of neuroradiology membership on the use and value of intracranial vessel wall MRI. AJNR Am J Neuroradiol 2022;43(7):951–7.
10. de Havenon A, Mossa-Basha M, Shah L, et al. High-resolution vessel wall MRI for the evaluation of intracranial atherosclerotic disease. Neuroradiology 2017;59(12):1193–202.
11. de Havenon A, Yuan C, Tirschwell D, et al. Nonstenotic culprit plaque: the utility of high-resolution vessel wall MRI of intracranial vessels after ischemic stroke. Case Rep Radiol 2015;2015:356582.
12. Guo Y, Canton G, Chen L, et al. Multi-planar, multi-contrast and multi-time point analysis tool (MOCHA) for intracranial vessel wall characterization. J Magn Reson Imaging 2022;56(3):944–55.
13. Li X, Sun B, Wang L, et al. Association of type 2 diabetes mellitus and glycemic control with intracranial plaque characteristics in patients with acute ischemic stroke. J Magn Reson Imaging 2021; 54(2):655–66.
14. Shi Z, Li J, Zhao M, et al. Progression of plaque burden of intracranial atherosclerotic plaque predicts recurrent stroke/transient ischemic attack: a pilot follow-up study using higher-resolution MRI. J Magn Reson Imaging 2021;54(2):560–70.
15. Sun B, Wang L, Li X, et al. Intracranial atherosclerotic plaque characteristics and burden associated with recurrent acute stroke: a 3d quantitative vessel wall MRI study. Front Aging Neurosci 2021;13: 706544.
16. Sun J, Mossa-Basha M, Canton G, et al. Characterization of non-stenotic plaques in intracranial arteries with multi-contrast, multi-planar vessel wall image analysis. J Stroke Cerebrovasc Dis 2022; 31(10):106719.
17. Zhu C, Malhotra A, Mossa-Basha M. Imaging of vulnerable intracranial atherosclerotic plaque for embolic stroke of undetermined source. J Am Coll Cardiol 2021;77(24):3140.
18. Alexander MD, Yuan C, Rutman A, et al. High-resolution intracranial vessel wall imaging: imaging beyond the lumen. J Neurol Neurosurg Psychiatr 2016;87(6):589–97.
19. Mossa-Basha M, Hwang WD, De Havenon A, et al. Multicontrast high-resolution vessel wall magnetic resonance imaging and its value in differentiating intracranial vasculopathic processes. Stroke 2015; 46(6):1567–73.
20. Rutman AM, Vranic JE, Mossa-Basha M. Imaging and management of blunt cerebrovascular injury. Radiographics 2018;38(2):542–63.
21. Vranic JE, Huynh TJ, Fata P, et al. The ability of magnetic resonance black blood vessel wall imaging to evaluate blunt cerebrovascular injury following acute trauma. J Neuroradiol 2020;47(3):210–5.
22. Wu L, Christensen D, Call L, et al. Natural history of blunt cerebrovascular injury: experience over a 10-year period at a level I trauma center. Radiology 2020;297(2):428–35.
23. Mossa-Basha M, Wasserman BA. Low-grade carotid stenosis: implications of MR imaging. Neuroimaging Clin N Am 2016;26(1):129–45.
24. Saba L, Mossa-Basha M, Abbott A, et al. Multinational survey of current practice from imaging to treatment of atherosclerotic carotid stenosis. Cerebrovascular Diseases (Basel, Switzerland) 2021; 50(1):108–20.
25. Saba L, Yuan C, Hatsukami TS, et al. Carotid artery wall imaging: perspective and guidelines from the ASNR vessel wall imaging study group and expert consensus recommendations of the american society of neuroradiology. Am J Neuroradiol 2018;39(2):E9–31.
26. Brinjikji W, DeMarco JK, Shih R, et al. Diagnostic accuracy of a clinical carotid plaque MR protocol

using a neurovascular coil compared to a surface coil protocol. J Magn Reson Imaging 2018;48(5): 1264–72.

27. Mandell DM, Mossa-Basha M, Qiao Y, et al. Intracranial vessel wall mri: principles and expert consensus recommendations of the american society of neuroradiology. Am J Neuroradiol 2017;38(2):218–29.

28. Mossa-Basha M, Huynh TJ, Hippe DS, et al. Vessel wall MRI characteristics of endovascularly treated aneurysms: association with angiographic vasospasm. J Neurosurg 2018;131(3):859–67.

29. Mossa-Basha M, Watase H, Sun J, et al. Inter-rater and scan-rescan reproducibility of the detection of intracranial atherosclerosis on contrast-enhanced 3D vessel wall MRI. Br J Radiol 2019;92(1097): 20180973.

30. Zhang C, Dou W, Jiang S, et al. High-resolution vessel wall MR imaging in diagnosis and length measurement of cerebral arterial thrombosis: a feasibility study. J Magn Reson Imaging 2022; 56(4):1267–74.

31. Balu N, Zhou Z, Hippe DS, et al. Accelerated multi-contrast high isotropic resolution 3D intracranial vessel wall MRI using a tailored k-space undersampling and partially parallel reconstruction strategy. Magma 2019;32(3):343–57.

32. Sannananja B, Zhu C, Colip CG, et al. Image-quality assessment of 3D Intracranial vessel wall MRI using DANTE or DANTE-CAIPI for blood suppression and imaging acceleration. Am J Neuroradiol 2022;43(6): 837–43.

33. Zhou Z, Chen S, Balu N, et al. Neural network enhanced 3D turbo spin echo for MR intracranial vessel wall imaging. Magn Reson Imaging 2021; 78:7–17.

34. Zhu C, Tian B, Chen L, et al. Accelerated whole brain intracranial vessel wall imaging using black blood fast spin echo with compressed sensing (CS-SPACE). Magma 2018;31(3):457–67.

35. Ospel JM, Marko M, Singh N, et al. Prevalence of Non-Stenotic (<50%) Carotid Plaques in Acute Ischemic Stroke and Transient Ischemic Attack: A Systematic Review and Meta-Analysis. J Stroke Cerebrovasc Dis 2020;29(10):105117.

36. Ospel JM, Singh N, Marko M, et al. Prevalence of ipsilateral nonstenotic carotid plaques on computed tomography angiography in embolic stroke of undetermined source. Stroke 2020;51(6):1743–9.

37. Kamtchum-Tatuene J, Wilman A, Saqqur M, et al. Carotid plaque with high-risk features in embolic stroke of undetermined source: systematic review and meta-analysis. Stroke 2020;51(1):311–4.

38. Zhao X, Hippe DS, Li R, et al. Prevalence and characteristics of carotid artery high-risk atherosclerotic plaques in chinese patients with cerebrovascular symptoms: a chinese atherosclerosis risk evaluation II study. J Am Heart Assoc 2017;6(8).

39. Kopczak A, Schindler A, Sepp D, et al. Complicated carotid artery plaques and risk of recurrent ischemic stroke or TIA. J Am Coll Cardiol 2022;79(22): 2189–99.

40. Schindler A, Schinner R, Altaf N, et al. Prediction of stroke risk by detection of hemorrhage in carotid plaques: meta-analysis of individual patient data. JACC Cardiovascular imaging 2020;13(2 Pt 1): 395–406.

41. Mark IT, Nasr DM, Huston J, et al. Embolic stroke of undetermined source and carotid intraplaque hemorrhage on MRI : a systemic review and meta-analysis. Clin Neuroradiol 2021;31(2):307–13.

42. Ota H, Yarnykh VL, Ferguson MS, et al. Carotid intraplaque hemorrhage imaging at 3.0-T MR imaging: comparison of the diagnostic performance of three T1-weighted sequences. Radiology 2010;254(2): 551–63.

43. Kopczak A, Schindler A, Bayer-Karpinska A, et al. Complicated carotid artery plaques as a cause of cryptogenic stroke. J Am Coll Cardiol 2020;76(19): 2212–22.

44. Wasserman BA, Smith WI, Trout HH 3rd, et al. Carotid artery atherosclerosis: in vivo morphologic characterization with gadolinium-enhanced double-oblique MR imaging initial results. Radiology 2002; 223(2):566–73.

45. Mitsumori LM, Hatsukami TS, Ferguson MS, et al. In vivo accuracy of multisequence MR imaging for identifying unstable fibrous caps in advanced human carotid plaques. J Magn Reson Imaging 2003;17(4):410–20.

46. Gutierrez J, Elkind MS, Virmani R, et al. A pathological perspective on the natural history of cerebral atherosclerosis. Int J Stroke : official journal of the International Stroke Society 2015;10(7):1074–80.

47. Wang Y, Liu X, Wu X, et al. Culprit intracranial plaque without substantial stenosis in acute ischemic stroke on vessel wall MRI: A systematic review. Atherosclerosis 2019;287:112–21.

48. Schaafsma JD, Rawal S, Coutinho JM, et al. Diagnostic impact of intracranial vessel wall MRI in 205 Patients with ischemic stroke or TIA. Am J Neuroradiol 2019;40(10):1701–6.

49. Tao L, Li XQ, Hou XW, et al. Intracranial Atherosclerotic Plaque as a Potential Cause of Embolic Stroke of Undetermined Source. J Am Coll Cardiol 2021;77(6):680–91.

50. Tian B, Zhu C, Tian X, et al. Baseline vessel wall magnetic resonance imaging characteristics associated with in-stent restenosis for intracranial atherosclerotic stenosis. J Neurointerventional Surg 2022.

51. Yang WJ, Abrigo J, Soo YO, et al. Regression of plaque enhancement within symptomatic middle cerebral artery atherosclerosis: a high-resolution MRI study. Front Neurol 2020;11:755.

52. Qiao Y, Zeiler SR, Mirbagheri S, et al. Intracranial plaque enhancement in patients with cerebrovascular

events on high-spatial-resolution MR images. Radiology 2014;271(2):534–42.

53. Song JW, Pavlou A, Xiao J, et al. Vessel wall magnetic resonance imaging biomarkers of symptomatic intracranial atherosclerosis: a meta-analysis. Stroke 2021;52(1):193–202.

54. Jiang Y, Zhu C, Peng W, et al. Ex-vivo imaging and plaque type classification of intracranial atherosclerotic plaque using high resolution MRI. Atherosclerosis 2016;249:10–6.

55. Hajj-Ali RA, Singhal AB, Benseler S, et al. Primary angiitis of the CNS. Lancet Neurol 2011;10(6): 561–72.

56. Torres J, Loomis C, Cucchiara B, et al. Diagnostic yield and safety of brain biopsy for suspected primary central nervous system angiitis. Stroke 2016; 47(8):2127–9.

57. Muraoka S, Taoka T, Kawai H, et al. Changes in vessel wall enhancement related to the recent neurological symptoms in patients with moyamoya disease. Neurol Med -Chir 2021;61(9):515–20.

58. Macleod MR, Amarenco P, Davis SM, et al. Atheroma of the aortic arch: an important and poorly recognised factor in the aetiology of stroke. Lancet Neurol 2004;3(7):408–14.

59. Amarenco P, Duyckaerts C, Tzourio C, et al. The prevalence of ulcerated plaques in the aortic arch in patients with stroke. N Engl J Med 1992;326(4): 221–5.

60. Ntaios G, Pearce LA, Meseguer E, et al. Aortic arch atherosclerosis in patients with embolic stroke of undetermined source: an exploratory analysis of the NAVIGATE ESUS Trial. Stroke 2019;50(11):3184–90.

61. Harloff A, Dudler P, Frydrychowicz A, et al. Reliability of aortic MRI at 3 Tesla in patients with acute cryptogenic stroke. J Neurol Neurosurg Psychiatr 2008; 79(5):540–6.

62. Harloff A, Strecker C, Dudler P, et al. Retrograde embolism from the descending aorta: visualization by multidirectional 3D velocity mapping in cryptogenic stroke. Stroke 2009;40(4):1505–8.

Imaging Approach to Venous Sinus Thrombosis

Francesco Carletti, PhD[a],*, Pedro Vilela, MD[b,c], Hans Rolf Jäger, MD[a,d]

KEYWORDS

- Venous sinus thrombosis • Dural sinus thrombosis • Venous thrombosis • Venous stroke
- Cerebral edema • MRV • CTV • Venography • Venogram

KEY POINTS

- Cerebral venous thrombosis (CVT) is a rare but important cause of stroke in young and middle-aged adults.
- The clinical presentation is highly variable, and the diagnosis of CVT depends on rapid and appropriate neuroimaging.
- Prompt diagnosis and treatment are key to good outcomes and preventing complications.
- Mortality among patients with CVT is low. Most patients achieve a good functional recovery but some experience long-term residual symptoms.
- Heparin is the mainstay treatment, even in the presence of intracerebral hemorrhage. Endovascular therapy does not improve the clinical outcome of patients with severe CVT.

Abbreviations	
CVT	Cerebral venous thrombosis
DVST	Deep venous sinus thrombosis
CoVT	Cortical venous thrombosis
CVST	Cortical and venous sinus thrombosis
dAVF	Dural arteriovenous fistula
SARS-CoV-2	Severe acute respiratory syndrome coronavirus 2
VITT	Vaccine-induced thrombotic thrombocytopenia
SSS	Superior Sagittal sinus
ISS	Inferior Sagittal sinus
SS	Straight sinus
TS	Transverse sinus
CS	Cavernous sinus
ESP	Entry slice phenomenon
VENC	Velocity-encoding

INTRODUCTION

Cerebral venous thrombosis (CVT) accounts for approximately 1% to 2% of all strokes[1] with an estimated incidence in adults of 1.32 to 1.57 per 100,000 person-years.[2,3] The more widespread availability of computed tomography (CT) and MR scanners and advances in imaging techniques has led to an earlier and more frequent diagnosis of CVT, particularly in less severe cases.[2] CVT is more common in young women during the peripartum and postpartum periods and those taking oral

[a] Lysholm Department of Neuroradiology, National Hospital for Neurology and Neurosurgery, Queen Square, London WC1N 3BG, UK; [b] Neuroradiology Department. Lisbon Western University Center (Centro Hospitalar Lisboa Ocidental -CHLO), Lisbon Portugal; [c] Imaging Department, Hospital da Luz Lisbon, Portugal; [d] Neuroradiological Academic Unit, Department of Brain Repair and Rehabilitation, UCL Queen Square Institute of Neurology, London WC1N 3BG, UK

* Corresponding author.

E-mail address: francesco.carletti@nhs.net

Radiol Clin N Am 61 (2023) 501–519
https://doi.org/10.1016/j.rcl.2023.01.011
0033-8389/23/© 2023 Elsevier Inc. All rights reserved.

contraception, as well as in patients with hypercoagulable states due to hematological disorders or malignancies (Table 1—Risk factors and conditions associated with CVT).[1]

Clinically, CVT can mimic other acute neurological disorders. Prompt and adequate neuroimaging is important to confirm or refute the diagnosis, as early diagnosis and treatment improve the prognosis.

The mortality rate is 8% to 10% and higher in severe cases, adult men, and/or those presenting with coma, brain hemorrhages, deep cerebral vein thrombosis, and those associated with infection and malignancy.[4] Up to 20% of patients with CVT will experience residual chronic symptoms.[5]

Intravenous heparin or low molecular weight heparin is the first-line treatment, even in the presence of hemorrhagic infarction.[6,7] The treatment should start as soon as the diagnosis is confirmed with the aim to recanalize occluded vein(s) or sinus(es) and prevent thrombus propagation.

Normal Anatomy of Venous Drainage of the Brain

A detailed description of the anatomy of the intracranial venous system is beyond the scope of this article.

The major dural sinuses and cortical veins are illustrated in Fig. 1, and cerebral venous drainage

Table 1
Risk factors and conditions associated with CVT

Risk Factors	Category
Risk pregnancy and puerperium	
Dehydration	
Obesity	
Immobilization	
Surgery and medical procedures	Neurosurgical procedures Lumbar puncture Jugular catheter occlusion
Trauma	Head injury
Infection	Systemic infections Ear, sinuses, face, and orbits infections central nervous system (CNS) infections Immunosuppression may increase the risk for septic CVT
Drugs	Oral contraceptives Hormone replacement therapy Cancer drugs (asparaginase, tamoxifen, and thalidomide) Hormone stimulation Glucocorticoids
Inflammatory and autoimmune disorders	Vasculitides Antiphospholipid syndrome Inflammatory bowel disease Sarcoidosis
Malignancy	CNS neoplasms (meningioma, glomus tumor, medullablastoma) Hematologic neoplasms Metastases and carcinomatosis Non-CNS tumors
Hematologic disorders	Protein C, S, Antithrombin and Factor V (Leiden) deficiency G20210 A prothrombin gene mutation Polycythemia Thrombocythemia Vaccine-induced thrombotic thrombocytopenia Sickle cell disease Hemolytic anemia Paroxysmal nocturnal hemoglobinuria

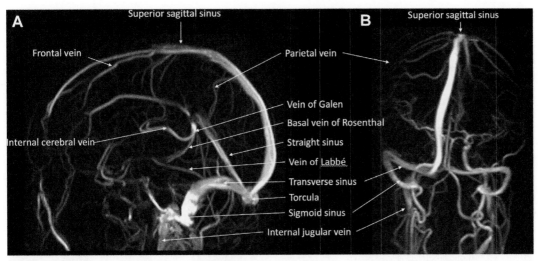

Fig. 1. Anatomy of the cerebral veins and dural venous sinuses (A,B).

patterns in **Fig. 2**. It is important to be aware of the fact that there is great interindividual variability in the number, size, and disposition of cerebral venous structures. Flow is potentially multidirectional because the intracranial veins have no valves. Several potential anastomoses exist among extracranial–intracranial, superficial–deep, and infrasupratentorial venous systems. This wide variability explains the different clinical outcomes in similar intracranial venous thromboses.

Protocols

The recommended imaging protocols include brain and vessel (venous) imaging using nonenhanced CT (NECT) and CT Venogram (CTV) or brain MR imaging and MR Venogram (MRV), depending on availability.[8] MR imaging is recommended if it does not delay the diagnosis.[7]

Brain MR imaging should include T1-weighted and T2-weighted, a hemorrhage-sensitive sequence (susceptibility-weighted imaging [SWI] or T2* gradient recalled echo [GRE]) and diffusion-weighted imaging (DWI).[7] T1-weighted and T2-weighted images are helpful in the characterization of the age of the thrombus (**Table 2**— Signal characteristics of the thrombus in different stages of CVT) and detection of edema. DWI allows differentiating vasogenic from cytotoxic edema.[9,10] SWI is superior to the T2* GRE sequence in detecting subtle thrombosis and accurate localization of the clot or bleeding.[11]

Depending on the local availability, several vascular imaging techniques can be used to diagnose CVT.[12]

CTV is a widely available and fast. Dual-energy CT, due to its ability to discriminate between calcifications and iodine contrast media based on their unique energy-dependent attenuation profiles, can be used to remove bone from CTV, facilitating the evaluation of intracranial veins and CVT.[13,14] Additionally, virtual-unenhanced images of the brain can be generated from a DE CTV. Dynamic 4D CTA/V visualizes arterial, capillary, and venous phases reducing the chance of error. It is suited for evaluating the venous collateral circulation and the presence of dural arteriovenous fistulae (dAVF). Generally, CT and CTV should be avoided in radiation-sensitive populations (such as children or pregnant women) and techniques requiring gadolinium injection in pregnant and postpartum women and patients with severe kidney insufficiency.

MRV techniques used for the diagnosis of CVT may vary but the techniques most used include phase-contrast MRV (PC MRV), time-of-flight MRV (TOF MRV), and 3D contrast-enhanced MRV (CE MRV).

Magnetic resonance black-blood thrombus imaging has shown excellent sensitivity for CVT[15–18] with direct visualization of thrombi without requiring intravenous gadolinium.

CEMRV can accurately depict recanalized or partially recanalized chronically thrombosed dural sinus segments.[19] This sequence is not sensitive to flow-related phenomena such as TOF MRV but can be challenging to interpret in case of enhancing lesions in close topographic proximity with dural sinuses/cortical veins.

Dynamic MRA (time-resolved MRA or 4D-MRA) may be very effective for diagnosing CTV[20] and can distinguish between slow flow and thrombosis. In imaging follow-up of patients with CVT, dynamic 4D MRA can detect recanalization, CVT recurrence and exclude dAVF.

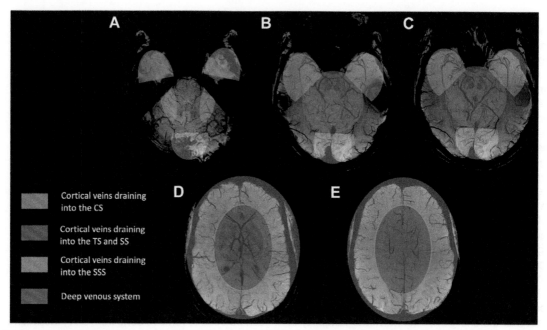

Fig. 2. Susceptibility-weighted imaging axial images (7T) with color overlay representing the major venous drainage territories A-E.

Nowadays, digital subtraction angiography (DSA) is seldom needed and is reserved for patients requiring endovascular treatment.

Imaging Findings of Cerebral Venous Thrombosis

In the radiological diagnosis of CTV, both direct and indirect signs must be identified. Direct signs of CVT include the visualization of the thrombus and/or the venous occlusion. Indirect signs include intracranial complications such as brain edema with swelling, decreased CSF absorption with hydrocephalus, parenchymal and subarachnoid hemorrhage, and venous infarction. Additionally, it is important to look for the possible origin of the thrombosis and any underlying associated pathologic condition.

Table 2
Signal characteristics of the thrombus in different stages of cerebral venous thrombosis

Stage	Time Course	Signal Intensity and Vein Appearance
Acute	Day 1–5	Intermediate T1WI, low T2WI, and T2* or SWI signal due deoxyhemoglobin Enlarged veins
Subacute (early)	Day 5–14	High T1WI, low signal on T2WI due to the conversion of deoxyhemoglobin into methemoglobin In large vessels, the changes proceed centripetally
Subacute (late)	Day 14–21	High signal in all sequences due to extracellular methemoglobin Intense peripheral dural enhancement with central filling defect after gadolinium administration (empty delta analog)
Chronic	After day 21	Variable signal intensity (SI) depending on the degree of clot organization. Organized and vascularized thrombus may show intense enhancement but minimal or no enhancement may also occur Veins are no longer enlarged

Thrombus visualization

The intravenous thrombus may be detected on CT and MR imaging. NECT may often show subtle findings or seem normal[21,22] but has relatively high sensitivity in deep venous thrombosis.[23] Fresh thrombus on NECT appears as hyperdensity in the occluded sinus or vein, which is enlarged. The thrombus can seem rounded in veins perpendicular to the imaging plane or tubular in those parallel to the imaging plane (cord sign). An increase in fibrinogen and proteins within the thrombus cause hyperdensity. As the clot ages, its density decreases. After 7 to 14 days, the thrombus progressively becomes isodense to the brain parenchyma.

MR imaging is more sensitive for detecting venous thrombi than NECT.[24] As with CT, the signal intensity of the thrombus depends on its age and varies according to the paramagnetic effect of hemoglobin breakdown products present in the thrombus (see **Table 2**—Signal characteristics of the thrombus in different stages of CVT, **Figs. 8** and **11**).

These dynamic temporal changes also affect the DWI signal and apparent diffusion coefficient (ADC) values. Acute thrombus will be hypointense on DWI and ADC maps due to the T2 "blackout" effect of deoxyhemoglobin, whereas subacute thrombus may seem as hyperintense on DWI (**Fig. 3**). Fravole and colleagues[25] reported that patients with a thrombus returning a high DWI signal have a low short-term recanalization rate after anticoagulation. DWI signal changes of the thrombus are often similar to concomitant T1 and/or fluid attenuated inversion recovery (FLAIR) signal abnormalities[25,26] (see **Fig. 3**). DWI might establish the diagnosis in patients who need a fast scan for various reasons. A recent meta-analysis showed that, albeit its high specificity for CTV, DWI has low sensitivity for hyperintense venous thrombus.[27]

On T2*w GRE and SWI sequences, the thrombus may exhibit a strong magnetic susceptibility effect with signal loss (blooming effect). The T2* GRE was shown to be key for detecting cortical venous thrombosis (CoVT), with a sensitivity greater than 90%.[28] SWI shows similar or even more pronounced signal loss due to increased deoxyhemoglobin in thrombus, venous stasis, and slow collateral flow.

Venous occlusion

CTV or MRV can be used to demonstrate venous occlusion. A correctly performed CTV has high sensitivity and specificity for CVT (greater than 90%), visualizing the presence or absence of filling defects in the venous system.[29] A comparison between NECT and CECT is essential, especially in cases where the thrombosed vein/sinuses are spontaneously hyperdense and may mimic enhancement. A careful review of source images in multiple planes is required to avoid false negatives, particularly in assessing cortical veins adjacent to the bone and difficult to visualize. CEMRV (static or time-resolved) is comparable to CTV in demonstrating a thrombus as a filling defect.[11] Besides, CEMRV is preferable to the TOF and PC MRV because it is less sensitive to flow-related artifacts.

Intracranial complications

Indirect signs of CVT, such as brain edema, venous infarction, hemorrhage, and decreased CSF absorption with hydrocephalus, can be diagnosed with CT and MR imaging, the latter being more sensitive for detecting small parenchymal lesions, cerebral edema, and microhemorrhages.

Edema. Both vasogenic and cytotoxic edema occur in CVT,[9,10] showing a high signal on T2-weighted and FLAIR sequences and a low signal on T1-WI. DWI allows for differentiation between the two: ADC values in primarily vasogenic edema are increased but decreased in primarily cytotoxic edema. Patients with regions of increased or normal ADC values typically have a good prognosis. Unlike in arterial stroke, where restricted diffusion implies mostly irreversible brain tissue damage, diffusion restriction carries a variable prognosis in CVT and can disappear completely with the restoration of venous drainage (**Fig. 4**).

Venous infarction. A venous infarct may follow cerebral edema. Increased venous and capillary pressure reduces cerebral perfusion pressure and blood flow. Venous infarcts follow the topography of venous and not arterial territories, are mostly subcortical and frequently hemorrhagic and can enhance following BBB disruption. Adjacent prominent cortical venous enhancement is caused by venous congestion and tentorial enhancement due to dural venous collaterals. The term "venous infarction" has often been used interchangeably with "venous edema." However, since the parenchymal changes in CVT are often reversible with appropriate treatment, the term "venous infarction" should be used with caution.

Perfusion-weighted imaging is not routinely performed in CTV as perfusion parameters are not directly related to triage for treatment or outcome such as in arterial stroke. Limited arterial spin-labeling (ASL) data showed a reduced CBF in the hypoperfused parenchyma drained by a thrombosed sinus in the acute phase.[30,31] Serial increases in perfusion in patients responding to

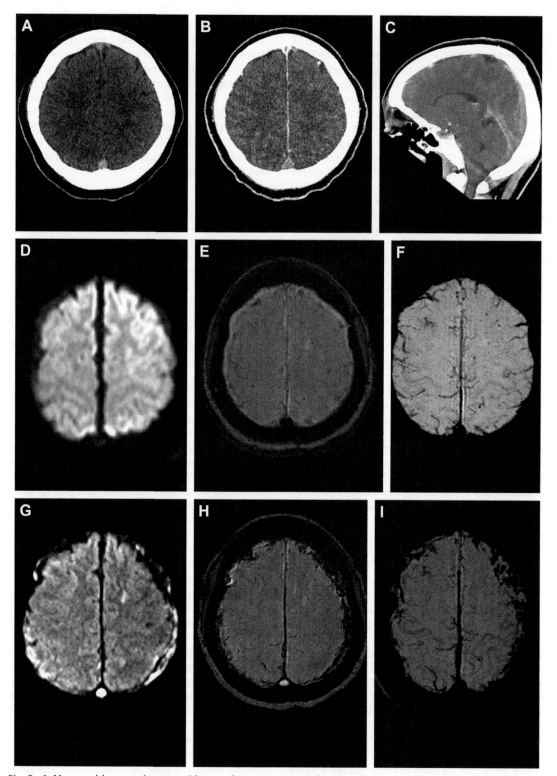

Fig. 3. A 41-year-old presenting to accident and emergency unit (A&E) with worsening headache and clumsiness. NECT (*A*) shows a hyperdense thrombus in the superior sagittal sinus (SSS) and CTV (*B*, *C*) shows a filling defect (empty delta sign in *B*). In the acute phase, the thrombus seems hypointense on DWI (*D*), magnitude (*E*) and maximum-intensity-projection (MIP) images (*F*) of SWI due to the T2 "blackout" effect of deoxyhemoglobin. On the MR imaging performed 10 days later (*G–I*), the subacute thrombus is hyperintense on DWI (*G*) and magnitude images of SWI (*H*). Please note that the hyperintense signal of the subacute thrombus is not visible on the MIP projection of SWI (*I*).

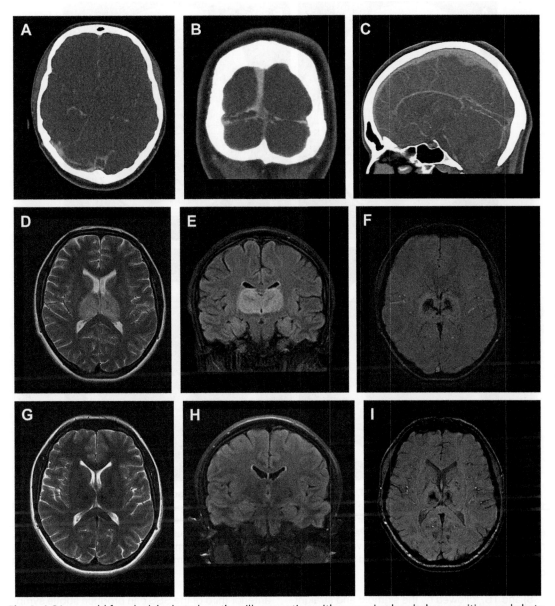

Fig. 4. A 21-year-old female dehydrated, on the pill, presenting with worsening headaches, vomiting, and photophobia. CTV (*A–C*) shows a filling defect in the deep cerebral veins (internal cerebral vein [ICV], vein of Galen, SS, and TS). MR imaging at baseline (*D, F*) and 6 months (*G–I*). Almost complete reversal of thalamic edema on T2-WI and FLAIR (*G, H*), with minor residual bilateral thalamic hypointensity on SWI and FLAIR images likely caused by microhemorrhages (*I*).

treatment suggest a potential role of ASL in disease monitoring.[31]

Brain hemorrhage. A brain hemorrhage can be seen in one-third of cases of CVT.[32] Small juxtacortical hemorrhages, with a concavity toward the adjacent sulcus (cashew nut sign), are typical of CVT (**Fig. 5**). Irregularly shaped or flame-shaped hemorrhages in the parasagittal frontal and parietal lobes are characteristics of SSS thrombosis (see **Fig. 5**A, B). Hemorrhage in the temporal or occipital lobes or infratentorial

hemorrhages is typical of transverse sinus (TS) occlusion (see **Fig. 5**C, D). Intraventricular and thalamic hemorrhages are typically observed in deep venous thrombosis (see **Fig. 4**F, I). Cortical subarachnoid hemorrhage is usually caused by CoVT but can be seen in up to 10% of venous sinus thrombosis.

Clinical and radiological features
Location of cerebral venous thrombosis The most common sites of CVT are the superior sagittal

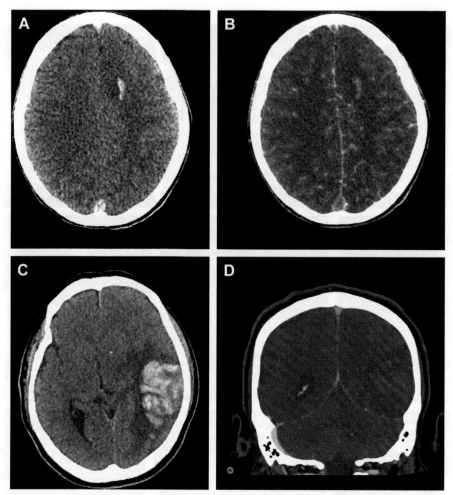

Fig. 5. Parenchymal hemorrhages in CVT. Patient 1 (*A, B*): NECT shows a small area of hemorrhage in the left fron-tal white matter and hyperdensity in the SSS. Irregularly shaped or flame-shaped hemorrhage in the parasagittal frontal white matter is typical of SSS thrombosis. There is a contrast-filling defect (empty delta sign) on CTV in keeping with an acute SSS thrombosis. Patient 2 (*C, D*): 56-year-old patient presenting with headache, confusion, and abdominal pain diagnosed with AZ vaccine-induced thrombosis and thrombocytopenia (VITT). On admission, NECT showed thrombosis of the sigmoid and transverse sinuses with large temporoparietal hemorrhage causing edema and mass effect.

(SSS) and TS, followed by the sigmoid and straight sinus. Thrombosis of the deep venous sinuses is less frequent than cortical vein thrombosis (10% and 17% of CVT). Cavernous sinus (CS) throm-bosis is rare (1% of cases of CVT).[4] In about one-third of cases, CVT can involve multiple venous sinuses or sinuses and cortical veins.[33] Isolated cortical vein thrombosis is rare,[34] although it may be underdiagnosed as the imaging findings can be subtle and easily overlooked.

Superior sagittal sinus thrombosis SSS throm-bosis is frequently associated with hypercoagula-ble states and represents a rare complication of infections (**Table 3**—Causes of septic dural throm-bosis). Intracranial hypertension is the main clinical presentation in patients with SSS. Occlusion of the

anterior third of the SSS can produce subtle symp-toms. Thrombosis may extend to the cortical veins causing focal deficits and seizures. Bilateral neurological deficits are typically late signs of SSS thrombosis.

On the axial CT images, the contrast void in the torcular region and surrounding enhancement is known as the "empty delta" sign (see **Figs. 5** and **11**). MR imaging and MRV offer greater imaging details (see **Fig. 11**).

Lateral sinus thrombosis
Sigmoid and transverse thromboses are rare com-plications of otitis media. Symptoms of ear infec-tion are followed by headache, nausea, vomiting, and neurological signs such as vertigo and fifth or sixth nerve impairment.

Table 3
Causes of septic dural thrombosis

Dural Sinus Thrombosis	Sites of Primary Infection	Microbiology
Superior sagittal sinus	Meningitis Frontal sinusitis (anterior SSS) Facial and oral surgical infection	*Staphylococcus pneumoniae* *Staphylococcus aureus,* Streptococci, *Klebsiella* *Pseudomonas*
Lateral sinus	Middle ear and mastoid	*Proteus* *S aureus* *Escherichia coli* Anaerobes *Pseudomonas*
Cavernous sinus	Sphenoid sinus Ethmoid sinusitis Teeth and supporting structures Facial infections Middle ear and mastoid	*S aureus* Streptococci Anaerobes Fungal pathogens

NECT allows the visualization of bony details of the middle ear and mastoid space (**Fig. 6**D). A CECT scan may detect abscess formation, sigmoid sinus thrombosis (**Fig. 6**A, B), cavernous sinus thrombosis (**Fig. 6**C) and ophthalmic vein thrombosis (**Fig. 6**E). MR imaging is better for assessing intracranial complications, such as subdural empyema and cerebritis and allows a detailed view of the meningeal inflammation and enhancement.

Deep venous sinus thrombosis
Occlusion of the deep cerebral venous system is seen in a minority of patients with CVT[24]

(**Figs. 7–9**) presenting with severe diencephalic dysfunction (coma, disturbances of eye movements, and pupillary reflexes) and altered mental status. Some patients might present with mild symptoms without decreased consciousness level or brainstem signs.[35]

NECT head is often the initial examination, particularly in comatose patients, demonstrating hyperdense deep veins and thalamic edema with possible extension to the caudate nuclei and deep white matter. Edema is often bilateral and can lead to obstruction of the foramen of Monro with hydrocephalus. CTV demonstrates the extent of filling defects in the straight sinus (SS), the vein

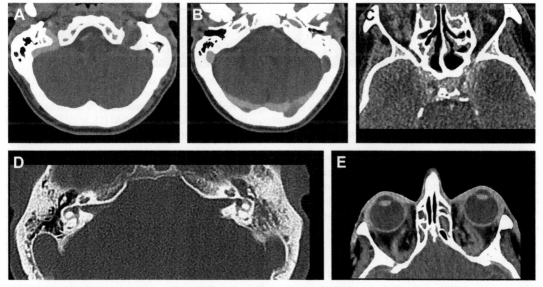

Fig. 6. A 50-year-old man presented to A&E with a severe headache. The patient had a septic thrombosis of the CS, left sigmoid sinus and internal jugular vein thrombosis. CECT shows filling defects in the left internal jugular vein (*A*), sigmoid sinus (*B*) and CS (*C*). Note the dilatation and lack of internal enhancement of the left superior ophthalmic vein due to thrombosis (*E*). Findings were secondary to sinusitis (not shown) and ear infection (*D*).

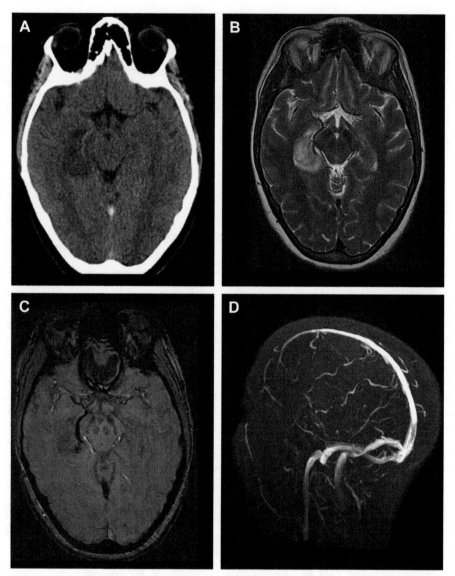

Fig. 7. Thrombosis of the right basal vein of Rosenthal. NECT (*A*) shows an area of low attenuation in the right mesial temporal lobe and hyperdensity in the right basal vein of Rosenthal and the SS, suggestive of acute deep vein thrombosis. T2-WI (*B*) demonstrates venous edema in the right medial temporal lobe. A thrombus in the right basal vein of Rosenthal and the SS causes a hypointense signal and blooming on SWI (*C*). MRV (*D*) confirms the diagnosis of a deep venous thrombosis with nonvisualization of the right basal vein of Rosenthal and SS.

of Galen, or ICVs. MR imaging is often performed in patients with milder symptoms or to corroborate CT findings. MRA and MRV are useful to distinguish between a top of basilar artery occlusion or thalamic hemorrhage and deep venous sinus thrombosis (DVST).[36]

Cortical venous thrombosis
Thrombosis of the cerebral cortical veins can be seen in conjunction with a dural venous sinus thrombosis or, less frequently, in isolation (**Fig. 9**).[34] It can be asymptomatic or cause seizures and other neurological symptoms depending on the presence and location of associated parenchymal lesions.

CoVT may present as hyperintense tubular structure (cord sign) on NECT or with indirect signs such as focal cortical edema, intra-axial or subarachnoid hemorrhage with effacement of the neighboring sulci.[34] CTV may demonstrate a filling defect in a vein overlying the cerebral cortex, with multiplanar reconstructions (MPRs) being particularly helpful. Gyral enhancement may occur in case of blood–brain barrier breakdown.

MR imaging has a higher sensitivity than CT for detecting parenchymal changes. CoVT is best

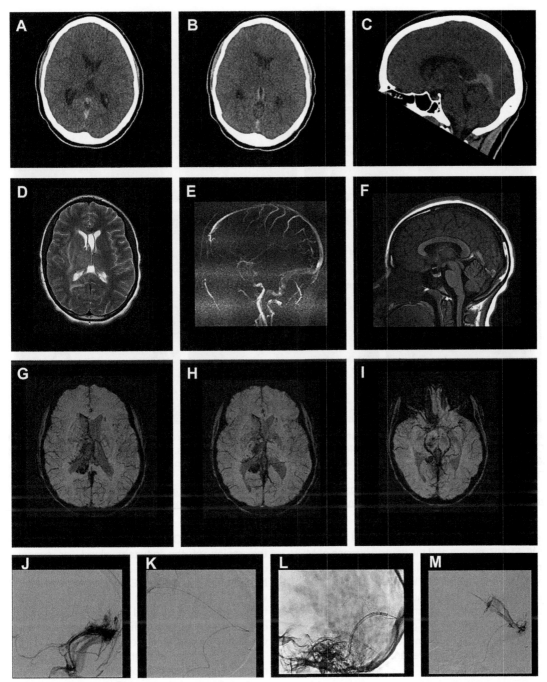

Fig. 8. A 22-year-old woman with 5 days history of headache and vomiting, with right eye lateral gaze deviation and progressive confusion NECT show high density in the ICVs, vein of Galen and SS (*A–C*). MR imaging shows DVST (*E, F*) with thalamic edema (*D*) and microhemorrhages (*G–I*). The edema has extended to the surrounding deep white matter (*D*). The clot is in the early subacute phase (hyperintense on T1-WI and hypointense on T2-WI). The extension of the clot is clearly demonstrated on SWI (*G–I*). Thrombectomy procedure (*J–M*): preprocedure angiogram (*J*), during the procedure using 6-mm stent retriever and multiple passes (*K, L*) and postprocedure selective DSA showing partial recanalization of the straight sinus (*M*).

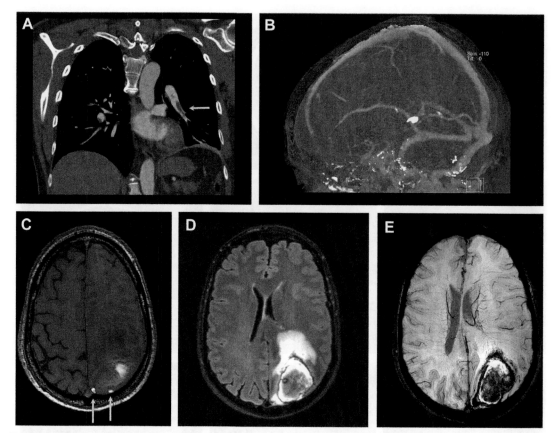

Fig. 9. A 50-year-old gentleman presenting 18 days after the Oxford-AstraZeneca coronavirus disease 2019 (COVID-19) vaccine with transient breathlessness, swollen right leg, fogginess, and slurred speech. Platelet count 30, anti-PF4 antibody positive. CT pulmonary angiography (*A*) showed acute pulmonary embolism (*white arrow*). CTV (*B*) demonstrates patency of the major dural venous sinuses. T1-WI (*C*) was able to detect an isolated cortical vein thrombosis (*white arrows*) in the proximity of a large left parieto-occipital hematoma (*C–E*). The mass effect from hemorrhage and surrounding edema is moderate but does not cause hydrocephalus.

demonstrated with a combination of T1-WI, T2-WI, DWI, FLAIR images and the source images of MRV and SWI or T2*WI (**Fig 9**). The hypointensity of a thrombosed vein on T2*WI (or SWI) is of great value for the early diagnosis of isolated cortical vein thrombosis.[37] Volumetric sequences and MPR views allow for the detection of thrombosis in small cortical veins and offer a more precise assessment of the recanalization following treatment.

Cavernous sinus thrombosis

Clotting within the CS may have a septic or aseptic cause. Patients with CS thrombosis present with a rapid onset of severe headache, nausea and vomiting, unilateral or bilateral proptosis, chemosis, reduced vision, and signs of a compromised function of the third to sixth cranial nerves.

NECT of the head may show engorgement or dilation of the superior and/or inferior ophthalmic veins, enlargement and bowing of the lateral

margins of the CS, sinusitis or mass lesions in the region of the pituitary gland, or osseous changes involving the sphenoid or temporal bones. High-resolution CECT orbits may be useful when the patient cannot have MR imaging and typically shows a bilateral enlargement of the CS, convexity, and linear enhancement of its lateral walls and venous filling defects (see **Fig. 6**C).

MR imaging offers higher soft tissue contrast resolution and is preferable for investigating suspected CS thrombosis. MR imaging and MRV enable direct visualization of the thrombus/filling defect in the CS. Additionally, MR imaging depicts cerebral infarcts, empyema, meningitis, cerebritis, and abscess associated with infections and helps differentiate inflammatory from neoplastic lesions infiltrating the CS and mimicking thrombosis (**Fig. 10**).

MRA is not routinely required for the diagnosis of CS thrombosis. However, three-dimensional (3D) TOF MRA can show the degree of extrinsic

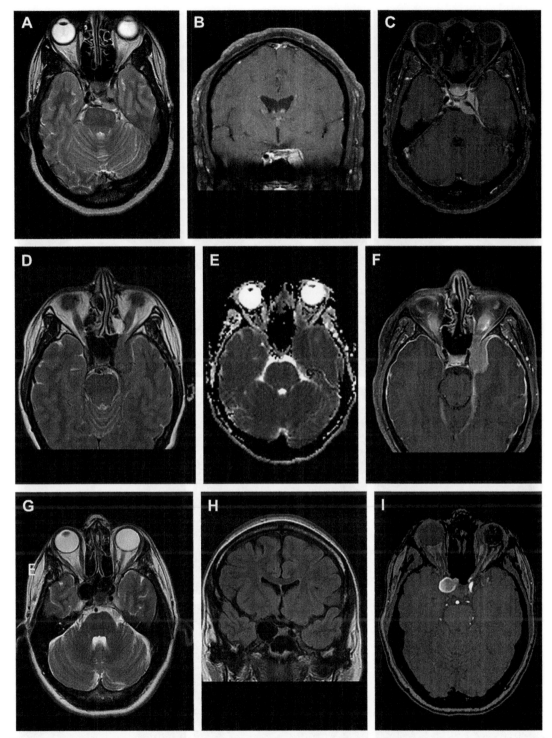

Fig. 10. Examples of CS lesions mimicking thrombosis. Meningioma (*A–C*) involving the posterior part of the left CS, Meckel cave, and tentorium bulging in the prepontine cistern. Biopsy proven marginal zone CNS lymphoma (*D-F*) in a 40-year-old woman presenting with headache, double vision (left sixth nerve palsy), and dizziness. The MR imaging scan demonstrates pachymeningitis with an enhancing mass behind the right orbit and in the cavernous sinuses (left greater than right). The differential diagnosis included IgG4-related disease. Large right cavernous ICA aneurysm (*G–I*) in a young patient with headache and visual disturbance.

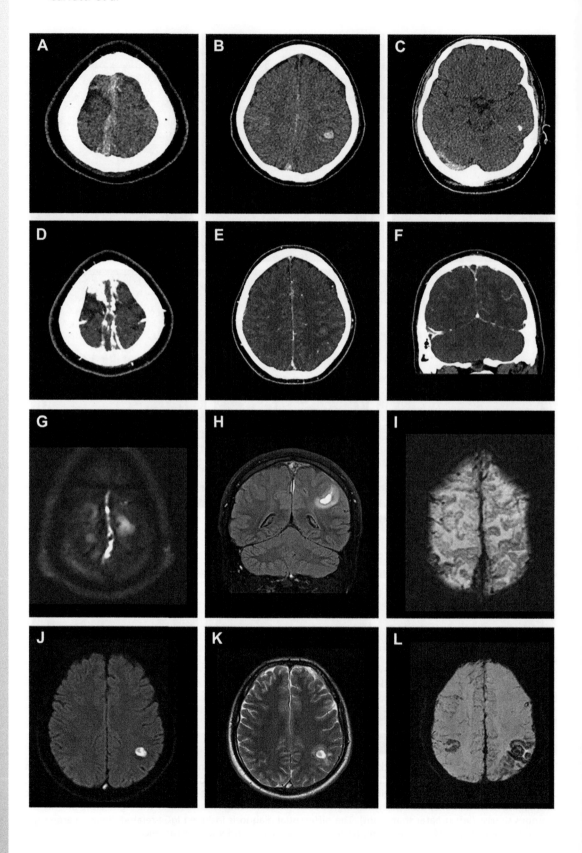

narrowing of the cavernous ICAs or rule out a CS aneurysm as a cause of an enlarged CS (see **Fig. 10G–I**). Time-resolved (4D) CEMRA is highly specific and sensitive for the diagnosis of carotid-cavernous fistulas secondary to venous thrombosis.

Coronavirus disease 2019 infection and vaccine-associated thrombosis

CVT rarely occurs in patients with severe acute respiratory syndrome coronavirus 2 without other predisposing risk factors.[38] There are reports of patients immunized with the adenovirus-vector ChAdOx1 nCov-19 (AstraZeneca, N1C 4AG, London, United) and Ad26.COV2.S (Janssen, 1000 US-202, Raritan, United States) COVID-19 vaccines[39–43] who developed CVT and thrombocytopenia. These patients developed CVT and VITT between 5 and 30 days after the vaccination date and had higher mortality than those with other causes of CVT.[41,42,44,45] Although most cases were triggered by the first dose of the ChAdOx1 nCov-19 vaccine, some cases occurred after the second dose of the vaccine.[46] Vaccine-associated thrombosis can involve venous sinuses or cortical veins (**Fig. 9**, and **Fig. 11**).

Diagnostic Pitfalls

False positives

False-positive cases on nonenhanced computed tomography *Increased hematocrit.* Arterial and venous vessels may be hyperdense in patients with an increased hematocrit. This can occur in polycythemia (erythrocytosis) or relative polycythemia due to hemoconcentration (volume contraction caused by diuretics, vomiting, diarrhea, or smoking). A careful comparison of the arterial and venous density allows differentiating patients with high hematocrit from patients with CVT.[47]

Beam hardening artifact. Beam-hardening artifacts, particularly in the posterior fossa, can mimic an acute thrombosis of the TS.

False-positive cases on MR imaging *Slow venous blood flow in the plane of image acquisition.* A slow venous blood flow may cause a loss of the normal venous flow voids and generate MR signal.[48] This occurs when the imaging plane is oriented parallel to the venous sinus. The same sequence obtained in a plane perpendicular to the vessel allows differentiating flow voids related to slow flow from a thrombus.

Entry slice phenomenon (ESP). It refers to the high intraluminal signal on the initial slices of T1-WI.[49] An additional SE sequence in a different plane is enough to differentiate this artifact from a true thrombus. Alternatively, a PC MRV visualizes the venous flow independently from the T1-weighted signal and allows for the distinction between a subacute thrombus and an ESP artifact.

False-positive cases on contrast-enhanced computed tomography or MR imaging On CECT or CEMRI, normal anatomical structures within venous sinuses, such as arachnoid granulations, Willis cords and fenestrations, can produce venous filling defects that could be misinterpreted as venous sinus thrombosis.

Normal anatomical structures. Arachnoid granulations, which are normally rounded, can occasionally elongate along the long axis of a dural sinus, simulating a thrombus.[50] Unlike thrombi, arachnoid granulations have sharp margins, are isointense to the CSF, do not expand the dural sinus, and do not extend into more than one dural sinus. A vein may be seen entering the dural sinus next to an arachnoid granulation.

Willis cords are linear structures that normally exist within the dural venous sinuses[51] and can be mistaken for a thrombus where partial recanalization has occurred. However, Willis cords differ from thrombi: they are thin (1–2 mm) linear or curvilinear filling defects with sharp margins and a broad base of attachment to the dural sinus wall, whereas thrombi have irregular margins and are thicker than septa.

Anatomical variants. Fenestrated or split dural venous sinuses can be mistaken for thrombotic filling defects. Bifurcation of the SSS before the occipital protuberance can resemble a venous sinus thrombosis with a "pseudo-empty delta sign."[52] A "pseudo-empty delta sign" can also result from delayed scanning after contrast administration.[53]

Fig. 11. A 23-year-old patient presenting to A&E with headaches, dizziness, nausea, and then right upper and lower limb weakness. The patient received the AZ vaccine 14 days before the CT scan and developed CVT and VITT. NECT and CTV in A&E showed right TS and SSS thrombosis with left parietal hemorrhage. The thrombus is mildly hyperdense on the NECT scan (*A–C*) and causes a filling defect on the CTV (*D–F*). The thrombus in the SSS is hyperintense in DWI (*G*), FLAIR (*H, I*), and T2-weighted (*J*) images due to the presence of extracellular methemoglobin (late subacute phase). SWI (*K, L*) shows susceptibility artifacts in the occluded SSS, a left parietal hematoma, and hemosiderin staining from subarachnoid hemorrhage.

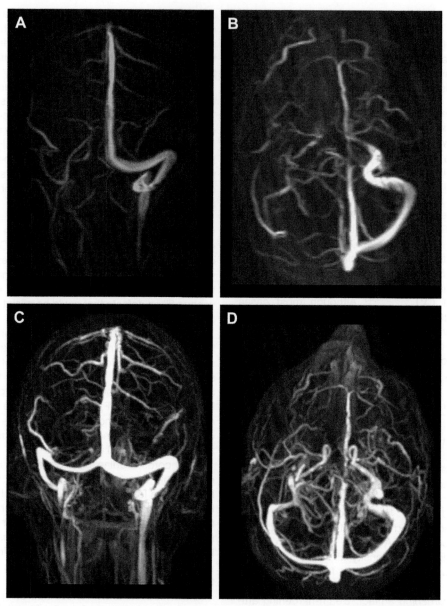

Fig. 12. Nonvisualization of TS on PC MRV (*A, B*) mimicking thrombotic occlusion. Dynamic CEMRA (*C, D*) allows a correct diagnosis and shows patency of the right TS. Unlike PC-MRV, time-resolved (4D) MRV does not require any prior knowledge of the flow velocity within the TS. Moreover, dynamic CEMRA is not vulnerable to many artifacts affecting noncontrast MRV techniques.

False-Positive Cases on MR Venogram *Anatomical variants.* Hypoplasia or aplasia of the TS,[54] hypoplasia of the anterior third of the SSS, or duplication of the SSS can cause a lack of flow-related signal on MRV.

Slow flow and flow gaps. "Flow gaps" on MRV are artifactual signal voids caused by slow venous flow. They represent a common occurrence in nondominant TSs of healthy individuals[55] but they are rarely seen in the dominant TS or other dural sinuses. MIP image reconstruction of MRV tends to underestimate the vessel caliber and overestimate venous hypoplasia and flow gaps. Therefore, it is important to accurately assess source images to prevent a misdiagnosis. The presence of a persistent occipital sinus and mastoid emissary veins, a small jugular foramen, or a sigmoid sinus groove further indicates the presence of hypoplastic TS. Similarly, arachnoid granulations and Willis cords can produce flow defects on MRV.

In-plane saturation in TOF-MRV. In-plane saturation in TOF-MRV can induce an apparent absence of flow in the anterior and middle portions of the SSS. This happens when the dural sinus lies parallel (or "in-plane") to the imaging plane and is generated by an inferior saturation band used to saturate arterial signal on TOF MRV obtained using source images in the axial plane. Acquisitions in an orthogonal acquisition, or without inferior saturation band, or PC MRV, will demonstrate the patency of the SSS.

Nonvisualization of TS on PC MRV. PC MRV requires that an optimal velocity-encoding variable (VENC) is predicted a priori. When the selected VENC value does not match the flow velocity of the TS, the latter is not visualized, mimicking an occlusion (**Fig. 12**).[56]

False negatives

False-negative cases on nonenhanced computed tomography *Subacute or chronic thrombosed dural sinus.* A thrombosed dural sinus in the subacute or chronic phase may seem isodense to the brain parenchyma and could be mistaken for normal brain tissue.

Thrombosed cortical vein against the skull. A small thrombosed cortical vein can be difficult to detect against the adjacent skull. However, multiplanar reformations may help to demonstrate the thrombosed vein.

Acute thrombosis versus hemorrhage. Sometimes, a thrombus expanding a venous sinus may be mistaken for an acute subdural or epidural hemorrhage or subarachnoid hemorrhage.[57] CTV, MR, and MRV may aid the final diagnosis by showing an abnormal signal within a cortical vein or venous sinus rather than outside the vessel.

False-negative cases on MR imaging *T2-weighted hypointense thrombus.* An acute thrombus returns a low signal on T2-WI, simulating a normal flow void of patent sinuses.[58] An acute thrombus containing paramagnetic deoxyhemoglobin returns an intermediate signal on T1-WI simulating normal brain tissue. The clue to the correct diagnosis comes from T2*GRE/SWI sequences, where the magnetic susceptibility of deoxyhemoglobin causes hypointensity and "blooming."

False-negative cases on contrast-enhanced computed tomography/MR imaging *Wrong timing of CTV.* When CTV images are acquired shortly after contrast administration, the cerebral veins will be poorly visualized, decreasing the chances of detecting venous thrombosis.

Chronic thrombus enhancement. Chronic venous sinus thrombosis can demonstrate intense gadolinium enhancement of the thrombosed segments mimicking a patent dural sinus.[59] The thrombus changes structure with time and develop capillary channels in the chronic phase. In this stage, susceptibility artifacts on GRE or SWI images can reduce significantly, increasing the chances of false positives.[49] MRV can demonstrate the presence of a chronic thrombus.

False-negative cases on MR Venogram *"T1 shine-through" effect on TOF-MRV.* When the thrombus moves from the acute to the subacute phase, the methemoglobin returns a high T1-weighted signal (T1 shine-through effect) on TOF-MRV and mimics flow signal. However, on MRV source images, the thrombus signal is not as intense as the flow-related signal.[24] Besides, the subacute thrombus is hyperintense on T1-WI. In cases of diagnostic uncertainty, PC MRV, which is not affected by the hyperintensity of methemoglobin, can be helpful.

SUMMARY

CTV is an uncommon but important cerebrovascular disorder. The patient outcome depends on a timely diagnosis and treatment, the former relying heavily on diagnostic imaging. Radiologists must be able to identify features of CVT, which can be subtle. We reviewed the imaging findings of CVT on CT- and MR-based techniques, highlighting the strengths, limitations, and diagnostic pitfalls of various neuroimaging techniques.

CLINICS CARE POINTS

- CVT is a potentially reversible condition when promptly recognized and treated. The clinical diagnosis may be challenging. Therefore, patients with suspected CVT require urgent neuroimaging to confirm CVT.

- Imaging findings include direct (clot visualization or demonstration of vein/dural venous sinus filling defect) and indirect signs (edema, hydrocephalus, hemorrhage, and venous infarction) of CVT.

- MR imaging is the preferred imaging modality for diagnosing CVT (if it does not delay the diagnosis) and monitoring treatment response.

- SWI or GE T2-WI combined with other sequences improve the accuracy of CVT diagnosis and facilitate the detection of subtle CVT (eg, acute and subacute CoVT).

- CEMRV is comparable to CTV in demonstrating a thrombus as a filling defect and is less prone to artifacts than TOF or PC MRV. Dynamic CEMRA helps to detect veins/sinus recanalization and CVT recurrence and can exclude dAVF.

DECLARATION OF INTERESTS

The authors have nothing to disclose.

REFERENCES

1. Stam J. Cerebral venous and sinus thrombosis: incidence and causes. Adv Neurol 2003;92:225–32.

2. Devasagayam S, Wyatt B, Leyden J, et al. Cerebral venous sinus thrombosis incidence is higher than previously thought: a retrospective population-based study. Stroke 2016;47:2180–2.

3. Coutinho JM, Zuurbier SM, Aramideh M, et al. The incidence of cerebral venous thrombosis: a cross-sectional study. Stroke 2012;43:3375–7.

4. Ferro JM, Canhão P, Stam J, et al. Prognosis of cerebral vein and dural sinus thrombosis: results of the International Study on Cerebral Vein and Dural Sinus Thrombosis (ISCVT). Stroke 2004;35:664–70.

5. Silvis SM, de Sousa DA, Ferro JM, et al. Cerebral venous thrombosis. Nat Rev Neurol 2017;13:555–65.

6. Ferro JM, Bousser MG, Canhão P, et al. European stroke organization guideline for the diagnosis and treatment of cerebral venous thrombosis - endorsed by the european academy of neurology. Eur Stroke J 2017;2:195–221.

7. Saposnik G, Barinagarrementeria F, Brown RD, et al. Diagnosis and management of cerebral venous thrombosis: a statement for healthcare professionals from the American Heart Association/American Stroke Association. Stroke 2011;42:1158–92.

8. van Dam LF, van Walderveen MAA, Kroft LJM, et al. Current imaging modalities for diagnosing cerebral vein thrombosis - A critical review. Thromb Res 2020;189:132–9.

9. Ducreux D, Oppenheim C, Vandamme X, et al. Diffusion-weighted imaging patterns of brain damage associated with cerebral venous thrombosis. AJNR Am J Neuroradiol 2001;22:261–8.

10. Forbes KP, Pipe JG, Heiserman JE. Evidence for cytotoxic edema in the pathogenesis of cerebral venous infarction. AJNR Am J Neuroradiol 2001;22:450–5.

11. Dmytriw AA, Song JSA, Yu E, et al. Cerebral venous thrombosis: state of the art diagnosis and management. Neuroradiology 2018;60:669–85.

12. Vilela P. Imaging of cerebral venous and sinus thrombosis. Clinical Neuroradiology. Cham: Springer International Publishing; 2019. p. 325–52.

13. Morhard D, Fink C, Graser A, et al. Cervical and cranial computed tomographic angiography with automated bone removal: dual energy computed tomography versus standard computed tomography. Invest Radiol 2009;44:293–7.

14. Lell MM, Ruehm SG, Kramer M, et al. Cranial computed tomography angiography with automated bone subtraction: a feasibility study. Invest Radiol 2009;44:38–43.

15. Niu PP, Yu Y, Guo ZN, et al. Diagnosis of non-acute cerebral venous thrombosis with 3D T1-weighted black blood sequence at 3T. J Neurol Sci 2016;367:46–50.

16. Wang G, Yang X, Duan J, et al. Cerebral venous thrombosis: mr black-blood thrombus imaging with enhanced blood signal suppression. AJNR Am J Neuroradiol 2019;40:1725–30.

17. Yang Q, Duan J, Fan Z, et al. Early detection and quantification of cerebral venous thrombosis by magnetic resonance black-blood thrombus imaging. Stroke 2016;47:404–9.

18. Yang X, Wu F, Liu Y, et al. Diagnostic performance of MR black-blood thrombus imaging for cerebral venous thrombosis in real-world clinical practice. Eur Radiol 2022;32:2041–9.

19. Leach JL, Wolujewicz M, Strub WM. Partially recanalized chronic dural sinus thrombosis: findings on MR imaging, time-of-flight MR venography, and contrast-enhanced MR venography. AJNR Am J Neuroradiol 2007;28:782–9.

20. Meckel S, Reisinger C, Bremerich J, et al. Cerebral venous thrombosis: diagnostic accuracy of combined, dynamic and static, contrast-enhanced 4D MR venography. AJNR Am J Neuroradiol 2010;31:527–35.

21. Linn J, Brückmann H. Cerebral venous and dural sinus thrombosis* : state-of-the-art imaging. Clin Neuroradiol 2010;20:25–37.

22. Linn J, Michl S, Katja B, et al. Cortical vein thrombosis: the diagnostic value of different imaging modalities. Neuroradiology 2010;52:899–911.

23. Linn J, Pfefferkorn T, Ivanicova K, et al. Noncontrast CT in deep cerebral venous thrombosis and sinus thrombosis: comparison of its diagnostic value for both entities. AJNR Am J Neuroradiol 2009;30:728–35.

24. Leach JL, Fortuna RB, Jones BV, et al. Imaging of cerebral venous thrombosis: current techniques, spectrum of findings, and diagnostic pitfalls. Radiographics 2006;26:S19–41.

25. Favrole P, Guichard J-P, Crassard I, et al. Diffusion-weighted imaging of intravascular clots in cerebral venous thrombosis. Stroke 2004;35:99–103.

26. Patel D, Machnowska M, Symons S, et al. Diagnostic performance of routine brain MRI sequences for dural venous sinus thrombosis. AJNR Am J Neuroradiol 2016;37:2026–32.

27. Lv B, Jing F, Tian CL, et al. Diffusion-weighted magnetic resonance imaging in the diagnosis of cerebral venous thrombosis : a meta-analysis. J Korean Neurosurg Soc 2021;64:418–26.

28. Altinkaya N, Demir S, Alkan O, et al. Diagnostic value of T2*-weighted gradient-echo MRI for segmental evaluation in cerebral venous sinus thrombosis. Clin Imaging 2015;39:15–9.

29. Rodallec MH, Krainik A, Feydy A, et al. Cerebral venous thrombosis and multidetector CT angiography: tips and tricks. Radiographics 2006; 26(Suppl 1):S5–18 [discussion: S42].

30. Kang JH, Yun TJ, Yoo RE, et al. Bright sinus appearance on arterial spin labeling MR imaging aids to identify cerebral venous thrombosis. Medicine (Baltim) 2017;96:e8244.

31. Furuya S, Kawabori M, Fujima N, et al. Serial arterial spin labeling may be useful in assessing the therapeutic course of cerebral venous thrombosis: case reports. Neurol Med -Chir 2017;57:557–61.

32. Pongmoragot J, Saposnik G. Intracerebral hemorrhage from cerebral venous thrombosis. Curr Atheroscler Rep 2012;14:382–9.

33. Ameri A, Bousser M-G. Cerebral venous thrombosis. Neurol Clin 1992;10:87–111.

34. Coutinho JM, Gerritsma JJ, Zuurbier SM, et al. Isolated cortical vein thrombosis: systematic review of case reports and case series. Stroke 2014;45:1836–8.

35. van den Bergh WM, van der Schaaf I, van Gijn J. The spectrum of presentations of venous infarction caused by deep cerebral vein thrombosis. Neurology 2005;65:192–6.

36. Bell DA, Davis WL, Osborn AG, et al. Bithalamic hyperintensity on T2-weighted MR: vascular causes and evaluation with MR angiography. AJNR Am J Neuroradiol 1994;15:893–9.

37. Boukobza M, Crassard I, Bousser MG, et al. MR imaging features of isolated cortical vein thrombosis: diagnosis and follow-up. AJNR Am J Neuroradiol 2009;30:344–8.

38. Baldini T, Asioli GM, Romoli M, et al. Cerebral venous thrombosis and severe acute respiratory syndrome coronavirus-2 infection: A systematic review and meta-analysis. Eur J Neurol 2021;28:3478–90.

39. Schulz JB, Berlit P, Diener HC, et al. COVID-19 vaccine-associated cerebral venous thrombosis in germany. Ann Neurol 2021;90:627–39.

40. See I, Su JR, Lale A, et al. Us case reports of cerebral venous sinus thrombosis with thrombocytopenia after Ad26.COV2.S vaccination, March 2 to April 21, 2021. JAMA 2021;325:2448–56.

41. Krzywicka K, Heldner MR, Sánchez van Kammen M, et al. Post-SARS-CoV-2-vaccination cerebral venous sinus thrombosis: an analysis of cases notified to the European Medicines Agency. Eur J Neurol 2021;28: 3656–62.

42. Pavord S, Scully M, Hunt BJ, et al. Clinical features of vaccine-induced immune thrombocytopenia and thrombosis. N Engl J Med 2021;385:1680–9.

43. Furie KL, Cushman M, Elkind MSV, et al. Diagnosis and management of cerebral venous sinus thrombosis with vaccine-induced immune thrombotic thrombocytopenia. Stroke 2021;52:2478–82.

44. Perry RJ, Tamborska A, Singh B, et al. Cerebral venous thrombosis after vaccination against COVID-19 in the UK: a multicentre cohort study. Lancet 2021;398:1147–56.

45. Sánchez van Kammen M, Aguiar de Sousa D, Poli S, et al. Characteristics and outcomes of patients with cerebral venous sinus thrombosis in SARS-CoV-2 vaccine-induced immune thrombotic thrombocytopenia. JAMA Neurol 2021;78:1314–23.

46. Krzywicka K, van de Munckhof A, Zimmermann J, et al. Cerebral venous thrombosis due to vaccine-induced immune thrombotic thrombocytopenia after a second ChAdOx1 nCoV-19 dose. Blood 2022;139: 2720–4.

47. Poon CS, Chang JK, Swarnkar A, et al. Radiologic diagnosis of cerebral venous thrombosis: pictorial review. AJR Am J Roentgenol 2007;189:S64–75.

48. Pandey S, Hakky M, Kwak E, et al. Application of basic principles of physics to head and neck MR angiography: troubleshooting for artifacts. Radiographics 2013;33:E113–23.

49. Pai V, Khan I, Sitoh YY, et al. Pearls and pitfalls in the magnetic resonance diagnosis of dural sinus thrombosis: a comprehensive guide for the trainee radiologist. J Clin Imaging Sci 2020;10:77.

50. Liang L, Korogi Y, Sugahara T, et al. Normal structures in the intracranial dural sinuses: delineation with 3D contrast-enhanced magnetization prepared rapid acquisition gradient-echo imaging sequence. AJNR Am J Neuroradiol 2002;23:1739–46.

51. Farb RI. The dural venous sinuses: normal intraluminal architecture defined on contrast-enhanced MR venography. Neuroradiology 2007;49:727–32.

52. Zouaoui A, Hidden G. Cerebral venous sinuses: anatomical variants or thrombosis. Acta Anat 1988; 133:318–24.

53. Ulmer JL, Elster AD. Physiologic mechanisms underlying the delayed delta sign. AJNR Am J Neuroradiol 1991;12:647–50.

54. Alper F, Kantarci M, Dane S, et al. Importance of anatomical asymmetries of transverse sinuses: an MR venographic study. Cerebrovasc Dis 2004;18: 236–9.

55. Ayanzen RH, Bird CR, Keller PJ, et al. Cerebral MR venography: normal anatomy and potential diagnostic pitfalls. AJNR Am J Neuroradiol 2000;21: 74–8.

56. Chang Y-M, Kuhn AL, Porbandarwala N, et al. Unilateral nonvisualization of a transverse dural sinus on phase-contrast MRV: frequency and differentiation from sinus thrombosis on noncontrast MRI. Am J Neuroradiol 2020;41:115–21.

57. Akins PT, Axelrod YK, Ji C, et al. Cerebral venous sinus thrombosis complicated by subdural hematomas: case series and literature review. Surg Neurol Int 2013;4:85.

58. Hinman JM, Provenzale JM. Hypointense thrombus on T2-weighted MR imaging: a potential pitfall in the diagnosis of dural sinus thrombosis. Eur J Radiol 2002;41:147–52.

59. Provenzale JM, Kranz PG. Dural sinus thrombosis: sources of error in image interpretation. AJR Am J Roentgenol 2011;196:23–31.

The Use of Intracranial Vessel Wall Imaging in Clinical Practice

Abderrahmane Hedjoudje, MD, MSE[a,b,*], Jean Darcourt, MD[c], Fabrice Bonneville, MD, PhD[c], Myriam Edjlali, MD, PhD[b,d]

KEYWORDS

• Atherosclerosis • Vasculitis • Aneurysm • Stroke • Vessel wall MR imaging

KEY POINTS

- 3D Vessel Wall MRI is increasingly used in clinical practice to diagnose and manage patients with cerebrovascular disease.
- Vessel Wall MRI provides a unique perspective by focusing on the pathology of the vessel wall rather than the vessel lumen, making it powerful in detecting vessel wall changes.
- The article reviews the imaging principles and pitfalls of Vessel Wall MRI, and describes how imaging patterns of vessel wall enhancement can improve the specificity of traditional angiographic imaging in detecting, characterizing, and monitoring intracranial vascular disease.

INTRODUCTION

For a wide spectrum of vascular, inflammatory, or tumoral diseases, post-contrast three-dimensional (3D) T1-weighted imaging of the brain is frequently used. The increased detection of visual contrast uptake and reduction in the static field inhomogeneity artifacts are some advantages that support the use of 3D fast spin echo (FSE) sequences over gradient echo sequences, for example, helping a better detection of brain metastases[1] or multiple sclerosis lesions enhancement.[2] In addition, due to their variable flip angle, 3DT1 FSE sequence used with an optimized spatial resolution and also includes an inherent black-blood effect enabling it to analyze vessel wall. An early application in that field was the detection of cervical artery dissections.[3]

In adjunction with MR angiography (MRA) sequences, vessel wall MR imaging (VW-MR imaging) using 3DT1 FSE sequences bring useful information about presence, degrees, and patterns of vessel wall enhancement. Its application helps to detect, characterize, and follow over time intracranial vascular disorders such as cerebral vasculitis, reversible cerebral vasoconstriction syndrome (RCVS), arterial dissection, intracranial atherosclerosis disease (ICAD),[4,5] moyamoya disease (MMD), and intracranial aneurysms.

In this article, we review the imaging principles and pitfalls of VW-MR imaging, we describe imaging patterns of the vessel wall enhancement that improve the specificity of conventional angiographic imaging to detect, characterize and follow intracranial vascular disease.

Technical Considerations, Pitfalls, and Limits

Three-dimensional VW-MR imaging has gained popularity in the diagnosis and management of patients with cerebrovascular disease in clinical practice. The technique can, however, generate

[a] Department of Diagnostic and Interventional Neuroradiology, Sion Hospital, CHVR, Sion, Switzerland; [b] Laboratoire D'imagerie Biomédicale Multimodale (BioMaps), Université Paris-Saclay, CEA, CNRS, Inserm, Service Hospitalier Frédéric Joliot, Orsay, France; [c] Department of Diagnostic and Therapeutic Neuroradiology, Hôpital Purpan, Toulouse, France; [d] Department of Radiology, APHP, Hôpitaux Raymond-Poincaré & Ambroise Paré, DMU Smart Imaging, GH Université Paris-Saclay, Paris, France
* Corresponding author. Department of Diagnostic and Interventional Neuroradiology, Sion Hospital, CHVR, Sion, Switzerland.
E-mail address: abderrahmane.hedjoudje@hopitalvs.ch

Radiol Clin N Am 61 (2023) 521–533
https://doi.org/10.1016/j.rcl.2023.01.007
0033-8389/23/© 2023 Elsevier Inc. All rights reserved.

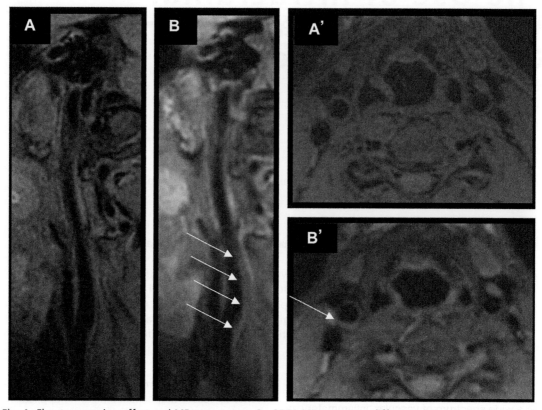

Fig. 1. Flow suppression effect and MR parameters: On 3DT1 FSE sequence, different parameters play a role in flow suppression effect. In this example, an increase of echo train length (low ETL: *A, A'*; long ETL: *B, B'*) makes a slow flow artifact seems against the posterior wall of the internal carotid artery (*arrows*). ETL, echo train length.

artifacts that arise from the technical caveats (eg, slow or recirculated flow or inadequate spatial resolution).

The slow flow in small veins can be misinterpreted as arterial wall enhancement after contrast injection. The simplest way to avoid this trap is to recognize the linear morphology of veins on VW-MR imaging in several planes. A recirculating or a disturbed flow may also yield plaque-mimicking flow artifacts due to incomplete flow suppression, which is commonly seen in the curved and large vessel segments (**Fig. 1**). It can also be seen when imaging intracranial aneurysm or close to the vessel wall or within the aneurysmal lumen when flow is turbulent.

An expert consensus Guideline from the American Society of Neuroradiology provides recommendations for the clinical implementation of intracranial VW-MR imaging.[6] Several technical aspects need to be considered when implementing VW-MR imaging in intracranial vessels, including flow suppression, in blood and in cerebrospinal fluid (CSF), spatial resolution, and signal-to-noise ratio.

Motion-induced intra-voxel dephasing[7] drives a part of blood flow suppression effect as phase dispersion and signal loss are caused by a large range of blood flow velocities. Low and variable flip-angle refocusing pulses promote phase dispersion and hence increase blood flow suppression. This phenomenon is increased when the flow direction is along with the frequency encoding axis.[8] Acquiring VW-MR imaging in multiple orientations may help to discern the artifacts caused by orientation-related incomplete flow suppression.[9]

Because of the motion-induced intra-voxel dephasing phenomenon, the spatial resolution of the sequence plays a role in flow suppression effect. Inadequate spatial resolution can lead to inadequate flow suppression on slow flow velocities, especially close to the vessel wall, and may lead to an overestimation of wall thickness[9] on VW-MR imaging and to a post-gadolinium slow flow enhancement artifact that could be misinterpreted as a presence of a vessel wall disorder such as ICAD or vasculitis. Spatial resolution should be optimized to have access to ≤ 0.7 mm and ideally ≤ 0.5 mm spatial resolution.[7]

Some technical options can also help to increase a black-blood effect, such as DANTE preparation module (Delay Alternating with Nutation for Tailored Excitation) or motion-sensitive driven equilibrium preparation module. However, their impact is less important with slow flow velocities less than 0.1 cm/s, and very slow flow, especially close to the wall, or in disturbed flows with high vorticity areas (eg, intra-aneurysmal) can therefore still present some flowing artifacts due to incomplete flow suppression.[7]

Whereas in the intracranial anterior circulation, vessel wall enhancement is considered abnormal, vertebrobasilar axis can present thin wall enhancement due to the presence of vasa vasorum. Vasa vasorum can also be present at the cervical level of internal carotid arteries. Thin enhancement of those portions should not be considered as abnormal.[10] At the cervical level, passive enlargement of the internal carotid vasa vasorum plexus secondarily to an internal carotid artery severe stenosis can also mimic wall enhancement (Fig. 2).

Finally, parietal wall of internal carotid artery within their cavernous portions or close to the dura cannot be analyzed. After contrast has been administered, the dura enhances, so as the cavernous sinuses, and the pituitary gland. Therefore, wall enhancement of vessels of this location cannot be analyzed.

Distinguishing Enhancement Patterns of Intracranial Artery Diseases

The different etiologies and their enhancement patterns are summarized in **Table 1**.

Intracranial atherosclerosis disease

ICAD lesions can range from slight wall thickening with plaques that are angiographically occult secondary to positive remodeling to severe stenotic lesions. Pre-Gd and post gadolinium (post-Gd) VW-MR imaging enables imaging beyond the lumen to characterize the vessel wall and allows better assessment of ICAD burden and identification of vulnerable plaque. Wall thickening, eccentricity index, enhancement distribution, metrics of enhancement length, volume, signal intensities on pre-contrast T2-weighted, pre-contrast/post-contrast T1-weighted acquisitions and per-patient burden are different metrics originating from pre-Gd and post-Gd VW-MR imaging analysis.

The typical appearance of ICAD on VW-MR imaging is an eccentric, heterogeneous mild to moderate enhancing, outward remodeling lesion with heterogeneous T2 signal, and juxtaluminal T2 hyperintensity that typically involves proximal intracranial branches or bifurcation points.

Although earlier studies have used eccentric vessel wall thickening patterns to identify intracranial plaque, an increasing number of studies report an overlap of eccentric and concentric wall thickening as plaque features.[11]

As ICAD plaques are very thin compared with cervical carotid plaques, VW-MR imaging using T2w, T2*w, and T1w images lacks spatial resolution to correctly differentiate lipid core from fibrous component and calcification.[12,13] However, intraplaque hemorrhage is an interesting marker of vulnerability of intracranial arteries. It seems as a high signal intensity on pre-Gd VW-MR imaging defined as an intraplaque T1 hyperintensity brighter than the signal intensity of internal reference muscle tissue[14] (**Fig. 3**). Intraplaque hemorrhage is attributed to fragile neovascularity with endothelial disruption that increases plaque wall shear stress and hence vulnerability.[15] It has proved to be an important risk factor for plaque vulnerability, with increased rates of plaque complications and stroke.[16]

Inflammatory plaque enhancement has been also widely studied.

Contrast enhancement characterization is useful for prognostic and diagnostic purposes (see **Fig. 3**). ICAD enhancement has been associated with its likelihood to have caused a recent ischemic event, independently of the plaque thickness.[17] Several studies have shown that intracranial plaque enhancement strongly correlates with ischemic stroke independent of the degree of stenosis.[18] Both degree and persistence of enhancement at follow-up imaging[19] strengthen diagnostic confidence in identifying culprit plaque and future risk for stroke recurrence.[18] The plaque is unlikely to be a culprit lesion if no enhancement or decrease in the degree of enhancement at follow-up imaging is seen.[20] As vessel wall enhancement may occur in generalized inflammatory diseases, as well as in ICAD plaques arterial, wall enhancement in equivocally suspected intracranial atherosclerosis cannot be conclusively excluded as another inflammatory vascular pathology. High-field High resolution vessel wall imaging (HR-VWI) allows the identification of ICAD in stroke patients with suspected underlying vasculopathy but otherwise classified as cryptogenic.[21] A recent meta-analysis showed that plaque enhancement, positive remodeling, T1 hyperintensity, and surface irregularity are strong imaging biomarkers of symptomatic plaque in patients with ischemic events.[22]

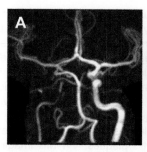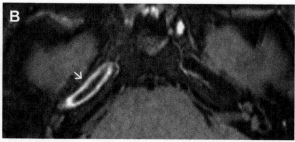

Fig. 2. A 35-year-old man with multiple transient ischemic attacks in the right internal carotid artery (ICA) territory. (*A*) TOF MRA revealed a severe stenosis of the right terminal ICA, with subsequent collapse of the diameter of the cervical and petrous ICA. (*B*) Vessel wall imaging did not show any enhancement at the level of the stenosis itself (not shown) but concentric enhancement within the carotid canal (*arrow*). This tricky image does not represent carotid walls enhancement, arteritis, or focal inflammation, but rather corresponds to the passive enlargement of the pericarotid plexus secondarily to the ICA collapse.

Finally, concerning radiation-chemotherapy (RCT)-induced arteriopathy, VW-MR imaging may help to identify patients at an increased risk for later ICAD-related complications requiring closer follow-up. Investigations of premature ICAD after RCT may lead to an improvement of actual cranial radiation protocols, aiming to decrease late sequelae[23] (**Fig. 4**).

Intracranial artery dissections

Spontaneous intracranial artery dissection is an uncommon (2.6–3.0 per 1,00,000 people per year)[24,25] and probably underdiagnosed cause of stroke, defined by the occurrence of a hematoma in the wall of an intracranial artery. Although far less common than cervical artery dissection, it remains a cause of ischemic stroke especially in children and young adults.[26] The conventional radiological findings of arterial dissection include intimal flap, double lumen, intramural hematoma, aneurysmal dilatation, tapered stenosis, and occlusion. In HR-MR studies, intimal flap and double lumen are common findings seen in patients with middle cerebral artery (**Fig. 5**) dissection along with intramural hematoma.[27] If HR-MR imaging indicates intramural hematoma without intimal flap or double lumen, intracranial artery dissection should first be included as part of the differential diagnosis. Intramural hematoma can demonstrate various signal intensities, such as intraplaque hemorrhage. Although a high signal intensity on T1-weighted imaging is the most common finding associated with intramural hematoma, isointensity and hypointensity can also be observed in the early stages[28] and requires a control at 5 to 7 days or more to look for a signal change that could positive the diagnosis of dissection.

The differentiation between intramural hematoma and intraplaque hemorrhage may sometimes be challenging. Clinical information such as age, ICAD risk factors, and radiologic findings such as

a clear geometric change seen on follow-up (arterial dissection is being indeed a dynamic vascular pathology) and wall calcifications (see **Fig. 4**) are crucial elements to help differentiate the conditions.[29]

In intracranial artery dissection, vessel wall enhancement may not be an uncommon finding.[30] Although vessel wall enhancement is not completely understood, it has been considered to result from inflammation,[31] slow blood flow in the false lumen, or enhancement of the vasa vasorum[30] (**Fig. 6**).

Reversible cerebral vasoconstriction syndrome/cocaine-induced vasculopathy

RCVS is characterized by reversible smooth muscle shortening and increased wall redundancy resulting in wall thickening and transient luminal narrowing.[8] RCVS may be diagnosed in the presence of sudden-onset headache with or without evidence of concomitant hemorrhage. Intracranial luminal abnormalities on MRA are the primary diagnostic feature of RCVS but could be normal in the early stage of the disease.[32] MRA abnormalities report multiple focal stenosis progressing over time from distal to proximal vessels of the circle of Willis arteries and their branches. Smooth, tapered narrowing followed by abnormal dilated segments of second- and third-order branches of the cerebral arteries is the most characteristic abnormality.[33] Reversibility within 3 month is considered the most specific feature of RCVS.

More than half the cases occur postpartum or after exposure to adrenergic or serotonergic drugs. It can be difficult to distinguish RCVS from other arteriopathies as most lack a gold standard diagnostic test and are similarly associated with headache and stroke. Because of management differences between RCVS and vasculitis, early discrimination is important; in RCVS, CSF examination and brain biopsy have

Table 1
Vessel wall imaging characteristics according to pathologies

Characteristics	Atherosclerosis	Vasculitis	RCVS	MMD	A-MMS	V-MMS	Dissection	Radiation Induced	Primary Angiitis
				Pathologies					
Pattern of the lesion	Eccentric, rarely circumferential	Circumferential, rarely eccentric	If present, circumferential thin, rarely eccentric	Circumferential	Rarely eccentric	Eccentric	Eccentric, rarely circumferential	Circumferential concentric	Concentric
Enhancement	++	++	+/–	-	+/–	++	+/–	+	+
Distribution	Variable degree of stenosis	Stenosis, often multifocal	Multifocal stenosis, reversible, posterior circulation often involved	Progressive stenosis of ICA and proximal middle cerebral artery (MCA). Outer vessel diameter may be reduced.	Like MMD, concomitant atherosclerotic stenosis of other intracranial vessels may be present.	Like MMD but may involve other vessels atypical for MMD.	Often focal	Often multifocal	Multiple arterial involvement
T1 hyperintensity	+/–	-	-	-	-	-	+	+/–	-
T2 signal	Heterogeneous, juxtaluminal hyperintensity	Isointense, homogeneous	Isointense, homogeneous	N/A	N/A	N/A	Variable	N/A	Isointense
Outer remodeling	++	-	-	-	+/–	+	+	-	-
Potential overlap in findings	Vasculitis	RCVS, atherosclerosis	Vasculitis	Vasculitis	Vasculitis	Atherosclerosis	Atherosclerosis	Atherosclerosis	Vasculitis

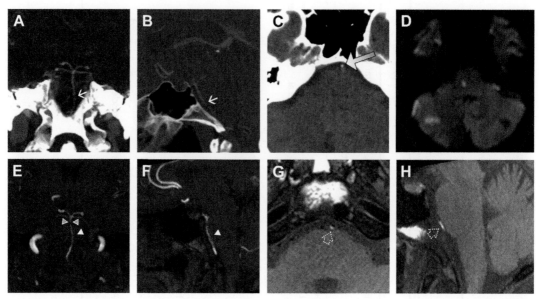

Fig. 3. A 54-year-old man with history of cerebellar and pontine infarcts. CT angiogram with maximal intensity projections (MIP) in (*A*) coronal and (*B*) sagittal views showed a basilar artery stenosis at the level of the anteroinferior cerebellar arteries (*white arrow*) with anterior calcification (*gray arrow*), as observed on (*C*) non-contrast axial CT. At the level of the stenosis, ischemic pontine lesions were visualized on (*D*) axial DWI. Surprisingly, the stenosis was less visible at this level on TOF MRA with MIP reformatted view in (*E*) coronal and (*F*) sagittal planes. On the contrary, another filling defect is demonstrated further (*double gray arrowhead*), just below the superior cerebellar arteries, where CTA was normal. This is interpreted as an artifact due to a competition of flow between antegrade flow coming from the basilar artery through the stenosis and a retrograde flow coming down from the PCOMs on this direction-sensitive TOF MRA (*white arrowhead*). (*G*) Axial and (*H*) sagittal views of vessel wall imaging performed without gadolinium injection revealed a spontaneous hyperintensity (*dot arrow*) of the plaque at the posterior wall of the basilar artery (opposite to the calcification) in relation with an acute intraplaque hemorrhage. This case illustrates that spontaneous hyperintensity of an hemorrhagic plaque might be misinterpreted or missed on TOF.

little utility other than to exclude mimics.[34] Both RCVS and vasculitis result in vessel wall thickening and luminal narrowing, but RCVS typically demonstrates little to no enhancement with only 31% to 47% of patients showing any enhancement with this disease whereas vasculitis presents in contrast more intense wall enhancement and moderate wall thickening.[5,35,36] Although inflammation is not considered to play a key role in the pathogenesis of RCVS,

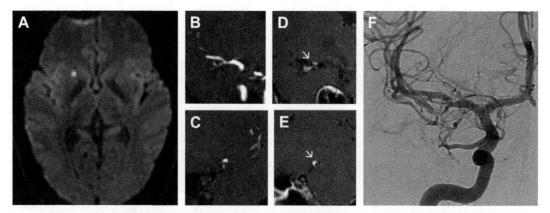

Fig. 4. A 37-year-old man with transient ischemic attack. (*A*) DWI showed a lacunar stroke in the right striatum. TOF MRA with (*B*) coronal and (*C*) sagittal reformatted images revealed an underlying stenosis of the right middle cerebral artery. Post-contrast vessel wall imaging with (*D*) coronal and (*E*) sagittal reformatted images demonstrated focal eccentric enhancement (*arrows*), suggestive of an inflammatory ICAD stenosis. On (*F*) digital subtracted angiogram performed as a follow-up 2 months later, the stenosis was unchanged. DWI, diffusion weitghed imaging; TOF, time of flight; PCOM, posterior communicant artery

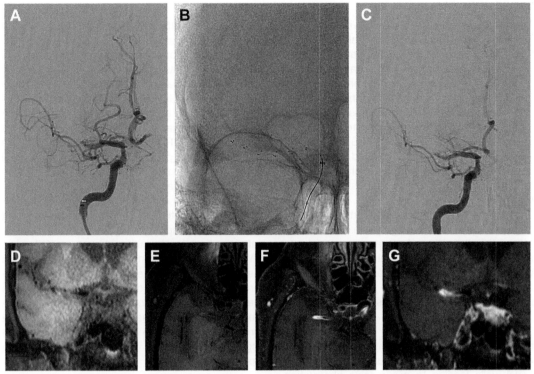

Fig. 5. A 78-year-old man with acute stroke due to right middle cerebral artery occlusion, treated by mechanical thrombectomy. (*A–C*) Antero posterior views of right internal carotid artery DSA that (*A*) initially confirms the distal M1 occlusion, (*B*) with four inefficient passes of a stentriever deployed in right middle cerebral artery, leading to (*C*) the absence of recanalization. A 48-hour follow-up MR imaging with vessel wall imaging (*D, E*) before and (*F, G*) after gadolinium injection with axial and coronal reformatted images showed marked enhancement of both the lumen and the proximal walls of the M1 segment at the level of the occlusion and site of thrombectomy. DSA, digital substracted arteriography.

prolonged vasoconstriction per se has been proposed to be associated with an inflammatory process,[37,38] with rare cases described of RCVS and strong enhancement.

Because cocaine-induced vasculitis is considered a spectral disorder of RCVS,[39–41] it is reasonable to deduce that vascular wall inflammation exists in at least some patients with secondary RCVS. Prolonged vasoconstriction has been hypothesized to contribute to the development of secondary angiitis; similar mechanisms might

also contribute to prolonged vascular wall enhancement.

Moyamoya disease
MMD is a chronic idiopathic cerebrovascular disorder characterized by stenosis of arteries around the circle of Willis with formation of aberrant collateral vessels. In cases where this phenomenon is associated with underlying disease such as sickle cell anemia, neurofibromatosis type 1, radiation therapy, or congenital syndromes, it is classified

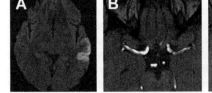
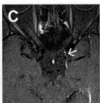
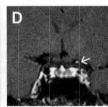
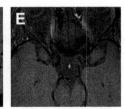

Fig. 6. A 30-year-old woman with acute speech disorder. (*A*) DWI showed cortical temporal hyperintensity suggestive of acute stroke, downstream a stenosis of the left terminal internal carotid artery, as seen on (*B*) TOF MRA. Post-contrast vessel wall imaging with (*C*) axial and (*D*) coronal reformatted images depicted eccentric enhancement of the left terminal internal carotid artery (*arrows*). After medical treatment, the vessel wall enhancement disappeared on (*E*) the 1-year follow-up VWI.

as moyamoya syndrome (MMS).[42] With the formation of strong compensating collaterals at the base of the brain, moyamoya vasculopathy leads to steno-occlusive processes of the carotid termini, proximal MCA, and anterior cerebral artery (ACA).[43] We also distinguish atherosclerotic-MMS and vasculitic-MMS when associated with aforementioned pathologies. MMD tends to have bilateral involvement, whereas MMS is often unilateral.[44,45] MMD often displayed concentric, non-enhancing lesions with wall shrinkage and often does not exhibit substantial wall thickening.[46]

When used in conjunction with conventional imaging methods, VW-MR imaging can considerably improve the distinction of moyamoya vasculopathies. When compared with luminal imaging alone, VW-MR imaging increases diagnostic accuracy and confidence in the ability to distinguish moyamoya illness from ICAD and vasculitic MMS.[46]

Primary and secondary CNS vasculitis

Cerebral vasculitis is defined as inflammation of arterial walls leading to progressive obstruction of the lumen, increased coagulation, and hence risk of stroke. Primary central nervous system (CNS) vasculitis is a rare disease (annual incidence of 2.4/1 million) caused by the direct involvement of vessels.[47] Secondary vascular inflammation is more frequent and can result from systemic connective tissue disorders or may be secondary to noninflammatory process such as infection, neoplasm, drugs, or radiation therapy.

Cerebral vasculitis is suspected on imaging when parenchymal ischemic lesions are associated to multifocal irregularities or stenoses detected on MRA with a concomitant presence of circumferential enhancement on VW-MR imaging. The ability of vascular MR imaging to identify vasculitis relates to the size of the affected vessels. Vasculitis in terms of size of the involved arteries is categorized in the 2012 Chapel Hill Consensus Conference.[48] On VW-MR imaging, intracranial vasculitis tends to present with segmental, concentric homogenous enhancement of the vessel wall, and/or circumferential, periadventitial enhancement following a vessel segment. The enhancement can be either pencil-thin or thick, extending beyond the margin of the vessel wall.[36,49]

The location[48] of VW-MR imaging enhancement lesions can help to identify the type of suspected vasculitis: proximal involvement will suggest giant cell arteritis (GCA), systemic sclerosis, primary angiitis of the central nervous system, and infectious disease, especially Varicella-zoster vasculitis that frequently affect M1 segment, responsible of basal ganglia infarcts.[50]

The location of vessel wall enhancement can also be used as a target for biopsy, greatly improving the diagnostic accuracy of biopsies.[49] Interestingly, in GCA, normal findings on scalp artery MR imaging are very strongly associated with negative temporal artery biopsy findings.[51] This suggests that MR imaging could be used as the initial diagnostic procedure in GCA, with temporal artery biopsy being reserved for patients with abnormal MR imaging findings (**Fig. 7**).

The degree of enhancement indicates the activity of vasculitis as concentric enhancement on VW-MR imaging might represent active inflammation in vasculitis. However, follow-up VW-MR imaging findings proved ambiguous as persisting enhancement despite immunosuppressive therapy and clinical remission has been reported as a frequent finding[52] In some situations, when decreased degree of enhancement on vasculitis follow-up is reported, VW-MR imaging findings confirm favorable treatment responses (**Fig. 8**).

Aneurysms and Vascular Malformations

Intracranial aneurysms

The presence of aneurysm wall enhancement (AWE) of intracranial aneurysm has initially been reported in ruptured aneurysms[53] (**Fig. 9**). Since then, a large majority (85%–100%) of ruptured intracranial aneurysms[54] have been described as harboring AWE on VW-MR imaging, with more prominent enhancement compared with unruptured aneurysms.[55–57]

Although there is considerable variation in how enhancement is graded or measured in terms of thickness, intensity, location, and homogeneity, all studies have been able to use enhancement characteristics to distinguish between "stable" and "unstable" aneurysms in a statistically significant way. In two meta-analyses of around 500 aneurysms, AWE has been shown to be connected to unstable or ruptured condition with an odds ratio (OR) of 20 to 34.[58,59]

Even when ruptured aneurysm was withdrawn from studies, AWE has been shown to be associated with size and instability, carrying an 11-fold OR for instability, that is, growing or symptomatic. Moreover, the lack of wall enhancement seems to strongly predict aneurysm stability.[60] The first studies with follow-up data have been published.[61–63] On these retrospective studies, increased AWE during follow-up has been described as a predictor of subsequent aneurysmal growth.[61] Hence, AWE may become a

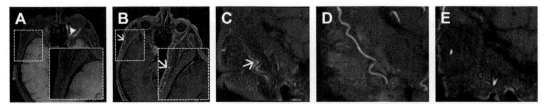

Fig. 7. A 64-year-old patient with right frontal orbital headaches. Vessel wall imaging performed (*A*) before and (*B, C*) after gadolinium injection showed concentric enhancement of superficial temporal artery, especially on (*C*) sagittal reformatted image (*arrow*). Of note, this artery was normal on (*D*) sagittal reformatted image of TOF MRA. (*E*) Follow-up VWI after 7 months of tocilizumab demonstrated regression of the vascular enhancement.

promising imaging marker to predict aneurysm behavior, identify high-risk aneurysms, and represent a potential target for clinical trials.[62] Prospective studies are now warranted to confirm this hypothesis.[63]

Brain arteriovenous malformations

Given the early evidence that VW-MR imaging may help in the identification of high-risk aneurysms, VW-MR imaging could also be a tool to improve the identification and characterization of high-risk intracranial arteriovenous malformations (AVMs). However, fewer VW-MR imaging studies have been performed on these more complex vascular malformations.[64] Moreover, a pilot study of VW-MR imaging in clinically unruptured brain AVMs demonstrated varying degrees of vessel wall hyperintensity, or

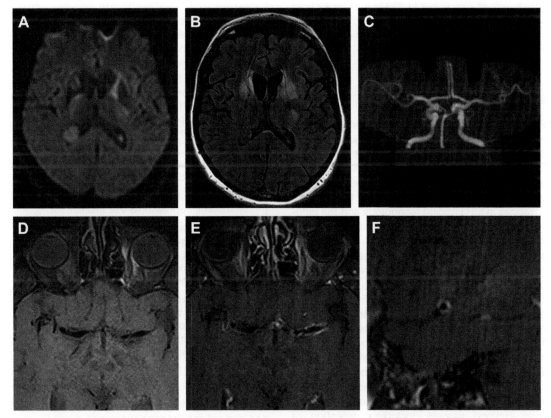

Fig. 8. A 52-year-old woman with transient right hemiparesis in a context of relapsing mood disorders and cognitive impairment since 3 weeks. MR imaging with (*A*) DWI and (*B*) FLAIR showed bilateral basal ganglia hyperintensities of uncertain origin, especially because (*C*) TOF MRA was normal, without intracranial stenosis. Vessel wall imaging performed (*D*) before and (*E* and *F*) after gadolinium injection with (*E*) axial and (*F*) sagittal reformatted images showed concentric enhancement of middle cerebral arteries, suggestive of cerebral arteritis. Basal ganglia lesions thus corresponded to subacute infarcts in this setting. FLAIR, fluid attenuated inversion recovery.

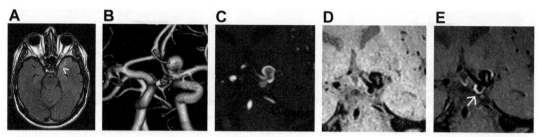

Fig. 9. A 71-year-old man, with acute headache. (*A*) Axial FLAIR showed hyperintensity in the left Sylvian fissure (*arrowhead*) suggestive of acute SAH. TOF MRA with (*B*) 3D volume rendering and (*C*) coronal MIP reformatted image depicted two left A1 aneurysms of different sizes facing each other. If the upper one was initially suspected of rupture because of its larger size, the small lower one was thought to be unruptured because of its tiny size and would only be followed up secondarily. Vessel wall imaging (*D*) before and (*E*) after contrast administration strikingly demonstrated marked circumferential enhancement of the lower one (*arrow*), witnessing some instability. Decision has been subsequently taken to embolize both aneurysms in emergency. SAH, subarachnoid haemorrhage.

enhancement, in the majority of the cases.[65] Although a portion of the hyperintensity could be due to incomplete blood suppression due to the complex hemodynamic of AVM, vessel wall enhancement can occur in AVMs with or without prior rupture.[64,65] Larger, longitudinal studies are needed to understand the implications of this intranidal enhancement.

SUMMARY

VW-MR imaging is an imaging technique that delivers a fundamentally different viewpoint by emphasizing on the pathology of the vessel wall as opposed to traditional descriptions that focus on vessel lumen. It is now routinely used in many MR imaging protocols in clinical practice. Recent advances in MR imaging technology and the diffusion of 3 Tesla (3T) magnetic field devices made VW-MR imaging widely available. It shows a crucial power in detecting vessel wall changes in patients with diseases including, but not limited to, central nervous system vasculitis, MMD, aneurysms, dissections, and ICAD. Radiologists must be familiar with the imaging appearance of normal vessel structures as well as the disease entities that may be encountered. It is also important to be familiar with the technique principles to be able to optimize image quality and to avoid potential pitfalls. Moreover, VW imaging is a promising technique for the exploration of intracranial pathologies beyond vessels, including detection of lepto- and pachymeningitis, punctuate pattern of parenchymal enhancement,[66] blood brain barrier rupture enhancement, and so forth. Demonstrating the full potential of VW-MR imaging will require larger prospective studies.

CLINICS CARE POINTS

- Intracranial vessel wall (VW) imaging offers advantages over lumen-based methods, detecting nonstenotic lesions and characterizing stenotic lesions that have been detected by common angiographic methods.

- A magnetic field strength of at least 3 T is necessary for intracranial VW imaging to achieve sufficient contrast-to-noise ratio (CNR) and spatial resolution for visualizing arterial VW and VW lesions.

- For optimal image assessment, radiologists need to be familiar with clinical patient information and the applied imaging parameters.

- Radiologists and clinicials can benefit from a systematic approach to VW assessment.

- Technical challenges in VW imaging include reducing acquisition time for pre- and post-contrast sequences without compromising signal-to-noise ratio and CNR, and the need for histopathologic validation.

- VWI can be useful in the work up of cryptogenic stroke by detecting intracranial culprit lesions but does not prevent from performing a complete stroke work-up to explore all potential etiologies.

DISCLOSURE

None of the authors have any relevant financial and/or nonfinancial relationships to disclose.

REFERENCES

1. Suh CH, Jung SC, Kim KW, et al. The detectability of brain metastases using contrast-enhanced spin-

echo or gradient-echo images: a systematic review and meta-analysis. J Neuro Oncol 2016;129(2): 363–71.

2. Ozturk A, Aygun N, Smith SA, et al. Axial 3D gradient-echo imaging for improved multiple sclerosis lesion detection in the cervical spinal cord at 3T. Neuroradiology 2013;55(4):431–9.

3. Edjlali M, Roca P, Rabrait C, et al. 3D Fast Spin-Echo T1 Black-Blood Imaging for the Diagnosis of Cervical Artery Dissection. AJNR Am J Neuroradiol 2013;34(9):E103.

4. Chen CY, Chen SP, Fuh JL, et al. Vascular wall imaging in reversible cerebral vasoconstriction syndrome – a 3-T contrast-enhanced MRI study. J Headache Pain 2018;19(1). https://doi.org/10.1186/S10194-018-0906-7.

5. Miller TR, Shivashankar R, Mossa-Basha M, et al. Reversible Cerebral Vasoconstriction Syndrome, Part 2: Diagnostic Work-Up, Imaging Evaluation, and Differential Diagnosis. AJNR Am J Neuroradiol 2015;36(9):1580–8.

6. Mandell DM, Mossa-Basha M, Qiao Y, et al. Intracranial Vessel Wall MRI: Principles and Expert Consensus Recommendations of the American Society of Neuroradiology. AJNR Am J Neuroradiol 2017;38(2):218.

7. Xie Y, Yang Q, Xie G, et al. Improved black-blood imaging using DANTE-SPACE for simultaneous carotid and intracranial vessel wall evaluation. Magn Reson Med 2016;75(6):2286.

8. Edjlali M, Qiao Y, Boulouis G, et al. Vessel wall MR imaging for the detection of intracranial inflammatory vasculopathies. Cardiovasc Diagn Ther 2020; 10(4):1108.

9. Antiga L, Wasserman BA, Steinman DA. On the overestimation of early wall thickening at the carotid bulb by black blood MRI, with implications for coronary and vulnerable plaque imaging. Magn Reson Med 2008;60(5):1020–8.

10. Portanova A, Hakakian N, Mikulis DJ, et al. Intracranial vasa vasorum: insights and implications for imaging. Radiology 2013;267(3):667–79.

11. Alexander MD, Yuan C, Rutman A, et al. High-resolution intracranial vessel wall imaging: imaging beyond the lumen. J Neurol Neurosurg Psychiatry 2016;87(6):589.

12. Yang WJ, Wong KS, Chen XY. Intracranial Atherosclerosis: From Microscopy to High-Resolution Magnetic Resonance Imaging. J Stroke 2017;19(3):249.

13. Zhao XQ, Dong L, Hatsukami T, et al. MR Imaging of Carotid Plaque Composition During Lipid-Lowering Therapy: A Prospective Assessment of Effect and Time Course. JACC Cardiovasc Imaging 2011; 4(9):977.

14. Song JW, Wasserman BA. Vessel wall MR imaging of intracranial atherosclerosis. Cardiovasc Diagn Ther 2020;10(4):982.

15. Zhu C, Tian X, Degnan AJ, et al. Clinical Significance of Intraplaque Hemorrhage in Low- and High-Grade Basilar Artery Stenosis on High-Resolution MRI. AJNR Am J Neuroradiol 2018; 39(7):1286.

16. Xu WH, Li ML, Gao S, et al. Middle cerebral artery intraplaque hemorrhage: prevalence and clinical relevance. Ann Neurol 2012;71(2):195–8.

17. Qiao Y, Zeiler SR, Mirbagheri S, et al. Intracranial Plaque Enhancement in Patients with Cerebrovascular Events on High-Spatial-Resolution MR Images. Radiology 2014;271(2):534.

18. Kim HJ, Choi EH, Chung JW, et al. Luminal and Wall Changes in Intracranial Arterial Lesions for Predicting Stroke Occurrence. Stroke 2020;51(8): 2495–504.

19. Zhou P, Wang Y, Sun J, et al. Assessment of Therapeutic Response to Statin Therapy in Patients With Intracranial or Extracranial Carotid Atherosclerosis by Vessel Wall MRI: A Systematic Review and Updated Meta-Analysis. Front Cardiovasc Med 2021; 0:1433.

20. Wu F, Ma Q, Song H, et al. Differential Features of Culprit Intracranial Atherosclerotic Lesions: A Whole-Brain Vessel Wall Imaging Study in Patients With Acute Ischemic Stroke. J Am Heart Assoc: Cardiovascular and Cerebrovascular Disease 2018; 7(15). https://doi.org/10.1161/JAHA.118.009705.

21. Fakih R, Roa JA, Bathla G, et al. Detection and Quantification of Symptomatic Atherosclerotic Plaques With High-Resolution Imaging in Cryptogenic Stroke. Stroke 2020;51(12):3623–31.

22. Song JW, Pavlou A, Xiao J, et al. Vessel Wall MR Imaging Biomarkers of Symptomatic Intracranial Atherosclerosis: A Meta-Analysis. Stroke 2021; 52(1):193.

23. Aoki S, Hayashi N, Abe O, et al. Radiation-induced arteritis: thickened wall with prominent enhancement on cranial MR images report of five cases and comparison with 18 cases of MMD. Radiology 2002; 223(3):683–8.

24. Labeyrie MA, Civelli V, Reiner P, et al. Prevalence and treatment of spontaneous intracranial artery dissections in patients with acute stroke due to intracranial large vessel occlusion. J Neurointerv Surg 2018; 10(8):761–4.

25. Debette S, Compter A, Labeyrie MA, et al. Epidemiology, pathophysiology, diagnosis, and management of intracranial artery dissection. Lancet Neurol 2015;14(6):640–54.

26. George MG. Risk Factors for Ischemic Stroke in Younger Adults. Stroke 2020;51(3):729–35.

27. Cho SJ, Choi BS, Bae YJ, et al. Image Findings of Acute to Subacute Craniocervical Arterial Dissection on Magnetic Resonance Vessel Wall Imaging: A Systematic Review and Proportion Meta-Analysis. Front Neurol 2021;12:586735.

28. Choi YJ, Jung SC, Lee DH. Vessel Wall Imaging of the Intracranial and Cervical Carotid Arteries. J Stroke 2015;17(3):238.

29. Dieleman N, van der Kolk AG, Zwanenburg JJM, et al. Imaging Intracranial Vessel Wall Pathology With Magnetic Resonance Imaging. Circulation 2014;130(2):192–201.

30. Sakurai K, Miura T, Sagisaka T, et al. Evaluation of luminal and vessel wall abnormalities in subacute and other stages of intracranial vertebrobasilar artery dissections using the volume isotropic turbo-spin-echo acquisition (VISTA) sequence: a preliminary study. J Neuroradiol 2013;40(1):19–28.

31. Pfefferkorn T, Saam T, Rominger A, et al. Vessel wall inflammation in spontaneous cervical artery dissection: a prospective, observational positron emission tomography, computed tomography, and magnetic resonance imaging study. Stroke 2011;42(6): 1563–8.

32. Ducros A, Boukobza M, Porcher R, et al. The clinical and radiological spectrum of reversible cerebral vasoconstriction syndrome. A prospective series of 67 patients. Brain 2007;130(Pt 12):3091–101.

33. Hamrick F, Havenon ADE, Taussky P, et al. Application of Vessel Wall Magnetic Resonance Imaging in Intracranial Cerebrovascular Pathology. Journal of Neurosonology and Neuroimaging 2019;11(2): 105–14.

34. Kontzialis M, Wasserman BA. Intracranial vessel wall imaging: current applications and clinical implications. Neurovascular Imaging 2016;2(1):1–6.

35. Miller TR, Shivashankar R, Mossa-Basha M, et al. Reversible Cerebral Vasoconstriction Syndrome, Part 1: Epidemiology, Pathogenesis, and Clinical Course. AJNR Am J Neuroradiol 2015;36(8):1392–9.

36. Mossa-Basha M, Shibata DK, Hallam DK, et al. Added Value of Vessel Wall Magnetic Resonance Imaging for Differentiation of Nonocclusive Intracranial Vasculopathies. Stroke 2017;48(11). https://doi.org/10.1161/STROKEAHA.117.018227.

37. Hajj-Ali RA. Primary angiitis of the central nervous system: Differential diagnosis and treatment. Best Pract Res Clin Rheumatol 2010;24(3):413–26.

38. Evaluation and treatment of central nervous system vasculitis - PubMed. Available at: https://pubmed.ncbi.nlm.nih.gov/7718420/. Accessed August 18, 2022.

39. Ducros A. Reversible cerebral vasoconstriction syndrome. Lancet Neurol 2012;11(10):906–17.

40. Singhal AB, Topcuoglu MA, Fok JW, et al. Reversible cerebral vasoconstriction syndromes and primary angiitis of the central nervous system: clinical, imaging, and angiographic comparison. Ann Neurol 2016;79(6):882–94.

41. Singhal AB, Hajj-Ali RA, Topcuoglu MA, et al. Reversible cerebral vasoconstriction syndromes:

analysis of 139 cases. Arch Neurol 2011;68(8): 1005–12.

42. Kuroda S, Fujimura M, Takahashi J, et al. Diagnostic Criteria for MMD - 2021 Revised Version. Neurol Med -Chir 2022;62(7):307.

43. Scott RM, Smith ER. MMD and MSS. N Engl J Med 2009;360(12):1226–37.

44. Yuan M, Liu ZQ, Wang ZQ, et al. High-resolution MR imaging of the arterial wall in MMD. Neurosci Lett 2015;584:77–82.

45. Suzuki J, Takaku A. Cerebrovascular "moyamoya" disease. Disease showing abnormal net-like vessels in base of brain. Arch Neurol 1969;20(3):288–99.

46. Mossa-Basha M, de Havenon A, Becker KJ, et al. Added Value of Vessel Wall MR Imaging in the Differentiation of Moyamoya Vasculopathies in a Non-Asian Cohort. Stroke 2016;47(7):1782.

47. Salvarani C, Brown RD, Christianson TJH, et al. Adult primary central nervous system vasculitis treatment and course: analysis of one hundred sixty-three patients. Arthritis Rheumatol 2015;67(6): 1637–45.

48. Jennette JC, Falk RJ, Bacon PA, et al. 2012 revised International Chapel Hill Consensus Conference Nomenclature of Vasculitides. Arthritis Rheum 2013;65(1):1–11.

49. Zeiler SR, Qiao Y, Pardo CA, et al. Vessel Wall MRI for Targeting Biopsies of Intracranial Vasculitis. AJNR Am J Neuroradiol 2018;39(11):2034–6.

50. Gilden D, Cohrs RJ, Mahalingam R, et al. Varicella zoster virus vasculopathies: diverse clinical manifestations, laboratory features, pathogenesis, and treatment. Lancet Neurol 2009;8(8):731–40.

51. Rhéaume M, Rebello R, Pagnoux C, et al. High-Resolution Magnetic Resonance Imaging of Scalp Arteries for the Diagnosis of Giant Cell Arteritis: Results of a Prospective Cohort Study. Arthritis Rheumatol 2017;69(1):161–8.

52. Patzig M, Forbrig R, Küpper C, et al. Diagnosis and follow-up evaluation of central nervous system vasculitis: an evaluation of vessel-wall MRI findings. J Neurol 2022;269(2):982–96.

53. Matouk CC, Mandell DM, Günel M, et al. Vessel wall magnetic resonance imaging identifies the site of rupture in patients with multiple intracranial aneurysms: proof of principle. Neurosurgery 2013;72(3): 492–6.

54. Edjlali M, Gentric JC, Régent-Rodriguez C, et al. Does aneurysmal wall enhancement on vessel wall MRI help to distinguish stable from unstable intracranial aneurysms? Stroke 2014;45(12):3704–6.

55. Nagahata S, Nagahata M, Obara M, et al. Wall Enhancement of the Intracranial Aneurysms Revealed by Magnetic Resonance Vessel Wall Imaging Using Three-Dimensional Turbo Spin-Echo Sequence with Motion-Sensitized Driven-

Equilibrium: A Sign of Ruptured Aneurysm? Clin Neuroradiol 2016;26(3):277–83.

56. Edjlali M, Guédon A, Hassen WB, et al. Circumferential thick enhancement at vessel wall MRI has high specificity for intracranial aneurysm instability. Radiology 2018;289(1):181–7.

57. Fu Q, Wang Y, Zhang Y, et al. Qualitative and Quantitative Wall Enhancement on Magnetic Resonance Imaging Is Associated with Symptoms of Unruptured Intracranial Aneurysms. Stroke 2020;52(1):213–22.

58. Wang X, Zhu C, Leng Y, et al. Intracranial Aneurysm Wall Enhancement Associated with Aneurysm Rupture: A Systematic Review and Meta-analysis. Acad Radiol 2019;26(5):664–73.

59. Texakalidis P, Hilditch CA, Lehman V, et al. Vessel Wall Imaging of Intracranial Aneurysms: Systematic Review and Meta-analysis. World Neurosurg 2018;117:453–8.e1.

60. Larson AS, Lehman VT, Lanzino G, et al. Lack of Baseline Intracranial Aneurysm Wall Enhancement Predicts Future Stability: A Systematic Review and Meta-Analysis of Longitudinal Studies. AJNR Am J Neuroradiol 2020;41(9). https://doi.org/10.3174/AJNR.A6690.

61. Gariel F, ben Hassen W, Boulouis G, et al. Increased Wall Enhancement During Follow-Up as a Predictor of Subsequent Aneurysmal Growth. Stroke 2020;51(6):1868–72.

62. Zhu C, Mossa-Basha M. Wall enhancement as an emerging marker of intracranial aneurysm stability: Roadmap toward a potential target for clinical trials. Eur J Neurol 2021;28(11):3550–1.

63. L'Allinec V, Chatel S, Karakachoff M, et al. Prediction of Unruptured Intracranial Aneurysm Evolution: The UCAN Project. Neurosurgery 2020;87(1):150–6.

64. Petridis AK, Dibue-Adjei M, Cornelius JF, et al. Contrast enhancement of vascular walls of intracranial high flow malformations in black blood MRI indicates high inflammatory activity. Chin Neurosurg J 2018;4(1):1–5.

65. Eisenmenger LB, Junn JC, Cooke D, et al. Presence of Vessel Wall Hyperintensity in Unruptured Arteriovenous Malformations on Vessel Wall Magnetic Resonance Imaging: Pilot Study of AVM Vessel Wall "Enhancement. Front Neurosci 2021;15:915.

66. Taieb G, Duran-Peña A, de Chamfleur NM, et al. Punctate and curvilinear gadolinium enhancing lesions in the brain: a practical approach. Neuroradiology 2016;58(3):221–35.

Imaging of Head Trauma
Pearls and Pitfalls

Aniwat Sriyook, MD[a,b,*], Rajiv Gupta, PhD, MD[b]

KEYWORDS

- Head trauma • Traumatic brain injury • Skull fracture • Intracranial hemorrhage • Brain contusion
- Diffuse axonal injury • Chronic traumatic encephalopathy

KEY POINTS

- Traumatic brain injury (TBI) is a major global health problem and needs immediate management to reduce morbidity and mortality.
- Imaging plays a vital role in triage, diagnosis, treatment planning, follow-up, and prognosis of patients with TBI.
- Non-contrast computed tomography with proper protocol and window setting acts as the first-line imaging with high sensitivity and specificity in detecting skull fractures and intracranial abnormalities.
- MR imaging has a role in a case of unremarkable computed tomography finding with a persistent unexplained cognitive or neurologic deficit due to its higher sensitivity in detecting some pathologies such as extra-axial hemorrhage, small or nonhemorrhagic brain contusion, posterior fossa injury, and diffuse axonal injury.

INTRODUCTION

Traumatic brain injury (TBI) is an alteration in brain function or other evidence of brain pathology caused by an external force.[1] TBI has been used to replace the former term, head injury because its more precise terminology highlights the importance of the damage to the brain. TBI is one of the most common causes of morbidity and mortality globally. An estimated 69 million patients suffer from TBI each year, with the highest annual incidence in North America and Europe and the most outstanding overall burden in Southeast Asia and western pacific regions.[2]

TBI can be classified into mild, moderate, and severe degrees based on the patient's consciousness using the Glasgow Coma Scale (GCS). There is a strong correlation between the GCS score and patient outcome after acute brain damage, particularly those with moderate and severe TBI (ie, the lower the GCS score, the poorer the outcome).[3] This correlation, however, may not hold for mild TBI. Approximately half of the patients with mild TBI report persistent symptoms one year after injury.[4] Although mild TBI occurs much more commonly than moderate and severe TBI, the damage to quality of life and socioeconomic status is still a significant burden.[5]

This article describes the indication for imaging, imaging modalities, recommended imaging protocols, and imaging findings of primary and secondary injuries, including pitfalls of each pathology.

IMAGING INDICATION AND MODALITIES

The imaging techniques have been improved considerably in recent years and play an essential role in traumatic patients, including TBI. Imaging

[a] Department of Radiology, King Chulalongkorn Memorial Hospital, The Thai Red Cross Society, and Faculty of Medicine, Chulalongkorn University, Bangkok 10330, Thailand; [b] Department of Radiology, Massachusetts General Hospital and Harvard Medical School, 55 Fruit Street, Boston, MA 02114, USA
* Corresponding author. Department of Radiology, King Chulalongkorn Memorial Hospital, The Thai Red Cross Society, and Faculty of Medicine, Chulalongkorn University, 1873 Rama IV Road, Pathum Wan, Pathum Wan, Bangkok 10330, Thailand
E-mail address: aniwat.s@chula.ac.th

Radiol Clin N Am 61 (2023) 535–549
https://doi.org/10.1016/j.rcl.2023.01.008
0033-8389/23/© 2023 Elsevier Inc. All rights reserved.

can assist clinicians in triage, diagnosis, treatment planning, follow-up, and prognosis of patients with TBI.

Various evidence-based guidelines attempt to standardize imaging indications for patients with TBI. With these guidelines, a non-contrast computed tomography (NCCT) of the head is considered an initial imaging modality in patients with moderate and severe TBI. However, in cases with mild TBI, NCCT is suggested only if indicated by the clinical decision rule, such as focal neurologic deficit and risk factors.[6]

NCCT has been accepted as first-line imaging in TBI cases due to its high sensitivity and specificity in detecting skull fractures and intracranial abnormalities such as hemorrhage, brain contusion, brain herniation, and hydrocephalus. Moreover, NCCT has benefits in the fast acquisition, widespread availability and accessibility, and no contraindication. The limitations of computed tomography (CT) are mainly about artifacts such as streak, partial volume averaging, and beam-hardening artifacts.

On the contrary, MR imaging takes more time for imaging acquisition with less availability and accessibility. Patients must be screened for metallic implants and foreign bodies before MR imaging scanning. However, the great advantage of MR imaging is its higher sensitivity than CT in detecting some pathologies such as extra-axial hemorrhage, small or nonhemorrhagic brain contusion, posterior fossa injury, and diffuse axonal injury (DAI). American College of Radiology (ACR) Appropriateness Criteria suggests that non-contrast MR imaging of the head usually has a role

as an initial modality in subacute or chronic head trauma with an unexplained cognitive or neurologic deficit. In addition, MR imaging may be appropriate as a follow-up imaging in case of acute head trauma with unchanged neurologic examination and unremarkable or positive findings on initial imaging, as well as in case of acute head trauma with new or progressive neurologic deficit.

IMAGING PROTOCOLS

The recommended head CT protocol for the adult is using multidetector CT at 120 kVp and 240 mAs with a section thickness of 5 mm. Coronal and sagittal image reconstructions at 5-mm section thickness are suggested. Reviewing images in all three planes is essential in detecting subtle intracranial abnormalities such as a thin extra-axial hemorrhage, and lesions at the vertex or along the skull base. It is also necessary to look at images in both standard brain (widths 80, level 40) and wide (widths 150 to 200, level 80) windows for maximizing pathology detection (**Fig. 1**). For detecting fractures, axial thin slice images (at least 1.25-mm slice thickness or thinner) with bone kernel should be obtained, as well as multiplanar and three-dimensional (3D) image reconstruction for better visualization.

The recommended head MR imaging protocol is axial T1-weighted, T2-weighted, T2-weighted-fluid-attenuated inversion recovery (FLAIR), T2*-gradient-recalled echo (GRE) or susceptibility-weighted imaging (SWI), and diffusion-weighted imaging (DWI) sequences. CT or MR angiography

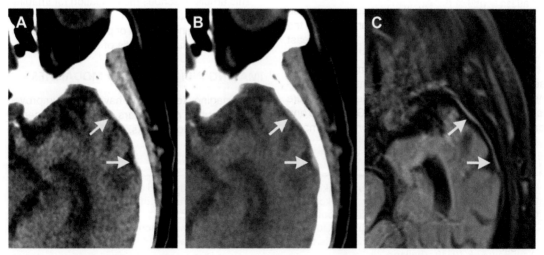

Fig. 1. Axial images of thin acute SDH (*arrow*) along the left temporal region in standard brain window (*A*), wide window (*B*), and FLAIR (*C*) images. The hematoma is better seen in wide window and FLAIR images than in standard brain window image.

should be added in cases with suspected intracranial arterial injury, as well as CT or MR venography for patients with suspected intracranial venous injury.

IMAGING FINDINGS

TBI can be classified into two main groups: primary and secondary. Primary injury results from direct impact to the head and occurs at the time of the initial head trauma, such as skull fracture, extra-axial hemorrhage, brain contusion, and DAI. Secondary injury develops later as complications, such as diffuse cerebral edema, brain herniation, and chronic traumatic encephalopathy (CTE).

It is crucial to understand the stages of intracranial hematoma before reviewing each pathology. On CT, the attenuation coefficient of the hematoma can be measured in Hounsfield units (HU) and interpreted as hypodensity, isodensity, and hyperdensity compared with cortex attenuation. The attenuation or density of hematoma is due to the protein component of hemoglobin.[7] Hyperacute hematoma is isodense, whereas acute hematoma is hyperdense (60 to 80 HU) due to clot retraction.[7,8] After that, the attenuation of the hematoma will decrease by approximately 1.5 HU per day and will be seen as isodense in the subacute stage and hypodense in the chronic stage.[9]

However, it should be noted that not all hematomas follow this rule. There is a linear relationship between the density of hematoma and hemoglobin concentration.[10] Thus, acute hematoma in an anemic patient (hemoglobin value less than 8 to 10 g/dL) or a coagulopathic patient can be visualized as isodense or even hypodense. Furthermore, acute hematoma can show a hematocrit fluid-fluid level in coagulopathic patients (eg, clotting disorder, on anticoagulant) as the blood does not form a clot and red cells settle dependently (Fig. 2).[11,12]

On MR imaging, the hematoma signal intensity depends on the blood's age, types of hemoglobin, and imaging sequences. The five stages of hematoma can be summarized in Table 1.

PRIMARY INJURIES
Skull Fracture

Skull comprises two main components: the calvaria and the skull base. Skull fractures can be mainly categorized into linear or depressed based on the mechanism of injury and management.

Linear fracture is a sharply marginated lucent line in the bone and could be either displaced or non-displaced. It results from low energy but a large area of blunt impact. Conservative treatment is often sufficient in the case of a linear fracture alone. However, if there are any associated intracranial injuries, the treatment is usually based on the other injuries (Fig. 3).

Depressed fracture occurs due to higher energy within a small impact area, resulting in the inward displacement of the bony fragment. It is frequently associated with tearing of the underlying meninges, as well as an increased chance of other intracranial injuries and infection, which require more aggressive or surgical treatment (Fig. 4).[12,13]

There are also some other fracture types that should be considered. Diastatic fractures are fractures that involve sutures, causing the widening of the affected sutures or synchondrosis (Fig. 5). Rarely, soft tissues (eg, meninges, brain parenchyma) and cerebrospinal fluid (CSF) may become trapped within the fractured site. Not only can the

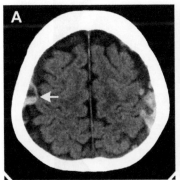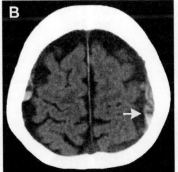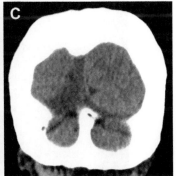

Fig. 2. Bilateral acute SDH in a 60-year-old woman with multiple myeloma, anemia, and thrombocytopenia (hemoglobin = 4.4 g/dL and platelet = 5000 cell/uL). Axial CT images (*A, B*) show hematocrit fluid–fluid levels (*arrows*) in the hematomas. Coronal image (*C*) at the posterior aspect of the head shows hypodense venous sinuses, corresponding with anemia.

Table 1
Signal intensity of hematoma on MR imaging

Stages of Hematoma	Types of Hemoglobin	T1WI	T2WI	DWI
Hyperacute	Oxyhemoglobin	Isointense	Hyperintense	Hyperintense on DWI and hypointense on ADC map
Acute (1 to 2 days)	Deoxyhemoglobin	Isointense	Hypointense	Hypointense on DWI and ADC map
Early subacute (2 to 7 days)	Intracellular methemoglobin	Hyperintense	Hypointense	Hypointense on DWI and ADC map
Late subacute (1 week to months)	Extracellular methemoglobin	Hyperintense	Hyperintense	Hyperintense on DWI and hypointense on ADC map
Chronic (months–years)	Hemosiderin	Hypointense	Hypointense	Hypointense on DWI and ADC map

fracture not heal, but also the bony gap progressively widens due to CSF pulsation. This expanding fracture is called a growing fracture. It is a delayed complication that usually presents months or years after the injury.

The location of the fracture is also an essential consideration, as it may be a clue to other associated symptoms or injuries. Fractures at the anterior skull base are commonly associated with dural tears and CSF leaks, particularly comminuted or oblique fractures.[14] Fractures that take place near the vessels may indicate associated vascular injuries, such as internal carotid artery (ICA) injury in middle cranial fossa fracture involving carotid canal, transverse-sigmoid dural venous sinus thrombosis in temporal or occipital bone fracture, and venous epidural hematoma (EDH) in sphenoid wing fracture or sagittal suture diastasis. Further vascular studies with CT angiography or venography should be ordered in these cases.

Fractures can be readily identified if they are depressed or obviously displaced. However, it can be problematic in non-displaced or minimally displaced linear fractures, which should keep normal sutures and vascular grooves in differential diagnoses. Calvarial and skull base sutures have sclerotic borders and zigzag patterns with interdigitations and are usually present in bilateral and somewhat symmetrical. Vascular grooves also have sclerotic borders and may have branching patterns. On the contrary, acute fractures

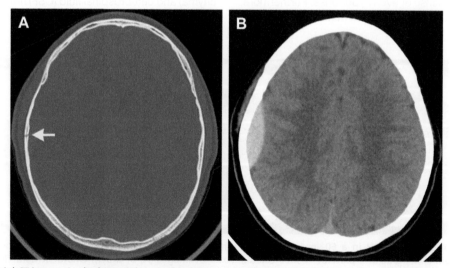

Fig. 3. Axial CT images in the bone (A) and wide (B) windows show a non-displaced linear fracture (arrow) at the right parietal bone, associated with a subjacent small acute EDH.

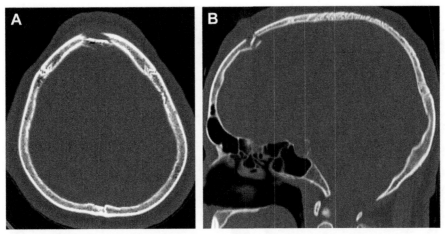

Fig. 4. Axial (*A*) and sagittal (*B*) CT images show a depressed fracture at the frontal bones.

present as sharply marginated lucent lines without sclerotic borders. Abnormal widening of the suture and synchondrosis should raise suspicion of a diastatic fracture. An overlying soft tissue swelling, underneath extra-axial hemorrhage, or brain contusion is also a piece of evidence that supports a diagnosis of acute fracture.[12,15]

Epidural Hematoma

EDH locates in the epidural space, between the inner table of the skull and the dura. It is highly associated with skull fractures (>90%) and can be classified by the origin of bleeding into two main categories: arterial (90% to 95%) and venous sites (5% to 10%).

Arterial EDH can occur in both supra- and infratentorium but predominated in the former,

particularly in the temporoparietal region due to the relatively thinning of the pterion (see **Fig. 3**). It is most related to the injury of the subjacent middle meningeal artery. The classic "lucid interval" is found in approximately 50% of patients with arterial EDH.[16]

Venous EDH occurs when the fractures involve dural venous sinuses, venous plexus, or veins. Typical locations are the anterior temporal region (due to sphenoparietal sinus injury) and vertex (due to superior sagittal sinus injury) (**Fig. 6**). Rarely, venous EDH can occur at the retroclival area due to basilar venous plexus injury from the clival fractures or the tectorial membrane stripping injury in pediatric cervical flexion-extension injury.[17]

Typical imaging appearances of the EDHs are the lens- or biconvex-shaped extra-axial

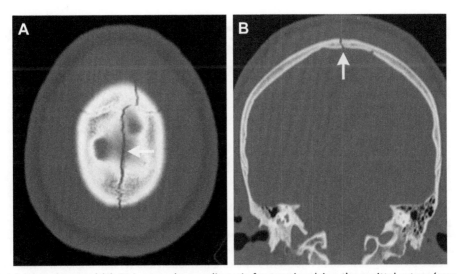

Fig. 5. Axial (*A*) and coronal (*B*) CT images show a diastatic fracture involving the sagittal suture (*arrow*).

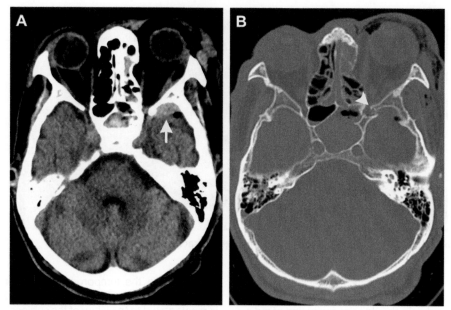

Fig. 6. Axial CT images in brain (*A*) and bone (*B*) windows of acute venous EDH along the left anterior temporal region (*arrow*) with a fracture at the greater wing of the left sphenoid bone (*arrowhead*).

hematomas that do not cross sutures due to the strong attachment of the dura around these areas except in cases with the presence of fractures across the sutures or diastatic fractures. However, these hematomas can cross the midline and tentorium cerebelli. Some hematomas may have the internal hypodense area (swirl sign), which suggests active bleeding (**Fig. 7**).[18]

Most arterial EDH requires surgical treatment; however, some cases can undergo conservative treatment depending on the location of the hematoma, initial and follow-up GCS, the volume of the hematoma, and degree of midline shift.[19] Unlike arterial EDH, most venous EDH needs only conservative treatment because venous bleeding has low pressure and is less likely to expand.

Subdural Hematoma

Subdural hematoma (SDH) occurs due to the tear of bridging cortical veins within the subdural space, between the dura and arachnoid. Unlike EDH, which is always related to significant traumatic head injury, SDH can occur even in minor injuries, especially in elderly patients. These patients are predilection for having brain atrophy, resulting

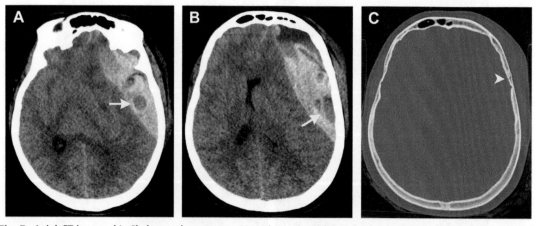

Fig. 7. Axial CT images (*A, B*) show a large acute EDH along the left cerebral convexity with swirl sign (*arrow*), suggesting active bleeding. Associated rightward subfalcine herniation and (*C*) non-displaced linear fracture at the left parietal bone are noted (*arrowhead*).

in more stretching of the bridging cortical veins and a more significant risk of tearing off these veins.

Imaging findings of SDHs appear to be crescent-shaped extra-axial hematomas along cerebral convexities, predominated in frontoparietal regions, falx cerebri, tentorium cerebelli, or rarely in the posterior fossa. SDHs can cross sutures but not cross the dural reflections such as falx cerebri and tentorium cerebelli. The density of the SDHs depends on the age and organization of hematomas. Acute SDHs usually show hyperdensity. Some of them have hypodense components, which may reflect the area of active bleeding (swirl sign), clot retraction, or mixed component between CSF and hematoma due to arachnoid tear (**Fig. 8**).[9,18] However, acute SDH may have isodensity in some circumstances, such as in anemic patients with hemoglobin levels of 8 to 10 g/dL, patients with coagulopathy, or a mixture with CSF.[9,10]

Subacute SDHs are iso-to-hypodensity to the cortex of the brain, making it easier to miss these hematomas, particularly when they appear as bilateral isodensity. The easy diagnostic clue is to identify the CSF. If CSF is inward displacement and not attached to the inner table of the skull, SDH should be considered (**Fig. 9**). Other methods include identifying the pressure effect such as midline shift, effacement of the ipsilateral sulci and ventricle, intravenous administration of the contrast media that reveals inward displacement of the enhanced cortical vessels, or using MR imaging.

Chronic SDHs are hypodensity with surrounding enhanced membranes and often have internal septations and loculations. These membranes are composed of granulation tissues with fragile capillaries, resulting in susceptibility to rebleeding and forming multistage SDHs (**Fig. 10**).[20]

Treatment of SDHs depends on the size of the SDHs, mass effects, and neurological status. If hematomas are large enough to cause mass effects and symptoms, the immediate surgical treatment seems to be the best option. Otherwise, conservative treatment with serial clinical and radiological follow-up should be enough.[21,22]

Traumatic Subarachnoid Hemorrhage

Subarachnoid hemorrhage (SAH) occurs in the subarachnoid space between the arachnoid and pia membranes. The most common cause of SAH is trauma.[23] Traumatic SAH may result from the tearing of vessels in the subarachnoid space, ruptured traumatic dissecting aneurysm, an extension from the intraparenchymal hematoma, or redistribution of the intraventricular hemorrhage (IVH). It is frequently associated with other intracranial injuries such as cerebral contusion, SDH, and EDH.

SAH appears as linear or serpentine hyperdensity on CT and FLAIR hyperintensity on MR imaging along the cortical sulci, most commonly near the impact site (coup) or opposite to the impact site (contrecoup), or in the cisterns (**Fig. 11**). It can be either focal or diffuse but prefer to be the former. SWI may have a benefit in detecting IVH or small amounts of SAH due to its higher sensitivity than the CT scan except for basilar cistern SAH.[23] Rarely, SAH can be seen as a focal

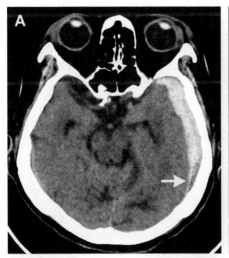
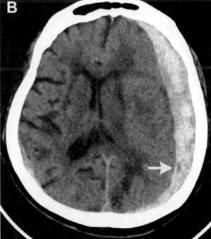

Fig. 8. Axial CT images (*A, B*) show acute SDH along the left cerebral convexity with some hypodense components (*arrows*), which may reflect the area of active bleeding (swirl sign), clot retraction, or mixed component between CSF and hematoma.

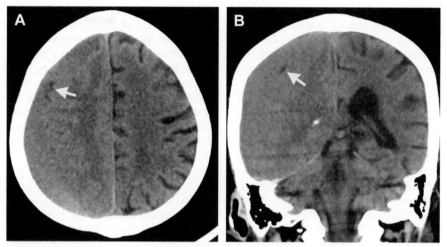

Fig. 9. Axial (A) and coronal (B) CT images show subacute SDH along the right cerebral convexity, which is isodense to the adjacent cortex. Inward displacement of CSF is noted (arrow).

hematoma and expresses the mass effect (Fig. 12). Midline SAH may suggest the presence of DAI, particularly when SAH occurs concomitantly with IVH, and is associated with poor outcomes.[24]

The complications of SAH are hydrocephalus and vasospasm. It could be either obstructive hydrocephalus by the hematoma in the cerebral aqueduct or fourth ventricular outlet or nonobstructive due to impaired CSF resorption. Vasospasm is a delayed complication, usually peaks at 7 to 10 days after injury, and can remain up to 2 weeks. Patients with extensive traumatic SAH are significantly more likely to have vasospasm.[25]

One of the most important pitfalls is that SAH could be either the cause or result of head injuries.

SAH can occur from other reasons, such as a ruptured aneurysm, which is the most common cause and accounts for approximately 85% of nontraumatic SAH.[26] The key point is to define the epicenter of the hemorrhage. The traumatic SAH is often focal and usually along the coup-contrecoup sites or adjacent to the concurrent cerebral contusion, SDH, and EDH. In ruptured aneurysms, the SAH is diffuse and centered in the suprasellar or central basal cisterns with diffuse peripheral extension (see Fig. 12). However, some traumatic SAH may present as a diffuse pattern, for example, severe skull base injury or acute arterial injury. Further CT or MR angiography should be obtained in these cases to exclude aneurysms or arterial injuries.

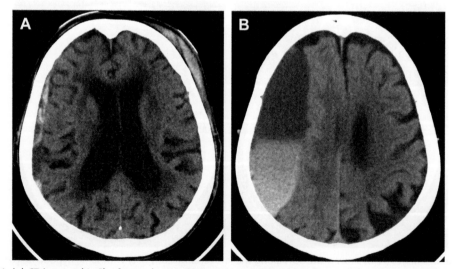

Fig. 10. Axial CT images (A, B) of two chronic SDH patients with rebleeding and forming acute ontop chronic appearances.

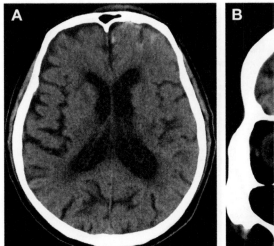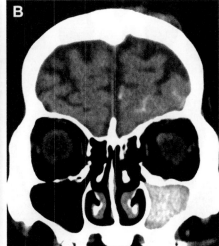

Fig. 11. Axial (*A*) and coronal (*B*) CT images show acute SAH along the left frontal cortical sulci.

Isolated traumatic SAH without other significant intracranial injuries usually has a favorable outcome. There is no need for aggressive treatment or routine CT scan follow-up. On the contrary, those with other concurrent intracranial injuries increase morbidity and mortality and may require surgical treatment.[23]

Brain Contusion

Brain contusions are superficial brain injuries involving gray and subjacent subcortical white matter. It can occur anywhere throughout the brain parenchyma in the manner of coup and contrecoup directions but predominantly in the areas adjacent to bony protuberance or dural fold. The most common locations are anterior inferior aspects of the frontal and temporal lobes.

Brain contusions appear as patchy hypodense areas (due to edema) with or without hemorrhagic foci in the early stage (**Fig. 13**). However, small or nonhemorrhagic contusions may not be visible in the CT image. MR imaging is more sensitive in detecting these lesions and better describes their extension. FLAIR image is the best for detecting the contusion or edematous areas, whereas T2*GRE or SWI is the best for detecting hemorrhagic areas. It usually has associated injuries such as overlying soft tissue injuries, skull fractures, or extra-axial hemorrhages.

A progression of the contusions can be detected in approximately 75% of patients and usually occurs within 24 to 48 h after injury. It can present as increased sizes or developed new areas of edema and hemorrhage with worsening mass effect. The small hemorrhagic spots may

coalesce into larger hematomas. The larger initial contusions show an increased likelihood of contusion progression.[27] Prompt surgical treatment is considered if the contusions cause a significant mass effect to decrease the intracranial pressure and improve cerebral perfusion.

Diffuse Axonal Injury

DAI refers to traumatic axonal stretch injury. This type of injury is frequently found in patients with TBI, particularly those with moderate and severe degrees, and is associated with poor outcomes. It occurs when patients get injured by acceleration-deceleration and rotational forces leading to the different rotational speeds of the cortex and underlying white matter (due to different densities), resulting in stretching and/or shearing of the axons. The typical clinical presentation is a sudden loss of consciousness that begins at the moment of injury with disproportionate to the imaging findings, for example, normal or minimal findings. Patients with DAI show significantly lower GCS scores than those who do not have DAI.[24]

MR imaging is the modality of choice for detecting DAI due to its higher sensitivity than CT. However, even MR imaging still underestimates the actual extension of DAI.[28] DAI can be nonhemorrhagic, hemorrhagic, or both. Imaging findings are summarized in **Table 2**. There are three successive stages of DAI based on their deeper locations and increasing severity of head injuries which are correlated with poorer clinical outcomes.[28,29] Stage 1 DAI (least severe) involves the gray-white matter junction, especially frontotemporal lobes. Stage 2 DAI occurs in the corpus callosum,

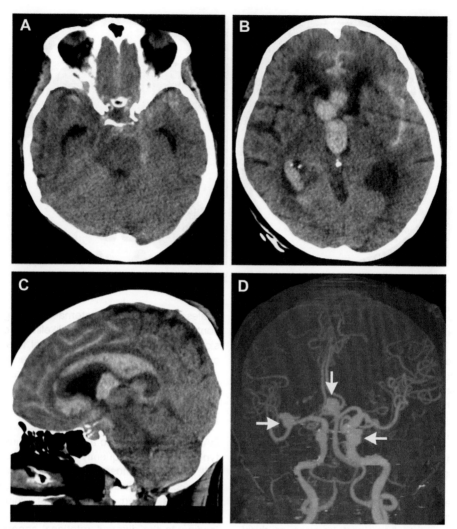

Fig. 12. A 78-year-old woman with head injury and alteration of consciousness. Her initial axial CT images (*A, B*) show diffuse acute SAH and IVH. Midsagittal CT images (*C*) show a thick interhemispheric SAH, forming like a focal hematoma and causing a mass effect on the posterior body of the corpus callosum. CT angiography image (*D*) shows three saccular aneurysms arising from the anterior communicating artery, right middle cerebral artery bifurcation, and left cavernous ICA. Intraoperative findings confirm a ruptured anterior communicating artery aneurysm.

especially the splenium and posterior body. Stage 3 DAI (most severe) involves the brainstem, especially the dorsolateral midbrain and upper pons (**Fig. 14**).

There is no current specific treatment of DAI, only supportive treatment and taking care of comorbidities. The patients with DAI show about a threefold higher risk of an unfavorable clinical outcome (Glasgow Outcome Scale 1 to 3 or Glasgow Outcome Scale-Extended 1 to 5) than those without DAI. Furthermore, the risk for an unfavorable clinical outcome increases about threefold for each increase in the DAI stage.[30]

SECONDARY INJURIES
Diffuse Cerebral Edema

Diffuse cerebral edema after a head injury is thought to be the result of several mechanisms and various mediators that leads to vasogenic and cytotoxic edema.[31] Diffuse cerebral edema also causes increased intracranial pressure and decreased cerebral perfusion, leading to further ischemia or infarction of the brain parenchyma. On CT, there is diffuse low attenuation of the cerebral hemispheres and loss of gray-white matter differentiation, associated with diffuse effacement of the cortical sulci, subarachnoid spaces,

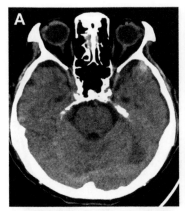 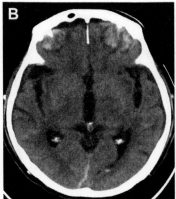 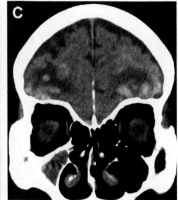

Fig. 13. Axial (*A*, *B*) and coronal (*C*) images show hemorrhagic brain contusions in anterior inferior aspects of the bilateral frontal and left temporal lobes, associated with a thin acute SDH along posterior falx cerebri and minimal bilateral acute SAH.

cisterns, and ventricles (**Fig. 15**). The cerebellum and brainstem are typically unaffected, giving the hyperdense appearance compared with the supratentorial structures (white cerebellum sign).

Brain Herniation

Brain herniation occurs when there is the space-taking lesion (eg, EDH, SDH, and intraparenchymal hematoma) within the closed intracranial space, resulting in the shifting of the brain tissue from its normal location to an adjacent space. There are many types of brain herniation, as described in **Table 3**, which can occur together at once or in isolation.

Chronic Traumatic Encephalopathy

CTE is one of the neurodegenerative diseases associated with repetitive head trauma, such as in collision sport athletes (eg, boxers and American football players) and military veterans with repetitive low-intensity blast exposures.[32] However, it is still unknown the threshold or severity degree

of the head injury or other predisposing factors to developing this disease; in other words, patients with CTE have a history of repetitive brain injury, but most of the repetitive brain injury patients will not develop CTE.[33] Patients with CTE show a progressive course of cognitive impairment and/or neurobehavioral dysregulation with not fully accounted for by other disorders. Currently, the definite diagnosis of CTE can be made by postmortem neuropathology only, which is revealed a unique pattern of hyperphosphorylated tau (p-tau) deposition. It also often exists with other pathologies, such as beta-amyloid (Aβ) plaques, alpha-synuclein, TDP-43 proteinopathies, and white matter rarefaction. There is an attempt to make a diagnosis during life through the patient's clinical syndrome using the term "Traumatic encephalopathy syndrome (TES)," which is developed by the National Institute of Neurological Disorders and Stroke (NINDS). However, these diagnostic criteria are primarily aimed for use in research settings and require future studies to determine clinicopathologic correlation.

Table 2
Imaging findings of DAI

Type of DAI	Imaging Modality	
	CT	MR Imaging
Nonhemorrhagic	• Normal (50% to 80%) • Small round, oval, or linear hypodense lesions with a long axis parallel to the axonal direction	• Small FLAIR hyperintensity foci ± restrict diffusion on DWI images
Hemorrhagic	• Small hyperdense foci (20% to 50%)	• Microbleeds on SWI and T2*GRE images (best visualized on SWI)

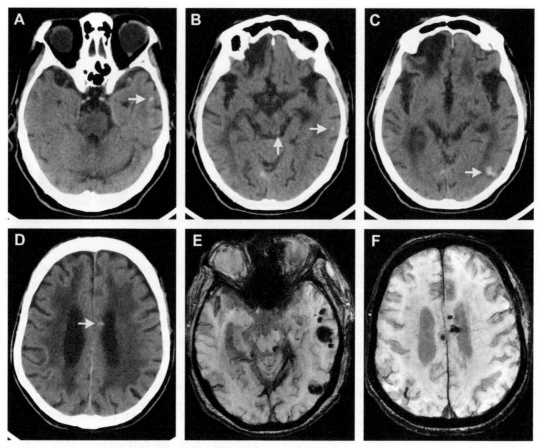

Fig. 14. Axial CT images (*A–D*) show multiple hemorrhagic DAI (*arrow*) involving the gray-white matter junction of the left temporal lobe (stage 1), the body of corpus callosum (stage 2), and the left-sided dorsolateral midbrain (stage 3). Axial SWI images (*E, F*) better visualize these DAI lesions.

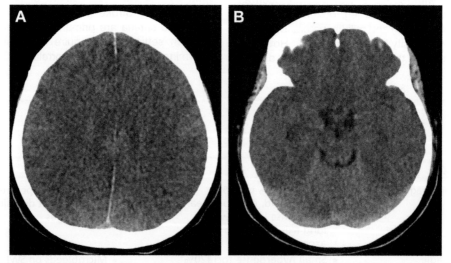

Fig. 15. Axial CT images (*A*) show diffuse hypodensity of the cerebral hemispheres with loss of gray-white matter differentiation and diffuse effacement of the cortical sulci, corresponding with diffuse cerebral edema. (*B*) The cerebellum is relatively spared (white cerebellum sign).

Table 3
Imaging findings and possible complications of brain herniations

Types of Brain Herniations	Imaging Findings	Complications
Subfalcine herniation	• Shifting the ipsilateral cingulate gyrus passing under the free edge of the falx cerebri to the contralateral side	• Acute cerebral infarction in the ipsilateral anterior cerebral artery (ACA) territory • Obstructive hydrocephalus of the contralateral lateral ventricle
Descending transtentorial herniation: Uncal herniation	• Downward displacement of the uncus, causing effacement of the ipsilateral suprasellar and crural cisterns • Contralateral displacement of the midbrain and cerebral peduncle against the tentorial free edge in more severe cases, resulting in the Kernohan notch phenomenon (false localizing sign)	• Acute cerebral infarction in the ipsilateral posterior cerebral artery (PCA) territory • Ipsilateral third cranial nerve palsy with pupillary involvement (dilated pupil) • Obstructive hydrocephalus (due to the cerebral aqueduct obliteration)
Descending transtentorial herniation: Central herniation	• Downward displacement of the diencephalon, midbrain, and pons • Effacement of the perimesencephalic cisterns • Flattening of the ventral pons against the clivus • Downward displacement of the basilar artery, quadrigeminal plate, and pineal gland	• Acute cerebral infarction in the PCA territory • Hydrocephalus (due to cerebral aqueduct obliteration) • Duret hemorrhage in the brainstem, usually in the central or paracentral region near the pontomesencephalic junction
Ascending transtentorial herniation	• Upward displacement of the cerebellum through the tentorial notch into the supratentorium • Effacement or obliteration of the quadrigeminal cistern • Flattening of the tectum • Anterior displacement of the midbrain	• Obstructive hydrocephalus (due to cerebral aqueduct obstruction) • Acute cerebral infarction in the superior cerebellar artery (SCA) or PCA territories
Tonsillar herniation	• Significant downward displacement of the cerebellar tonsil(s) (> 5 mm below the basion-opisthion or McRae line in adults) • Crowding of the foramen magnum • Effacement or obliteration of the cisterna magna • Anterior displacement of the brainstem	• Hydrocephalus (due to fourth ventricular outlet obstruction) • Acute cerebral infarction in the posterior inferior cerebellar artery (PICA) territory

The current role of neuroimaging is to rule out other diseases as it is no specific imaging features for the CTE diagnosis. Some structural imaging findings can be found at higher rates in patients with CTE, such as cerebral volume loss, encephalomalacia in the location that indicates prior trauma, such as in anteroinferior aspects of the frontal and temporal lobes, findings of chronic DAI, cavum septum pellucidum, and corpus callosum thinning.[32–34] No definite specific pattern of cerebral volume loss is detected, but some studies suggested that frontal-temporal lobes and diencephalon may be predominated in patients with CTE.

According to the CTE pathology, there are endeavors to use advanced imaging techniques, that is, PET with various tracers to detect patients with CTE during life, but it is very limited usefulness in the real world. FDG (2-deoxy-2-(18F)fluoro-deoxyglucose)-PET is used to evaluate patients at risk for CTE, but its results are rather inconsistent due to the heterogenous of underlying diseases and associated clinical syndromes. Some studies showed mild FDG hypometabolism corresponding with medial temporal and frontal atrophy. Beta-amyloid (Aβ)-PET imaging is aimed to rule out or identify comorbid Alzheimer's disease (AD) rather than the rule in CTE. Tau-PET is one of the most commonly used advanced imaging, but the major problem is the current Tau PET tracers which show off-target and non-specific binding properties. Most of these tracers are aimed for use in patients with suspected AD, whereas only some tracers such as 2-(1-{6-[(2-[fluorine-18]fluoroethyl) (methyl)amino]-2-naphthyl}-ethylidene)malononitrile (FDDNP) and flortaucipir (FTP) are used to study in patients with repetitive head trauma. FDDNP-PET is used in most early studies in repetitive head trauma patients, which may show uptake in white matter and subcortical structures along with limbic and brain stem regions, but its sensitivity and specificity in detecting CTE are severely limited due to nonspecific binding properties and low signal-to-noise ratio. FTP is a Tau PET tracer that FDA approves for evaluating patients with suspected AD but may show mild FTP uptake in the frontotemporal regions of patients with TES. Tau-PET may have an important role in the diagnosis of CTE during life if there is a new tracer that is more specific to CTE tau rather than AD tau.

SUMMARY

TBI is considered one of the significant health and socioeconomic problems globally. It can be classified into mild, moderate, and severe degrees by using the GCS, which may predict patient outcomes after acute brain damage. Imaging currently plays a vital role in TBI, particularly NCCT, which has been accepted as first-line imaging. In contrast, MR imaging has a role in the case of unremarkable CT finding with a persistent unexplained cognitive or neurologic deficit. Additional vascular studies (CT/MR angiography and CT/MR venography) should be performed in cases suspected of vascular injuries such as skull base fractures and skull fractures extending to dural venous sinus or jugular bulb. Familiar with the imaging findings of TBI, including primary and secondary injuries and pitfalls, is essential for radiologists as part of a trauma team, leading to prompt and precise diagnosis for the best patient care.

CLINICS CARE POINTS

- Imaging can assist clinicians in triage, diagnosis, treatment planning, follow-up, and prognosis of patients with traumatic brain injury (TBI).
- Non-contrast computed tomography is considered first-line imaging in TBI cases due to its high sensitivity and specificity in detecting skull fractures and intracranial abnormalities such as hemorrhage, brain contusion, brain herniation, and hydrocephalus.
- MR imaging shows higher sensitivity than computed tomography in detecting some pathologies such as extra-axial hemorrhage, small or nonhemorrhagic brain contusion, posterior fossa injury, and diffuse axonal injury.

DISCLOSURE

The authors have nothing to disclose.

REFERENCES

1. Menon DK, Schwab K, Wright DW, et al. Position statement: definition of traumatic brain injury. Arch Phys Med Rehabil 2010;91(11):1637–40.
2. Dewan MC, Rattani A, Gupta S, et al. Estimating the global incidence of traumatic brain injury. J Neurosurg 2019;130:1080–97.
3. Teasdale G, Maas A, Lecky F, et al. The Glasgow coma scale at 40 years: standing the test of time. Lancet Neurol 2014;13(8):844–54.
4. Nelson LD, Temkin NR, Dikmen S, et al. Recovery after mild traumatic brain injury in patients presenting to US Level I trauma centers: a transforming

research and clinical knowledge in traumatic brain injury (TRACK-TBI) study. JAMA Neurol 2019;76(9): 1049–59.

5. Perry DC, Sturm VE, Peterson MJ, et al. Association of traumatic brain injury with subsequent neurological and psychiatric disease: a meta-analysis. J Neurosurg 2016;124(2):511–26.

6. Shih RY, Burns J, Ajam AA, et al. ACR appropriateness criteria® head trauma: 2021 update. J Am Coll Radiol 2021;18(5s):S13–36.

7. New PF, Aronow S. Attenuation measurements of whole blood and blood fractions in computed tomography. Radiology 1976;121(3 Pt. 1):635–40.

8. Parizel PM, Makkat S, Van Miert E, et al. Intracranial hemorrhage: principles of CT and MRI interpretation. Eur Radiol 2001;11(9):1770–83.

9. Grelat M, Madkouri R, Bousquet O. Acute isodense subdural hematoma on computed tomography scan–diagnostic and therapeutic trap: a case report. J Med Case Rep 2016;10:43.

10. Smith WP Jr, Batnitzky S, Rengachary SS. Acute isodense subdural hematomas: a problem in anemic patients. AJR Am J Roentgenol 1981;136(3):543–6.

11. Cox M, Bisangwa S, Herpich F, et al. Fluid levels in the bleeding brain: a marker for coagulopathy and hematoma expansion. Internal and Emergency Medicine 2017;12(7):1071–3.

12. Rincon S, Gupta R, Ptak T. Imaging of head trauma. Handb Clin Neurol 2016;135:447–77.

13. Schweitzer AD, Niogi SN, Whitlow CT, et al. Traumatic brain injury: imaging patterns and complications. Radiographics 2019;39(6):1571–95.

14. Baugnon KL, Hudgins PA. Skull base fractures and their complications. Neuroimaging Clin 2014;24(3): 439–65. vii-viii.

15. Sanchez T, Stewart D, Walvick M, et al. Skull fracture vs. accessory sutures: how can we tell the difference? Emerg Radiol 2010;17(5):413–8.

16. Osborn AG, Harder SL. Epidural hematoma, classic. In: Osborn AG, Salzman KL, Jhaveri MD, editors. Diagnostic imaging: brain. 3rd ed. Philadelphia: Elsevier; 2016. p. 148–51.

17. Caglar YS, Erdogan K, Kilinc CM, et al. Retroclival epidural hematoma: a rare location of epidural hematoma, case report, and review of literature. J Craniovertebral Junction Spine 2020;11(4):342–6.

18. Al-Nakshabandi NA. The swirl sign. Radiology 2001; 218(2):433.

19. Zakaria Z, Kaliaperumal C, Kaar G, et al. Extradural haematoma–to evacuate or not? Revisiting treatment guidelines. Clin Neurol Neurosurg 2013;115(8): 1201–5.

20. Edlmann E, Giorgi-Coll S, Whitfield PC, et al. Pathophysiology of chronic subdural haematoma:

inflammation, angiogenesis and implications for pharmacotherapy. J Neuroinflammation 2017;14(1): 108.

21. Vega RA, Valadka AB. Natural history of acute subdural hematoma. Neurosurg Clin 2017;28(2): 247–55.

22. Feghali J, Yang W, Huang J. Updates in chronic subdural hematoma: epidemiology, etiology, pathogenesis, treatment, and outcome. World neurosurgery 2020;141:339–45.

23. Griswold DP, Fernandez L, Rubiano AM. Traumatic subarachnoid hemorrhage: a scoping review. J Neurotrauma 2022;39(1–2):35–48.

24. Mata-Mbemba D, Mugikura S, Nakagawa A, et al. Traumatic midline subarachnoid hemorrhage on initial computed tomography as a marker of severe diffuse axonal injury. J Neurosurg 2018;129(5): 1317–24.

25. Lin TK, Tsai HC, Hsieh TC. The impact of traumatic subarachnoid hemorrhage on outcome: a study with grouping of traumatic subarachnoid hemorrhage and transcranial Doppler sonography. J Trauma Acute Care Surgery 2012;73(1):131–6.

26. Marder CP, Narla V, Fink JR, et al. Subarachnoid hemorrhage: beyond aneurysms. Am J Roentgenol 2014;202(1):25–37.

27. Adatia K, Newcombe VFJ, Menon DK. Contusion progression following traumatic brain injury: a review of clinical and radiological predictors, and influence on outcome. Neurocritical Care 2021;34(1):312–24.

28. Gentry LR. Imaging of closed head injury. Radiology 1994;191(1):1–17.

29. Adams JH, Doyle D, Ford I, et al. Diffuse axonal injury in head injury: definition, diagnosis and grading. Histopathology 1989;15(1):49–59.

30. van Eijck MM, Schoonman GG, van der Naalt J, et al. Diffuse axonal injury after traumatic brain injury is a prognostic factor for functional outcome: a systematic review and meta-analysis. Brain Inj 2018; 32(4):395–402.

31. Unterberg AW, Stover J, Kress B, et al. Edema and brain trauma. Neuroscience 2004;129(4):1021–9.

32. Katz DI, Bernick C, Dodick DW, et al. National institute of neurological disorders and stroke consensus diagnostic criteria for traumatic encephalopathy syndrome. Neurology 2021;96(18):848–63.

33. Shetty T, Raince A, Manning E, et al. Imaging in chronic traumatic encephalopathy and traumatic brain injury. Sports Health 2016;8(1):26–36.

34. Alosco ML, Mian AZ, Buch K, et al. Structural MRI profiles and tau correlates of atrophy in autopsy-confirmed CTE. Alzheimer's Res Ther 2021;13(1): 193.

Cerebral Amyloid Angiopathy

Laszlo Szidonya, MD, PhD[a,b], Joshua P. Nickerson, MD[c,*]

KEYWORDS

- Cerebral amyloid angiopathy • Amyloid • MR imaging • Microhemorrhage
- Positron emission tomography

KEY POINTS

- As the global population ages, recognition of the imaging findings in the setting of cerebral amyloid angiopathy (CAA) is crucial for neuroimagers in that advancing age is the primary risk factor in this entity.
- Imaging hallmarks of CAA are peripherally located microhemorrhages that are best detected with susceptibility-weighted sequences. Lobar hemorrhages as well as superficial siderosis from earlier subarachnoid hemorrhages are also typical.
- Development of ^{18}F-labeled radiotracers for the detection of amyloid deposition in the brain has added to the early detection of both parenchymal and vascular amyloid deposits.
- There are a number of differential diagnostic considerations in the setting of cerebral microhemorrhage. Distribution, patient demographics, and earlier history are helpful in contrasting these processes from CAA.

INTRODUCTION

Cerebral Amyloid Prevalence and Demographics

Cerebral amyloid angiopathy (CAA) is a disease of cortical and leptomeningeal blood vessels, characterized by the deposition of amyloid proteins (most commonly β-amyloid, Aβ), which causes increased vascular fragility and permeability, leading to microscopic and macroscopic hemorrhages in a characteristic cortical and lobar distribution.[1] The gold standard for the diagnosis of CAA is histopathology from biopsy, sample from hematoma evacuation, or autopsy.[2] The prevalence of CAA increases with age, specifically 7.3% (mild, moderate, and severe CAA) between the ages 65 and 74 years, 17.6% between ages 75 and 84 years, and 34.6% for ages 85 years and older.[3] The most significant risk factor for the sporadic form of CAA is advancing age.[2] The world's population is getting older; the number of people aged 65 years or older is 771 million in 2022 (10% of the population) and projected to reach 1.6 billion by 2050 (16% of population) according to the United Nations World Population Prospects report.[4] Although definite diagnosis of CAA requires autopsy, probable or possible diagnosis can be made based on clinical features and neuroimaging demonstrating characteristic hemorrhages.[5,6] Susceptibility-weighted imaging (SWI) allows for accurate hemorrhage detection and is widely incorporated into clinical MR imaging protocols.[7] The combination of ageing populations and wide availability of more sensitive detection methods will increase detection in clinical practice.

Pathogenesis and Histology

The dominant feature of CAA is the deposition of vascular amyloid in the walls of small (<2 mm diameter) cortical and leptomeningeal vessels,

[a] Diagnostic Radiology, Oregon Health & Science University, L340, 3245 Southwest Pavilion Loop, Portland, OR 97239, USA; [b] Diagnostic Radiology, Heart and Vascular Center, Semmelweis University, Budapest, Hungary; [c] Diagnostic Radiology, School of Medicine, Oregon Health & Science University, 3181 Southwest Sam Jackson Park Road, Portland, OR 97239, USA
* Corresponding author.
E-mail address: nickerjo@ohsu.edu

Radiol Clin N Am 61 (2023) 551–562
https://doi.org/10.1016/j.rcl.2023.01.009
0033-8389/23/© 2023 Elsevier Inc. All rights reserved.

mainly arterioles, less commonly capillaries, and rarely venules.[1] The main component of vascular amyloid is a 40 amino acid fragment ($A\beta_{40}$), derived by proteolytic cleavage from the amyloid precursor protein, a transmembrane glycoprotein expressed by neurons. The general mechanism of amyloid deposition is similar to the formation of amyloid plaques in Alzheimer disease (AD) by the aggregation of $A\beta_{42}$ but $A\beta_{40}$ is more soluble than $A\beta_{42}$, causing differences in the location of the deposits and the resulting pathologic conditions.[8] The 4 major pathways of $A\beta$ elimination from the brain are proteolytic degradation, receptor-mediated uptake into glial cells and neurons, transcellular transport through the blood–brain barrier, and perivascular drainage with interstitial fluid.[9] When these clearance pathways are impaired, for example, in older age[10], the imbalance between $A\beta$ production and elimination causes these proteins to accumulate and aggregate, leading to cellular and tissue dysfunction. The $A\beta_{40}$:$A\beta_{42}$ ratio determines the location of the amyloid deposits, with a high ratio leading to vascular amyloid and CAA, and a low ratio causing parenchymal plaques and AD.[8]

Apolipoprotein E (APOE) has 3 major isoforms in humans, APOE2, APOE3, and APOE4, with single amino acid differences in 2 key positions. The different alleles encoding these proteins (ε2, ε3, and ε4) have varying degrees of association with AD and CAA, with ε4 increasing the risk of both.[11] Presence of the ε2 and/or ε4 allele reduces the risk of AD but increases CAA hemorrhage risk.

The histologic diagnosis of CAA is based on the detection of $A\beta$ in the affected vessel walls. The traditionally used Congo red stain shows amyloid as apple-green birefringence on polarized light microscopy but immunohistochemistry using anti-$A\beta$ antibodies offers more specific and sensitive visualization.[12] Amyloid deposits initially appear in the adventitia and outer part of the media, in a segmental distribution, which may cause biopsy diagnostic difficulties due to sampling variability.[3] In more severe CAA, deposits involve all vessel wall layers, can lead to both media thickening and thinning, and narrowing or dilation of the lumen, likely due to muscle degeneration and subsequent vessel wall weakening.

CAA preferentially affects leptomeningeal and cortical vessels, generally sparing white matter, basal ganglia, and thalami, an important difference compared with hypertension-related small vessel disease (HTN-SVD). The posterior brain (occipital, posterior temporal, and parietal lobes) is affected more commonly and more severely, with eventual involvement of the anterior brain as disease progresses. The cerebellum may also be involved in advanced stages.[1]

Clinical Presentation and Natural History

Hemorrhagic manifestations

Although only about 10% of all strokes are hemorrhagic, they have a high mortality (30%–40% in the first month) and morbidity.[13] CAA is the second most common cause of intracerebral hemorrhage (ICH) after hypertension in people aged older than 60 years. HTN-SVD preferentially affects the lenticulostriate, thalamic, and pontine perforators, resulting in deep hemorrhagic lesions in the basal ganglia, thalamus, and the pons. In contrast, CAA involves the cortical and subcortical vessels and causes lobar ICH with a posterior predilection, the occipital lobe being the most frequently and most severely affected[1,14] (Fig. 1).

The clinical manifestation of ICH caused by CAA is similar to hemorrhagic stroke attributed to bleeding arteriovenous malformations or tumors, and typically involves headache, nausea/vomiting, and altered level of consciousness, with focal neurological symptoms and/or seizures, depending on the size and location of the bleed.[13] The hemorrhages caused by CAA are more commonly recurrent, and the repeated episodes are frequently more severe.[15]

CAA may present in the form of convexity subarachnoid hemorrhage (cSAH), a result of CAA involving the leptomeningeal vessels, or extension from a lobar ICH.[16] Both the localization (convexity vs basal cisterns) and the clinical presentation are different from SAH caused by aneurysm rupture, commonly causing focal neurologic deficits instead of headaches. Over time, cSAH may lead to the development of cortical superficial siderosis (cSS), a gyriform deposition of hemosiderin involving the cerebral cortex, which is different from the classic superficial siderosis, which involves the brainstem, the cranial nerves, and the posterior fossa.[17]

Hemorrhagic manifestations can also be clinically occult, which is commonly the case with cerebral microbleeds (CMBs), caused by the rupture of vessels with a diameter less than 0.2 mm (Fig. 2). CMBs in CAA have a lobar predilection with a posterior predominance and are associated with a higher risk of recurrent ICH.[18]

Nonhemorrhagic manifestations

The involvement of small vessels by CAA can result in narrowing and occlusion of the lumen, and the development of acute ischemic infarcts, which may often occur in a clinically silent way in patients with CAA, and are associated with the

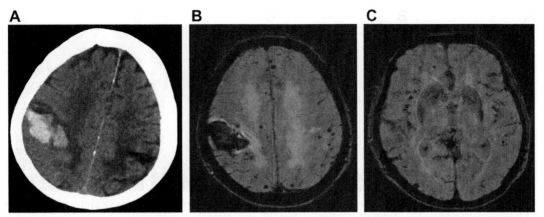

Fig. 1. A 74-year-old woman who presented to the emergency department with new left-sided motor and sensory deficits. A right-sided peripheral lobar parenchymal hemorrhage is evident on unenhanced head CT (*A*). Subsequent MR imaging also showed the hemorrhage (*B*) and revealed numerous peripheral susceptibility foci in the brain typical of CAA (*B, C*).

CMB burden.[19] In the acute phase, these lesions are best seen as foci of high signal intensity on diffusion-weighted images, and later as white matter hyperintensities (WMHs) on T2-weighted and FLAIR sequences. Over time, the accumulation of these small infarcts can be a cause of leukoaraiosis, characterized by a diffuse involvement of white matter with sparing of the subcortical U-fibers (**Fig. 3**A).

Cognitive decline
CAA is frequently seen in the brains of patients with dementia, and the prevalence of CAA is higher in demented patients compared with age-matched but nondemented controls.[20] CAA is associated with AD and cognitive decline, and this effect seems to be independent of the capillary involvement and cortical microinfarcts.[21] The significant overlap between the sporadic form of CAA and AD is presumably due to the shared role of Aβ in these processes.[22]

Sporadic Disease

Findings on computed tomography
The high sensitivity of computed tomography (CT) for acute intracranial bleeding makes it a robust modality for the detection of both lobar ICH (see **Fig. 1**) and cSAH. It is widely available and can be used to evaluate patients presenting with acute symptoms, when MR imaging may be less well tolerated. The Edinburgh CT diagnostic criteria use the presence or absence of SAH, APOE ε4 status, and finger-like projections from the ICH to rule in or rule out moderate or severe CAA.[23]

Findings on magnetic resonance
MR imaging provides the most sensitive tool for the depiction of hemorrhagic manifestations such as lobar ICH (see **Fig. 1**) and lobar CMB (see **Figs. 1** and **2**; **Fig. 3**),[24] in the form of SWI, which surpasses T2*-weighted gradient-recalled echo sequences in sensitivity for detecting CMBs.[25] The original Boston criteria (1.0) based the

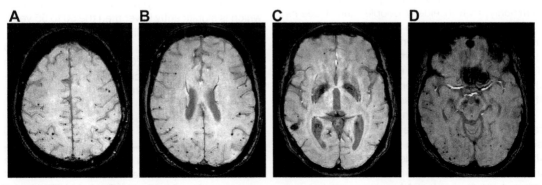

Fig. 2. SWI from of a 65-year-old man with progressive memory loss. Numerous peripheral susceptibility foci with a posterior predilection and sparing of the deep gray nuclei are typical of CAA (*A–D*).

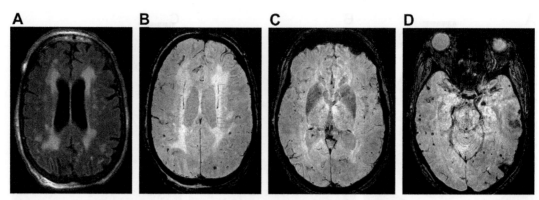

Fig. 3. An 87-year-old man with progressive memory loss. T2-FLAIR imaging reveals extensive and confluent areas of T2 prolongation throughout the deep white matter (*A*). SWI demonstrates characteristic peripheral microhemorrhages of amyloid angiopathy with notable sparing of the deep gray nuclei (*B–D*).

definition of probable CAA on the demonstration of multiple (≥2), strictly lobar hemorrhages (cortical, grey–white matter junction, and subcortical white matter) in patients aged 55 years or older and in the absence of other causes of hemorrhage.[26] The presence of deep territory hemorrhages, associated with HTN-SVD, precludes this diagnosis, whereas cerebellar hemorrhages are allowed but not counted to support CAA.[5] A recent study demonstrated that strictly superficial cerebellar CMBs (restricted to the cerebellar cortex and vermis) are associated with clinically diagnosed and pathologically verified CAA.[27]

The 2010 modified Boston criteria (1.5) added cSS as an additional hemorrhagic lesion when assessing the multiplicity of lesions for the diagnosis of probable CAA, increasing the sensitivity from 89.5% to 94.7% without affecting the specificity.[17]

MR imaging is also sensitive in the detection of silent ischemic and lacunar lesions. Lobar lacunes are associated with CAA, whereas deep lacunes are more frequent in HTN-SVD.[28] The use of the modified Boston criteria allowed the identification of new, nonhemorrhagic imaging biomarkers of CAA. Enlarged perivascular spaces (EPVS) are commonly seen in elderly people, and it seems that their presence in the centrum semiovale is associated with CAA, whereas EPVS in the basal ganglia are seen more commonly in HTN-SVD.[29] This may be related to the role of these spaces in the waste clearance systems of the brain and is the subject of intensive research.[30,31]

The most recent Boston criteria (2.0) incorporated 2 white matter features (EPVS in the centrum semiovale and WMHs in a multispot pattern) into the diagnosis of probable and possible CAA, increasing the sensitivity while keeping the specificity of the probable CAA category compared with the revised Boston criteria[6] (**Table 1**).

Cerebral Amyloid Angiopathy-Related Inflammation

Cerebral amyloid angiopathy-related inflammation (CAARI) is a rare syndrome in which amyloid deposits illicit a perivascular inflammatory response within the brain resulting in a pattern of vasogenic edema within the periphery of the brain on T2-weighted MR imaging[32] (**Fig. 4**). The pathogenesis is not well understood but the presence of a specific APOE ε4 allele may confer increased risk. A distinct but related entity, amyloid-beta related angiitis, may appear similar on imaging studies but is associated with direct vascular wall inflammation rather than perivascular abnormalities on microscopic examination.[33]

Iatrogenic Cerebral Amyloid Angiopathy

Iatrogenic transmission of Aβ was first reported in 2015, showing changes characteristic of AD and CAA during the autopsy study of patients with iatrogenic Creutzfeldt-Jakob disease, which suggested a prion-like transmission of Aβ-related pathologic conditions.[34] A recent case report and systematic review of 23 patients found a mean age of 37.7 years at first presentation, which is significantly lower than the 50 to 55 years or older in the current diagnostic criteria for sporadic CAA.[35] In addition, the iatrogenic cases had no association with APOE ε2 or ε4 alleles. The transmission likely occurred through contaminated surgical instruments and dural transplants.

Amyloid-Positron Emission Tomography Imaging

The amyloid hypothesis of AD suggests that the deposition of Aβ in the brain predates clinical symptoms by decades. ^{11}C-labeled Pittsburgh compound B (PiB) binds with high affinity to Aβ

Table 1
Boston criteria for the diagnosis of cerebral amyloid angiopathy

	Boston Criteria v2.0[6]	Modified Boston Criteria (v1.5)[17]
Definite CAA	Full brain postmortem with: • Spontaneous ICH, cSAH, transient focal neurological episodes, or cognitive impairment or dementia • Severe CAA with vasculopathy • Absence of other diagnostic lesion	Full brain postmortem with: • Lobar, cortical, or cortical-subcortical hemorrhage • Severe CAA with vasculopathy • Absence of other diagnostic lesion
Probable CAA with supporting pathologic condition	Clinical data and pathological tissue (evacuated hematoma or cortical biopsy) with: • Presentation with spontaneous ICH, cSAH, transient focal neurological episodes, or cognitive impairment or dementia • Some degree of CAA in specimen • Absence of other diagnostic lesion	Clinical data and pathological tissue (evacuated hematoma or cortical biopsy) with: • Lobar, cortical, or cortical-subcortical hemorrhage (ICH, CMB, or cSS) • Some degree of CAA in specimen • Absence of other diagnostic lesion
Probable CAA	Age ≥50 years, clinical data, and MR imaging with: • Presentation with spontaneous ICH, transient focal neurological episodes, or cognitive impairment or dementia • At least 2 of the following strictly lobar hemorrhagic lesions on T2*-w. MR imaging, in any combination: ICH, CMB, or cSS or cSAH Or • One lobar hemorrhagic lesion and one white matter feature (severe visible PVS in the centrum semiovale or WMH in a multispot pattern) • Absence of any deep hemorrhagic lesions (ICH or CMB) on T2*-w. MR imaging • Absence of other cause of hemorrhage • Cerebellar hemorrhagic lesions are considered neither lobar nor deep	Age ≥55 years, clinical data and MR imaging or CT with: • Multiple hemorrhages (ICH, CMB) restricted to lobar, cortical, or cortical-subcortical regions (cerebellar hemorrhage allowed) Or • Single lobar, cortical, or cortical-subcortical hemorrhage and cSS (focal or disseminated) • Absence of other cause of hemorrhage
Possible CAA	Age ≥50 years, clinical data and MR imaging with: • Presentation with spontaneous ICH, transient focal neurological episodes, or cognitive impairment or dementia • Absence of other cause of hemorrhage • One strictly lobar hemorrhagic lesion on T2*-w. MR imaging: ICH, CMB, or cSS or cSAH	Age ≥55 years, clinical data and MR imaging or CT with: • Single lobar, cortical or cortical-subcortical ICH, CMB, or cSS (focal or disseminated) • Absence of other cause of hemorrhage

(continued on next page)

Table 1
(continued)

Boston Criteria v2.0[6]	Modified Boston Criteria (v1.5)[17]
Or • One white matter feature (severe visible PVS in the centrum semiovale or WMH in a multispot pattern) • Absence of any deep hemorrhagic lesions (ICH or CMB) on T2*-w. MR imaging • Absence of other cause of hemorrhage • Cerebellar hemorrhagic lesions are considered neither lobar nor deep	

deposits was the first PET tracer to show Aβ in the brains of patients with AD, and it is still widely used in research applications.[36] It is however not Food and Drug Administration (FDA)-approved for clinical use, and the short half-life of [11]C (20 minutes) restricts its use to facilities with on-site cyclotron. The ^{18}F-labeled radiopharmaceuticals florbetapir, flutametamol, and florbetaben are all FDA-approved for clinical use in patients with AD, and their longer half-life (110 min) makes them clinically more useful for the detection of Aβ.[37]

Aβ deposition is a shared feature of AD and CAA, and the 2 conditions often overlap[22] (**Fig. 5**). PET imaging using ^{11}C-PiB and ^{18}F-florbetapir can measure both parenchymal (in AD) and cerebrovascular (in CAA) amyloid deposits and is able to detect CAA but its diagnostic utility in this setting is less clear. A

systematic review including 106 patients with CAA and 151 controls showed a moderate-to-good diagnostic accuracy for differentiating probable CAA patients from healthy controls and patients with deep ICH.[38] In a retrospective study of 38 patients with lobar ICH, 68% showed positivity on PiB-PET, and 13% of these did not fulfill the modified Boston criteria necessary for the probable CAA diagnosis, suggesting a use for amyloid PET in this patient population.[39]

Amyloid-Related Imaging Abnormality-E and Amyloid-Related Imaging Abnormality-H in the Setting of the New Alzheimer Drugs

There is close association between the pathologic processes of AD and CAA at the level of Aβ

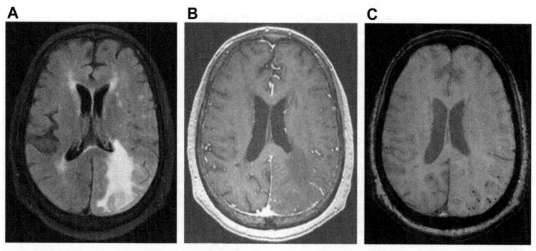

Fig. 4. A 63-year-old woman with seizures and cognitive decline. There is vasogenic edema in the left parietal and occipital white matter (*A*) surrounding foci of microhemorrhage on SWI (*C*) with a small amount of overlying leptomeningeal enhancement (*B*). Brain biopsy confirmed the diagnosis of inflammatory CAA. (*From* Kadam GH, Supple S, Jhaveri MD. Cerebral amyloid angiopathy-related inflammation: American Society of Neuroradiology 2020 case of the year. Neurographics 2022;12(2):98–102. Used with permission.)

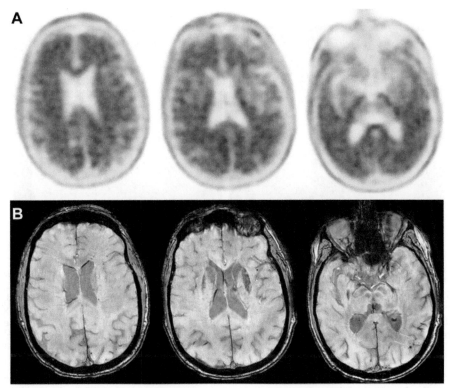

Fig. 5. A 70-year-old man with history of dementia. ^{18}F-florbetapir PET (*A*) shows abnormally increased cortical uptake, with obscuration of the gray-white differentiation. SWI (*B*) demonstrates multiple cortical-subcortical microhemorrhages (*arrows*) with sparing of the basal ganglia.

generation and brain clearance but they have a different mechanism of brain injury and resulting disease.[22] Antiamyloid monoclonal antibodies are emerging therapies for AD, with debated benefits, but a significant risk of side effects, most commonly manifesting as amyloid-related imaging abnormalities (ARIA).[40] The 2 patterns of imaging abnormality are (1) ARIA-E characterized by the presence of a vasogenic edema pattern throughout the subcortical white matter, similar in many respects to CAARI and (2) ARIA-H in which there is associated (microscopic or macroscopic) hemorrhage within the parenchyma. These side effects may be secondary to the overload of clearance pathways (including perivascular spaces [PVS]) by the amyloid mobilized by the antibodies from the brain parenchyma.[22]

Differential Considerations

Hypertensive hemorrhages

Patients with hypertension are at risk of intracranial hemorrhage, which is most frequently located within the basal ganglia, thalami, pons, and cerebellum. These are most often seen in the setting of essential hypertension but may also result from elevated blood pressure associated with the

use of vasoconstrictive drugs or other systemic conditions.[41] As with amyloid-related microhemorrhage, these are best demonstrated via the use of SWI sequences.[25] The central predominant pattern of hemosiderin deposition is the primary differentiating feature in hypertensive hemorrhage (**Fig. 6**). Of note, hypertension and CAA may be coexistent in older patients, which result in a mixed pattern of abnormality on imaging studies with both central and peripheral foci of susceptibility artifact.

A PiB-PET study showed significantly lower amyloid load in patients with a mixed pattern of CMBs compared with patients with CAA, similar to that of patients with HTN-SVD, suggesting that the latter may cause the mixed pattern.[42] Another study also found vascular risk factors in the background of mixed hemorrhages, with higher severity and recurrence rate compared with patients with purely deep microbleeds.[43]

Diffuse axonal injury

Axonal shear injuries result from high-energy forces acting on the brain often with a deceleration or rotational component. These often involve the junction between gray and white matter at the

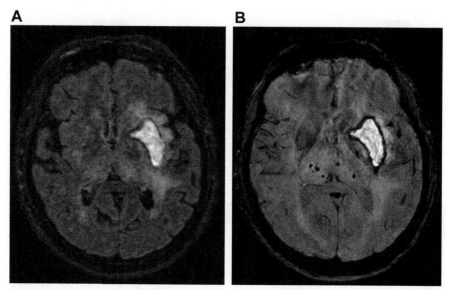

Fig. 6. A 55-year-old woman with new onset weakness is found to have a parenchymal hematoma centered within the left basal ganglia. T2-FLAIR (*A*) is notable for confluent areas of T2 hyperintensity involving deep white matter greater than expected for age. SWI (*B*) reveals additional susceptibility foci within the thalami. This pattern of deep gray hemorrhage with peripheral brain sparing is typical of hypertensive bleeds.

periphery of the brain due to the difference in density between the 2 regions of tissue because they respond to the same force. More significant shearing injuries may also occur in deeper white matter pathways including the corpus callosum, midbrain, and pons. Injury to the brainstem often portends a poor outcome. As with CAA, SWI following diffuse axonal injury may reveal extensive peripheral foci of artifact[44] (**Fig. 7**). Differentiating features include a history of trauma (especially high-velocity injury such as major

motor vehicle accident) as well as involvement of deeper white matter pathways, especially the corpus callosum.

Familial cavernomatosis syndromes

Although single incidentally discovered cerebral cavernous malformations are common, rarely these vascular malformations may be part of a familial syndrome in which numerous cavernous malformations may be present.[45] Although these are distributed randomly throughout the neural

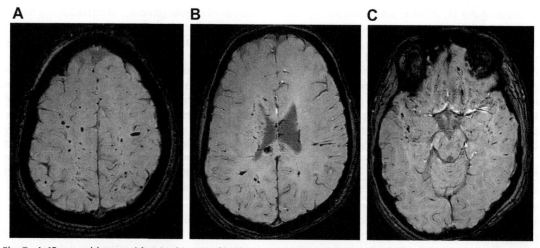

Fig. 7. A 42-year-old man with prior history of high-speed motor vehicle accident. The microhemorrhage pattern on SWI (*A–C*) from prior axonal shear injuries differs from CAA in the preferential involvement of major white matter pathways such as the corpus callosum (*B*) in a linear morphology paralleling the white matter tracts.

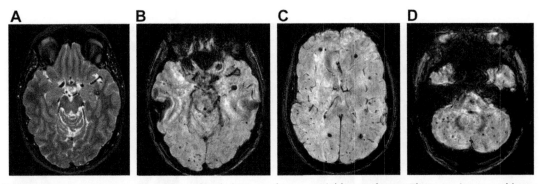

Fig. 8. A 59-year-old man with a strong family history of intracranial hemorrhages. There are innumerable susceptibility foci throughout the brain, including a few demonstrating central T2 hyperintense signal (*A*) without surrounding edema. These are present both in the supratentorial and infratentorial compartments (*B–D*). Given history and lack of earlier trauma or radiation, findings suggest familial cavernomatosis syndrome.

axis (including potentially in the spinal cord), if peripheral in location, imaging studies may share similarities with those seen in CAA (Fig. 8). However, patients with familial cavernomatosis typically present at a younger age when hemorrhage in association with one of the many malformations results in onset of symptoms. In addition, although small malformations may seem simply as discreet foci of susceptibility artifact on SWI, larger malformations will typically be associated with central areas of heterogenous T2 prolongation with a peripheral rim of susceptibility—the so-called popcorn appearance characteristic of these vascular abnormalities.

Encephalitis

A number of infectious diseases may result in hemorrhagic forms of encephalitis. Although these are often diffuse in nature, there may be extensive resulting microhemorrhage at the periphery of the brain simulating the pattern of CAA. Differentiating features should include a history of time spent in an endemic area as well as earlier febrile illness. These entities are asymptomatic and thus a thorough review of past medical history should illicit earlier infection. Perhaps, the most dramatic infectious encephalitis to result in microhemorrhage within the brain is cerebral malaria caused by the parasite plasmodium falciparum[46] (Fig. 9).

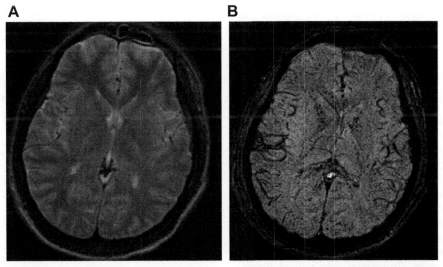

Fig. 9. A 31-year-old woman who recently returned from a 2-month trip to southeast Asia underwent MR imaging for recurrent headaches. Serology was positive for infection with *Plasmodium falciparum*. The extensive pattern of microhemorrhages on SWI (*B*) with normal T2-weighted imaging (*A*) is typical of cerebral malaria. (*From* Nickerson JP, Tong KA, Raghavan R. Imaging cerebral malaria with a susceptibility-weighted MR sequence. AJNR Am J Neuroradiol. 2009;30(6):e85-e86.)

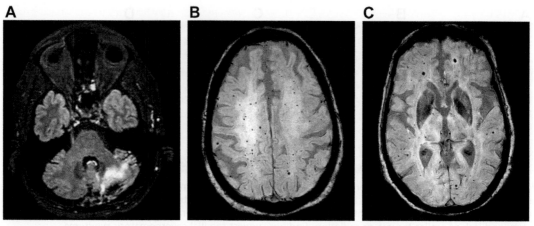

Fig. 10. A 35-year-old woman with a history of posterior fossa medulloblastoma who underwent craniospinal radiation therapy for disseminated tumor as a child. T2-FLAIR shows the site of the original tumor in the posterior fossa (*A*). Decades later numerous foci of susceptibility throughout the brain are reflective of radiation-induced capillary telangiectasias and cavernous venous malformations (*B, C*).

Radiation-induced vascular injury

Patients who have undergone radiation to the brain are at risk of developing vascular lesions including capillary telangiectasias and cerebral cavernous malformations. These are thought to be the result of injury to small blood vessels followed by an abnormal repair process after radiation exposure.[47] These lesions often occur several years after radiation therapy and are associated with foci of susceptibility artifact on susceptibility-weighted images in relative proximity to the radiation field. In patients who have received whole-brain radiation, these may occur diffusely and mimic the findings of CAA (**Fig. 10**). A history of radiation therapy should suggest this differential consideration.

SUMMARY

CAA is an important cause of intracranial hemorrhage particularly in older patients. As new pharmaceutical agents begin to become available for the treatment of amyloid-related brain disease, radiologists who interpret brain studies should be familiar with the hallmarks of this disease process. Close attention to SWI sequences for the presence of peripheral foci of hemosiderin deposition will allow for the appropriate early recognition of CAA in patients who may benefit from risk management or therapy to prevent recurrent hemorrhagic events. Correlation with patient demographics, history, and the distribution of signal abnormalities should facilitate differentiating CAA from a number of other causes of cerebral microhemorrhage.

CLINICS CARE POINTS

- As development of CAA increases with age, particular attention should be given to susceptibility-weighted image evaluation for cerebral microhemorrhages in patients of advanced age.
- SWI is the most sensitive sequence for microhemorrhage detection.
- CAA is primarily associated with peripheral or lobar hemorrhage. This is useful in differentiating from a number of other common causes of intracranial hemorrhage, most practically hypertensive hemorrhages that favor the deep gray nuclei and brainstem.
- Nonhemorrhagic markers of CAA such as prominent perivascular spaces in the centrum semiovale increase the diagnostic sensitivity and the usefulness of MR imaging.
- As pharmaceutical agents for the treatment of cerebral amyloid deposition become available, radiologists should become familiar with the potential complications of these medications including ARIA-E and ARIA-H.

DISCLOSURE

The authors have nothing to disclose.

REFERENCES

1. Charidimou A, Gang Q, Werring DJ. Sporadic cerebral amyloid angiopathy revisited: recent insights

into pathophysiology and clinical spectrum. J Neurol Neurosurg Psychiatr 2012;83(2):124–37.

2. Vinters HV. Cerebral amyloid angiopathy. A critical review. Stroke 1987;18(2):311–24.

3. Greenberg SM, Vonsattel JP. Diagnosis of cerebral amyloid angiopathy. Sensitivity and specificity of cortical biopsy. Stroke 1997;28(7):1418–22.

4. United Nations Department of Economic and Social Affairs PD. World Population Prospects 2022: Summary of Results. 2022. https://www.un.org/development/desa/pd/content/World-Population-Prospects-2022. Accessed 23 July, 2022.

5. Greenberg SM, Charidimou A. Diagnosis of cerebral amyloid angiopathy: evolution of the boston criteria. Stroke 2018;49(2):491–7.

6. Charidimou A, Boulouis G, Frosch MP, et al. The Boston criteria version 2.0 for cerebral amyloid angiopathy: a multicentre, retrospective, MRI-neuropathology diagnostic accuracy study. Lancet Neurol 2022; 21(8):714–25.

7. Sotoudeh H, Sarrami AH, Wang JX, et al. Susceptibility-weighted imaging in neurodegenerative disorders: a review. J Neuroimaging 2021;31(3):459–70.

8. Attems J, Lintner F, Jellinger KA. Amyloid beta peptide 1-42 highly correlates with capillary cerebral amyloid angiopathy and Alzheimer disease pathology. Acta Neuropathol 2004;107(4):283–91.

9. Herzig MC, Van Nostrand WE, Jucker M. Mechanism of cerebral beta-amyloid angiopathy: murine and cellular models. Brain Pathol 2006;16(1):40–54.

10. Kress BT, Iliff JJ, Xia M, et al. Impairment of paravascular clearance pathways in the aging brain. Ann Neurol 2014;76(6):845–61.

11. Verghese PB, Castellano JM, Holtzman DM. Apolipoprotein E in Alzheimer's disease and other neurological disorders. Lancet Neurol 2011;10(3):241–52.

12. Attems J, Jellinger K, Thal DR, et al. Review: sporadic cerebral amyloid angiopathy. Neuropathol Appl Neurobiol 2011;37(1):75–93.

13. Gil-Garcia CA, Alvarez EF, Garcia RC, et al. Essential topics about the imaging diagnosis and treatment of Hemorrhagic Stroke: a comprehensive review of the 2022 AHA guidelines. Curr Probl Cardiol 2022; 101328. https://doi.org/10.1016/j.cpcardiol.2022.101328.

14. Miller-Thomas MM, Sipe AL, Benzinger TL, et al. Multimodality review of amyloid-related diseases of the central nervous system. Radiographics 2016; 36(4):1147–63.

15. Passero S, Burgalassi L, D'Andrea P, et al. Recurrence of bleeding in patients with primary intracerebral hemorrhage. Stroke 1995;26(7):1189–92.

16. Sakurai K, Tokumaru AM, Nakatsuka T, et al. Imaging spectrum of sporadic cerebral amyloid angiopathy: multifaceted features of a single pathological condition. Insights Imaging 2014;5(3):375–85.

17. Linn J, Halpin A, Demaerel P, et al. Prevalence of superficial siderosis in patients with cerebral amyloid angiopathy. Neurology 2010;74(17):1346–50.

18. Greenberg SM, Vernooij MW, Cordonnier C, et al. Cerebral microbleeds: a guide to detection and interpretation. Lancet Neurol 2009;8(2):165–74.

19. Kimberly WT, Gilson A, Rost NS, et al. Silent ischemic infarcts are associated with hemorrhage burden in cerebral amyloid angiopathy. Neurology 2009;72(14):1230–5.

20. Keage HA, Carare RO, Friedland RP, et al. Population studies of sporadic cerebral amyloid angiopathy and dementia: a systematic review. BMC Neurol 2009;9:3.

21. Boyle PA, Yu L, Nag S, et al. Cerebral amyloid angiopathy and cognitive outcomes in community-based older persons. Neurology 2015;85(22):1930–6.

22. Greenberg SM, Bacskai BJ, Hernandez-Guillamon M, et al. Cerebral amyloid angiopathy and Alzheimer disease - one peptide, two pathways. Nat Rev Neurol 2020;16(1):30–42.

23. Rodrigues MA, Samarasekera N, Lerpiniere C, et al. The Edinburgh CT and genetic diagnostic criteria for lobar intracerebral haemorrhage associated with cerebral amyloid angiopathy: model development and diagnostic test accuracy study. Lancet Neurol 2018; 17(3):232–40.

24. Koren L, Hilario A, Salvador E, et al. Imaging Features in Cerebral Amyloid Angiopathy. Neurographics 2017;7(4):266–75.

25. Guo LF, Wang G, Zhu XY, et al. Comparison of ESWAN, SWI-SPGR, and 2D T2*-weighted GRE sequence for depicting cerebral microbleeds. Clin Neuroradiol 2013;23(2):121–7.

26. Knudsen KA, Rosand J, Karluk D, et al. Clinical diagnosis of cerebral amyloid angiopathy: validation of the Boston criteria. Neurology 2001;56(4):537–9.

27. Pasi M, Pongpitakmetha T, Charidimou A, et al. Cerebellar microbleed distribution patterns and cerebral amyloid angiopathy. Stroke 2019;50(7):1727–33.

28. Pasi M, Boulouis G, Fotiadis P, et al. Distribution of lacunes in cerebral amyloid angiopathy and hypertensive small vessel disease. Neurology 2017; 88(23):2162–8.

29. Charidimou A, Meegahage R, Fox Z, et al. Enlarged perivascular spaces as a marker of underlying arteriopathy in intracerebral haemorrhage: a multicentre MRI cohort study. J Neurol Neurosurg Psychiatr 2013;84(6):624–9.

30. Gouveia-Freitas K, Bastos-Leite AJ. Perivascular spaces and brain waste clearance systems: relevance for neurodegenerative and cerebrovascular pathology. Neuroradiology 2021;63(10):1581–97.

31. Bown CW, Carare RO, Schrag MS, et al. Physiology and clinical relevance of enlarged perivascular spaces in the aging brain. Neurology 2022;98(3):107–17.

32. Kadam GH, Supple S, Jhaveri MD. Cerebral Amyloid Angiopathy-related Inflammation: American Society of Neuroradiology 2020 Case of the Year. Neurographics 2022;12(2):98–102.

33. Chwalisz BK. Cerebral amyloid angiopathy and related inflammatory disorders. J Neurol Sci 2021; 424:117425.

34. Jaunmuktane Z, Mead S, Ellis M, et al. Evidence for human transmission of amyloid-β pathology and cerebral amyloid angiopathy. Nature 2015;525(7568): 247–50.

35. Banerjee G, Samra K, Adams ME, et al. Iatrogenic cerebral amyloid angiopathy: an emerging clinical phenomenon. J Neurol Neurosurg Psychiatr 2022. https://doi.org/10.1136/jnnp-2022-328792.

36. Rowe CC, Ng S, Ackermann U, et al. Imaging beta-amyloid burden in aging and dementia. Neurology 2007;68(20):1718–25.

37. Acuff SN, Mathotaarachchi S, Zukotynski K, et al. Clinical and technical considerations for brain PET imaging for dementia. J Nucl Med Technol. Mar 2020;48(1):5–8.

38. Charidimou A, Farid K, Baron JC. Amyloid-PET in sporadic cerebral amyloid angiopathy: a diagnostic accuracy meta-analysis. Neurology 2017;89(14): 1490–8.

39. Michiels L, Dobbels L, Demeestere J, et al. Simplified Edinburgh and modified Boston criteria in relation to amyloid PET for lobar intracerebral hemorrhage. Neuroimage Clin 2022;35:103107.

40. Withington CG, Turner RS. Amyloid-related imaging abnormalities with anti-amyloid antibodies for the treatment of dementia due to Alzheimer's disease. Front Neurol 2022;13:862369.

41. Henskens LH, van Oostenbrugge RJ, Kroon AA, et al. Brain microbleeds are associated with ambulatory blood pressure levels in a hypertensive population. Hypertension 2008;51(1):62–8.

42. Tsai HH, Pasi M, Tsai LK, et al. Microangiopathy underlying mixed-location intracerebral hemorrhages/microbleeds: a PiB-PET study. Neurology 2019; 92(8):e774–81.

43. Pasi M, Charidimou A, Boulouis G, et al. Mixed-location cerebral hemorrhage/microbleeds: Underlying microangiopathy and recurrence risk. Neurology 2018;90(2):e119–26.

44. Tong KA, Ashwal S, Obenaus A, et al. Susceptibility-weighted MR imaging: a review of clinical applications in children. AJNR Am J Neuroradiol 2008; 29(1):9–17.

45. Dammann P, Wrede K, Zhu Y, et al. Correlation of the venous angioarchitecture of multiple cerebral cavernous malformations with familial or sporadic disease: a susceptibility-weighted imaging study with 7-Tesla MRI. J Neurosurg 2017;126(2):570–7.

46. Nickerson JP, Tong KA, Raghavan R. Imaging cerebral malaria with a susceptibility-weighted MR sequence. AJNR Am J Neuroradiol 2009;30(6): e85–6.

47. Campbell BA, Lasocki A, Oon SF, et al. Evaluation of the Impact of Magnetic Resonance Imaging with Susceptibility-weighted Imaging for Screening and Surveillance of Radiation-induced Cavernomas in Long-term Survivors of Malignancy. Clin Oncol 2021;33(10):e425–32.

Moving?

Make sure your subscription moves with you!

To notify us of your new address, find your **Clinics Account Number** (located on your mailing label above your name), and contact customer service at:

Email: journalscustomerservice-usa@elsevier.com

800-654-2452 (subscribers in the U.S. & Canada)
314-447-8871 (subscribers outside of the U.S. & Canada)

Fax number: 314-447-8029

Elsevier Health Sciences Division
Subscription Customer Service
3251 Riverport Lane
Maryland Heights, MO 63043

*To ensure uninterrupted delivery of your subscription, please notify us at least 4 weeks in advance of move.

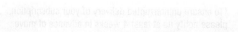

Printed and bound by CPI Group (UK) Ltd, Croydon, CR0 4YY

08/05/2025

01864717-0009